Praise for Ashtanga Yoga: Practice and Philosophy

"I love *Ashtanga Yoga: Practice and Philosophy*. At last there is a book that is not just on asana but coupled with that, the real beauty of asana and philosophy."

— Frances Liotta, founder of Yogamat

"Gregor Maehle's *Ashtanga Yoga: Practice and Philosophy* weaves philosophy and integrated knowledge of anatomy into our yoga practice to keep us centered in the heart of a profound tradition. He also gives us a brilliant translation and commentary on the Yoga Sutra, revealing a deep philosophical and historical context in which to ground and stimulate our entire lives."

— Richard Freeman, founder of the Yoga Workshop in Boulder, Colorado, and author of *The Yoga Matrix* CD

"A much-needed new tool for practicing the method with greater safety in the physical form and with much needed depth in the inner form of the practice. I especially appreciate the comprehensive approach, which includes philosophical perspectives, anatomy, vedic lore, a thorough description of the physical method itself as well as a complete copy of Patanjala Yoga Darshana. A valuable contribution to the evolving understanding of this profound system and method of yoga."

— Chuck Miller, Ashtanga Yoga teacher, senior student of Shri K. Pattabhi Jois since 1980 ii

ASHTANGA YOGA

Practice and Philosophy

ASHTANGA YOGA
Practice and Philosophy

A Comprehensive Description of the
Primary Series of Ashtanga Yoga,
Following the Traditional Vinyasa Count,
and an Authentic Explanation of
the Yoga Sutra of Patanjali

Gregor Maehle

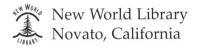

New World Library
Novato, California

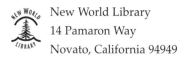

New World Library
14 Pamaron Way
Novato, California 94949

The material in this book is intended for education. Please consult a qualified health care practitioner before beginning any exercise program and learn yoga under personal supervision. This book is not a substitute for medical advice or instruction from a qualified yoga teacher. No expressed or implied guarantee as to the effects of the use of the recommendations can be given nor liability taken.

Every effort has been made to contact the holders of copyright of quoted material.

Originally published in Australia by Kaivalya Publications in 2006.
Text design and typography by Allan Watson
Photography by Adrian Kat
Illustrations by Steve Dance
Front cover photograph: Gregor Maehle and Monica Gauci performing *Kaundinyasana*, a posture dedicated to the sage Kaundinya, author of the commentary on Lakulisha's *Pashupata Sutra;* back cover photograph: Gregor Maehle and Monica Gauci performing *Yoga Mudra.*

Library of Congress Cataloging-in-Publication Data
Maehle, Gregor.
Ashtanga yoga : practice and philosophy : a comprehensive description of the primary series of ashtanga yoga and an authentic explanation of the Yoga sutra of Patanjali / Gregor Maehle.
      p.   cm.
Includes bibliographical references and index.
ISBN 978-1-57731-606-0 (pbk. : alk. paper)
1. Astanga yoga. 2. Patañjali. Yogasutra. I. Title.
RA781.68.M34 2007
613.7'046—dc22   2007022806

First New World Library edition, September 2007
ISBN-10: 1-57731-606-1
ISBN-13: 978-1-57731-606-0
Printed in Canada on partially recycled, acid-free paper

g New World Library is a proud member of the Green Press Initiative.

10   9   8   7   6   5   4   3   2   1

To the first and foremost of all teachers,
who has been known by various names,
such as the Brahman, the Tao, the Lord, and the Mother,
and who, after all names are left behind,
is still there as the incomprehensible, luminous,
vibrant, silent, vast emptiness in my heart.

Note

It is important to learn Ashtanga Yoga by the traditional method, according to which the next posture is added on only when the student has gained proficiency in the previous one. In this way excessive exertion, fatigue, and unwanted side effects are avoided. Proficiency in a posture can be assessed only by a qualified teacher.

The importance of learning the method from a qualified teacher cannot be stressed enough. It is not possible to learn yoga from a book or video, because these media cannot provide feedback when the student engages in a posture poorly. If this should be the case, little or no benefit would be gained from the practice; in fact damage could be done.

CONTENTS

INVOCATION

Om
Vande gurunam charanaravinde
sandarshita svatma sukhavabodhe
nih shreyase jangalikayamane
samsara halahala mohashantyai

Abahu purushakaram
shankhachakrasi dharinam
sahasra shirasam shvetam
pranamami patanjalim
Om

I bow to the lotus feet of the supreme teacher
who reveals the happiness of self-realization;
who like the jungle doctor removes the delusion
caused by the great poison of conditioned existence.

To Patanjali, who (representing the serpent of infinity)
has thousands of white, radiant heads,
who in his human form holds a conch (representing sound),
a discus (representing light), and a sword (representing discrimination),
I prostrate.

PREFACE

In the year 3102 BCE, the emperor Yudishthira stepped down and awaited the death of Krishna and the beginning of the dark age (Kali Yuga). Due to the increasing materialism and corruption of that age, the ancient sages (*rishis*) retreated into the recesses of the Himalayas.

However, as vedic teacher David Frawley has pointed out, the *rishi*s have not disappeared entirely: they are observing mankind from a distance. It depends on us whether it will become possible for them to return and with them much of the knowledge, wisdom, and intelligence of humankind. Through our combined efforts we must try to usher in a new golden age (Satya Yuga).

This book is an attempt to bring about a renaissance of ancient *dharma* and to play a part in restoring yoga to the glory it once was.

May all beings experience that which is auspicious.

Gregor Maehle
Perth, Australia
Ninth day of the bright fortnight in the lunar mansion of Phalguni, year 5108 Kali Yuga

ACKNOWLEDGMENTS

I extend my thanks to all the following:

To teachers who have influenced my work —

Yogasana Visharada Shri Krishna Pattabhi Jois of Mysore, who taught me this method, which he had received from his teacher Shri Tirumalai Krishnamacharya. Without the work of K. Pattabhi Jois, Ashtanga Vinyasa Yoga would have been lost. All modern practitioners of Ashtanga Yoga benefit directly or indirectly from his teaching.

Yoga Shastra Pundita Shri B. N. S. Iyengar of Mysore, student of T. Krishnamacharya and K. Pattabhi Jois, who instructed me in yoga philosophy.

Shri A. G. Mohan, student of T. Krishnamacharya, who answered my final questions regarding the *Yoga Sutra*.

Richard Freeman, Dena Wiseman, and Graeme Northfield, all students of K. Pattabhi Jois, who deepened my understanding of *asana*.

To my wife, Monica Gauci, for walking this path of yoga with me, for encouraging me to continue with this project in moments of doubt, for supplying valuable information for the practice section, and for being a model in the *asana* photographs.

To my editor and designer, Allan Watson, who, with his versatile expertise, has made a more than significant contribution to this book.

Also to —
Steve Dance — graphical illustrations and cover design
Adrian Kat — photography

To the following publishers and authors, who have given permission for the use of their material:
Advaita Ashrama, Kolkata
Sri Ramakrisna Math, Chennai
Hohm Press, Prescott, Arizona
Sri A. G. Mohan, Chennai
Motilal Banarsidass, Delhi
Kapil Math monastery, Madhupur

Finally, to everybody at 8limbs Ashtanga Yoga in Perth, Australia, for their work during the more than two years I was engaged in writing this text.

INTRODUCTION

During a study trip to the Ashtanga Yoga Research Institute in Mysore in 1996, I asked the Ashtanga master K. Pattabhi Jois about the relevance of different scriptures for the Ashtanga Vinyasa method. With the words "This is Patanjali Yoga," he pointed out that the text of prime importance for this school was the *Yoga Sutra* compiled by the ancient seer Patanjali. He said it was a difficult text, and only sincere study could lead to an understanding. He urged me to undertake daily study of the *Yoga Sutra* for a long time. The combination of these studies with daily Ashtanga Vinyasa practice led me eventually to realize that the *Yoga Sutra* and the *vinyasa* method are really only two sides of the same coin.

That is the central theme of this book. For yoga practice to be successful, there can be no separation of practice and philosophy. Indeed, new approaches to practice have always come out of philosophy, while practice prepares the intellect for philosophy. In fact the *Yoga Sutra* suggests that philosophical inquiry — *svadhyaya*, or *vichara* as Shankara calls it — is itself a form of practice, and an essential ingredient of the path to freedom.

This book is dedicated to bringing the two aspects back together and restoring what historically was one system, lost through the lapse of time.

The Rediscovery of the Ashtanga Vinyasa System

The notion that the *Yoga Sutra* and the *vinyasa* system are two sides of one coin has been strongly present from the beginning of the modern-day Ashtanga Yoga lineage. K. Pattabhi Jois received the *vinyasa* method from his master, T. Krishnamacharya; Krishnamacharya's own master, Ramamohan Brahmachary, instructed him to seek out what was understood to be the last remaining copy of an elusive scripture, the *Yoga Korunta*, thought to have been compiled by the ancient seer Vamana.

According to Krishnamacharya's biography,[1] the *Yoga Korunta* contained not only the *vinyasa* system but also the *Yoga Sutra* of Patanjali and its commentary, *Yoga Bhasya*, compiled by the Rishi Vyasa. These were bound together in one volume. We can see from this that, in ancient times, what are today regarded as two systems that only share the same name — the Ashtanga Yoga of Patanjali and the Ashtanga Vinyasa Yoga of the Rishi Vamana — were in fact one.

We see here also the idea that yogic philosophy is taught together with the practice. The practice of *asana* (posture) alone poses a danger. According to K. Pattabhi Jois, "Partial yoga methods out of line with their internal purpose can build up the 'six enemies' (desire, anger, greed, illusion, infatuation, and envy) around the heart. The full Ashtanga system practised with devotion leads to freedom within one's heart."[2]

Today, however, we are in the situation where on the one hand there are scholars who try to understand the *Yoga Sutra* without knowing its practices, while on the other hand there are many Ashtanga Vinyasa practitioners who are established in practice but do not know the philosophy of their system. Both aspects practiced together will make practice easy, because we know where it leads and how we get there. Without dedicated practice, philosophy can turn into mere theory. Once established in practice, we will swiftly internalize the philosophy and attain higher yoga.

The Relevance of Ashtanga Yoga Today

I do not claim here that Vinyasa Yoga is the only form of Patanjali Yoga. That would be absurd. It is, however, one of the authentic representations of Patanjali's sutra that is still alive.

1. *Krishnamacharya the Purnacharya*, Krishnamacharya Yoga Mandiram, Chennai.
2. *The Yoga Journal*, San Francisco, November/December 1995.

This system is precious — and relevant — today because it was conceived by the ancient seer Vamana, the author of the *Yoga Korunta*, especially for house-holders (*grihasta*). A householder is somebody who has a job and family, and lives and works in society, as opposed to a monk, hermit, or ascetic (*sannyasi*). Some forms of yoga are designed for hermits who have no social responsibility and therefore can be engaged with meditation techniques all day long.

Being a hermit or ascetic, however, was never a requirement for yoga. As the *Bhagavad Gita* explains, "One who outwardly performs his social duties but inwardly stays free is a yogi."[3] If every-body ceased performing their social responsibilities, the text continues,[4] this world would be ruined, for obvious reasons. So we need not be disturbed if responsibility for others keeps us from devoting more time to our practice, since fulfilling one's duty is practice. But what is important is *how* we practice. How do we spend the precious time we can allocate to practicing?

When T. Krishnamacharya had completed his training, his master, R. Brahmachary, proposed to him that he should get married, have a family, and teach yoga to city dwellers. This came as a surprise to the younger man: being so highly trained, he could have become a great scholar or the abbot of a monastery. But as a teacher of yoga to city dwellers he would have very low social status.

Brahmachary told Krishnamacharya to study the *Yoga Korunta*, as he knew this would equip him best for teaching householders. The Vinyasa Yoga described in that text was the ideal form of Patanjali Yoga for householders, since it required only around two hours of practice per day.

The Eight Limbs of Yoga, and How They Work Together

According to Patanjali there are eight "limbs" of yoga. How they work together can be understood from the following story:

Once upon a time a couple lived happily together in a country that had an unjust king. The king became jealous of their happiness and threw the

3. *Bhagavad Gita* III.7.
4. *Bhagavad Gita* III.24.

man into a prison tower. When his wife came to the tower at night to comfort him, the man called down to her that she should return the next night with a long silken thread, a strong thread, a cord, a rope, a beetle, and some honey. Although puzzled by the request, the wife returned the next evening with all the items. Her husband then asked her to tie the silken thread to the beetle and smear honey onto its antennae. She should then place the beetle on the tower wall with its head facing upward. Smelling the honey, the beetle started to climb up the tower in expectation of finding more of it, dragging the silken thread as it did so. When it reached the top of the tower the man took hold of the silken thread and called down to his wife that she should tie the strong thread to the other end. Pulling the strong thread up, he secured it also and instructed her further to tie the cord to the other end. Once he had the cord the rest happened quickly. With the rope attached to the cord he pulled it up, secured one end of it and, climbing down, escaped to freedom.

The couple are, of course, yogis. The prison tower represents conditioned existence. The silken thread symbolizes the purifying of the body through *asana*. The strong thread represents *pranayama*, breath extension, the cord symbolizes meditation, and the rope stands for *samadhi*, the state of pure being. Once this rope is held, freedom from conditioned existence is possible.

Patanjali's eight limbs of yoga relate to Ashtanga Vinyasa practice thus:

The first limb consists of a set of ethics, which ensures that the yogi interacts in a harmonious way with the surrounding community. The ethical precepts are: not to harm others, to be truthful, not to steal, to engage in intercourse only with one's partner, and to abstain from greed.

The second limb consists of observances, which ensure that body and mind are not polluted once they have been purified. Purification in yoga has nothing to do with puritanism. Rather it refers to the "stainability" of body and mind. "Stainability" is the propensity of the body / mind to take on a conditioning or imprint from the environment. The observances are physical and mental cleanliness, contentment, simplicity, study of sacred texts, and acceptance of the existence of the Supreme Being. The first two limbs are initially implemented from the outside, and they form a platform from which practice is undertaken. Once we are established in yoga they become our second nature: they will arise naturally.

The third limb is *asana*. Many obstacles to knowing one's true nature are manifested in the body, for example disease, sluggishness, and dullness. The body profoundly influences and, if in bad condition, impinges on the functioning of mind and intellect. Through the practice of yoga *asana*s the body is made "strong and light like the body of a lion," to quote Shri K. Pattabhi Jois. Only then will it provide the ideal vehicle on the path of yoga.

As the *Yoga Sutra* explains,[5] every thought, emotion, and experience leaves a subconscious imprint (*samskara*) in the mind. These imprints determine who we will be in the future. According to the *Brhad Aranyaka Upanishad*, as long as liberation is not achieved, the soul, like a caterpillar that draws itself from one blade of grass over to the next, will, by the force of its impressions in this life, reach out and draw itself over to a new body in a new life.

This means that the body we have today is nothing but the accumulation of our past thoughts, emotions, and actions. In fact our body is the crystallized history of our past thoughts. This needs to be deeply understood and contemplated. It means that *asana* is the method that releases us from past conditioning, stored in the body, to arrive in the present moment. It is to be noted that practicing forcefully will only superimpose a new layer of subconscious imprints based on suffering and pain. It will also increase identification with the body. In yoga, identification with anything that is impermanent is called ignorance (*avidya*).

This may sound rather abstract at first, but all of us who have seen a loved one die will remember the profound insight that, once death has set in, the body looks just like an empty shell left behind. Since the body is our vehicle and the storehouse of our past, we want to practice *asana* to the point where it serves us well, while releasing and letting go of the past that is stored in it.

Yoga is the middle path between two extremes. On the one hand, we can go to the extreme of practicing fanatically and striving for an ideal while denying

5. *Yoga Sutra* II.12.

the reality of this present moment. The problem with this is that we are only ever relating to ourselves as what we want to become in the future and not as what we are right now. The other extreme is advocated by some schools of psychotherapy that focus on highlighting past traumas. If we do this, these traumas can increase their grip on us, and we relate to ourselves as we have in the past, defining ourselves by the "stuff that's coming up" and the "process that we are going through." *Asana* is an invitation to say goodbye to these extremes and arrive at the truth of the present moment.

How do past emotions, thoughts, and impressions manifest in the body? Some students of yoga experience a lot of anger on commencing forward bending. This is due to past anger having been stored in the hamstrings. If we consciously let go of the anger, the emotion will disappear. If not, it will surface in some other form, possibly as an act of aggression or as a chronic disease. Other students feel like crying after intense backbending. Emotional pain is stored in the chest, where it functions like armor, hardening around the heart. This armor may be dissolved in backbending. If we let go of the armor, a feeling of tremendous relief will result, sometimes accompanied by crying.

Extreme stiffness can be related to mental rigidity or the inability to let oneself be transported into unknown situations. Extreme flexibility, on the other hand, can be related to the inability to take a position in life and to set boundaries. In this case, *asana* practice needs to be more strength based, to create a balance and to learn to resist being stretched to inappropriate places. *Asana* invites us to acknowledge the past and let it go. This will in turn bring us into the present moment and allow us to let go of limiting concepts such as who we think we are.

The fourth limb is *pranayama*. *Prana* is the life force, also referred to as the inner breath; *pranayama* means extension of *prana*. The yogis discovered that the pulsating or oscillating of *prana* happens simultaneously with the movements of the mind (*chitta vrtti*). The practice of *pranayama* is the study and exercise of one's breath to a point where it is appeased and does not agitate the mind.

In the *vinyasa* system, *pranayama* is practiced through applying the *Ujjayi* breath. By slightly constricting the glottis, the breath is stretched long. We learn to let the movement follow the breath, which eventually leads to the body effortlessly riding the waves of the breath. At this point it is not we who move the body, but rather the power of *prana*. We become able to breathe into all parts of the body, which is equivalent to spreading the *prana* evenly throughout. This is *ayama* — the extension of the breath.

The fifth limb is *pratyahara* — sense withdrawal. The *Maitri Upanishad* says that, if one becomes preoccupied with sense objects, the mind is fueled, which will lead to delusion and suffering.[6] If, however, the fuel of the senses is withheld, then, like a fire that dies down without fuel, the mind becomes reabsorbed into its source, the heart. "Heart" in yoga is a metaphor not for emotions but for our center, which is consciousness or the self.

In Vinyasa Yoga, sense withdrawal is practiced through *drishti* — focal point. Instead of looking around while practicing *asana*, which leads to the senses reaching out, we stay internal by turning our gaze toward prescribed locations. The sense of hearing is drawn in by listening to the sound of the breath, which at the same time gives us feedback about the quality of the *asana*. By keeping our attention from reaching out, we develop what tantric philosophy calls the center (*madhya*). By developing the center, the mind is eventually suspended and the *prana*, which is a manifestation of the female aspect of creation, the Goddess or Shakti, ceases to oscillate. Then the state of divine consciousness (*bhairava*) is recognized.[7]

The sixth limb is *dharana* — concentration. If you have tried to meditate on the empty space between two thoughts, you will know that the mind has the tendency to attach itself to the next thought arising. Since all objects have form, and the witnessing subject — the consciousness — is formless, it tends to be overlooked by the mind. It takes a great deal of focus to keep watching consciousness when distractions are available.

The practice of concentration, then, is a prerequisite and preparation for meditation proper. The

training of concentration enables us to stay focused on whatever object is chosen. First, simple objects are selected, which in turn prepare us for the penultimate "object," formless consciousness, which is nothing but pure awareness.

Concentration in Vinyasa Yoga is practiced by focusing on the *bandha*s. On an external level the focus is on *Mula* and *Uddiyana Bandha* (pelvic and lower abdominal locks), but on an internal level it is on the bonding together of movement, breath, and awareness (*bandha* = bonding). To achieve this bonding, we have to let go of the beta brain-wave pattern, which normally accompanies concentration. Instead we need to shift to an alpha pattern, which enables multiple focus and leads into simultaneous awareness of everything, or being in this moment, which is meditation.

The seventh limb is *dhyana* — meditation. Meditation means to rest, uninfluenced, between the extremes of the mind and suddenly just "be" instead of "becoming." The difference between this and the previous limb is that, in concentration, there is a conscious effort to exclude all thoughts that are not relevant to our chosen object. In meditation there is a constant flow of impressions from the object and of awareness toward the object, without any effort of the will. Typical objects chosen are the heart lotus, the inner sound, the breath, the sense-of-I, the process of perception, and intellect, one's meditation deity (*ishtadevata*) or the Supreme Being.

In Vinyasa Yoga, meditation starts when, rather than *doing* the practice, we are *being done* or *moved*. At this point we realize that, since we can watch the body, we are not the body but a deeper-lying witnessing entity. The *vinyasa* practice is the constant coming and going of postures, the constant change of form, which we never hold on to. It is itself a meditation on impermanence. When we come to the point of realizing that everything we have known so far — the world, the body, the mind, and the practice — is subject to constant change, we have arrived at meditation on intelligence (*buddhi*).

Meditation does not, however, occur only in *dhyana*, but in all stages of the practice. In fact the Ashtanga Vinyasa system is a movement meditation. First we meditate on the position of the body in space, which is *asana*. Then we meditate on the

6. *Maitri Upanishad* VI.35.
7. *Vijnanabhairava*, trans. and annot. Jaideva Singh, Motilal Banarsidass, Delhi, 1979, p. 23.

4

life force moving the body, which is *pranayama*. The next stage is to meditate on the senses through *drishti* and listening to the breath, which is *pratyahara*. Meditating on the binding together of all aspects of the practice is concentration (*dharana*).

The eighth limb, *samadhi*, is of two kinds — objective and objectless. Objective *samadhi* is when the mind for the first time, like a clear jewel, reflects faithfully what it is directed at and does not just produce another simulation of reality.[8] In other words the mind is clarified to an extent that it does not modify sensory input at all. To experience this, we have to "de-condition" ourselves to the extent that we let go of all limiting and negative programs of the past. Patanjali says, "Memory is purified, as if emptied of its own form."[9] Then all that can be known about an object is known.

Objectless *samadhi* is the highest form of yoga. It does not depend on an object for its arising but, rather, the witnessing subject or awareness, which is our true nature, is revealed. In this *samadhi* the thought waves are suspended, which leads to knowing of that which was always there: consciousness or the divine self. This final state is beyond achieving, beyond doing, beyond practicing. It is a state of pure ecstatic being described by the term *kaivalya* — a state in which there is total freedom and independence from any external stimulation whatsoever.

In the physical disciplines of yoga, *samadhi* is reached by suspending the extremes of solar (*pingala*) and lunar (*ida*) mind. This state arises when the inner breath (*prana*) enters the central channel (*sushumna*). Then truth or deep reality suddenly flashes forth.

Why a Traditional Practice is Still Applicable

A peasant once spoke to the sage Ramakrishna thus: "I am a simple villager. Please give me in one sentence a method by which I can obtain happiness." Ramakrishna's answer was: "Totally accept the fact that you are a machine operated upon by God." This needs to be deeply understood. It is through the belief that individuals exercise free will that ego is produced; and, in turn, ego produces suffering. In the *Bhagavad Gita* Lord Krishna states, "All actions are done in all cases by the *guna*s (qualities) of *prakrti* (nature). He whose mind is deluded through egoism thinks I am the doer."[10]

This means that the entire cosmos, including our body-mind complex, is an unconscious machine operated upon by God. Our self, who is pure consciousness, is forever inactive. It merely witnesses. The giving up of the idea that it is we who act is echoed in the *Yoga Sutra* by Patanjali's use of the term *kaivalya*. This final state of yoga is the realization of the complete independence of consciousness. Since it is completely independent, it has no way of influencing the world. Like a mirror, which simply reflects, consciousness can neither reject nor hold on to objects of its choice. Give up the sense of agency,[11] says Krishna: "Only a fool believes I am the doer."

The surrender of the illusion of free will is reflected in the *vinyasa* system by acceptance of the original system as expounded by the Rishi Vamana. Of course it is easy to make up our own sequences of *asana*s, and possibly commercial success and fame will result. But then we run the risk of falling for the ego, which says I am the doer and the creator. We are only pure consciousness — the seer, the witness, the self — which, as the *Samkhya Karika*[12] says, plays no active part in this world.

That does not mean we cannot adapt the practice for some time if difficulties are to be met or yoga therapy needs to be practiced. We need to return to the original system whenever possible, though. Rishi Vamana's system leads through outer structure and limitation to inner freedom. If we constantly practice self-made sequences, we create inner limitation through outer freedom.

The *rishi*s of old did not conceive the ancient arts and sciences by trial and error. The method they employed was *samyama*, which combines concentration (*dharana*), meditation (*dhyana*), and absorption (*samadhi*). In that way, deep knowledge of how things really are can be gained. Patanjali himself

8. *Yoga Sutra* I.41.
9. *Yoga Sutra* I.43, quoted from *The Yoga Sutras of Patanjali*, trans. C. Chapple, Sri Satguru Publications, Delhi, 1990, p. 53.
10. *Srimad Bhagavad Gita*, trans. Sw. Vireswarananda, Sri Ramakrishna Math, Madras, p. 79.
11. Frequently used in Indian texts, this word means "the condition of being in action or exercising power."
12. A text describing Samkhya, the ancient prototype of all Indian philosophies.

explains in the *Yoga Sutra* how he gained his knowledge. Knowledge of the mind, he says, is gained by doing *samyama* on the heart.[13]

He also explains how the body can be understood. Medical knowledge, he says,[14] is gained by practicing *samyama* on the navel *chakra*. This is how the science of *Ayurveda* came into being. It should be noted that Patanjali compiled the *Charaka Samhita*, an ayurvedic text. When we study and practice the ancient sciences today, we need to do this with a feeling of respect and devotion.

The teachings of the ancient masters have never been declared invalid. They have only ever been added to.

13. *Yoga Sutra* III.34.
14. *Yoga Sutra* III.29.

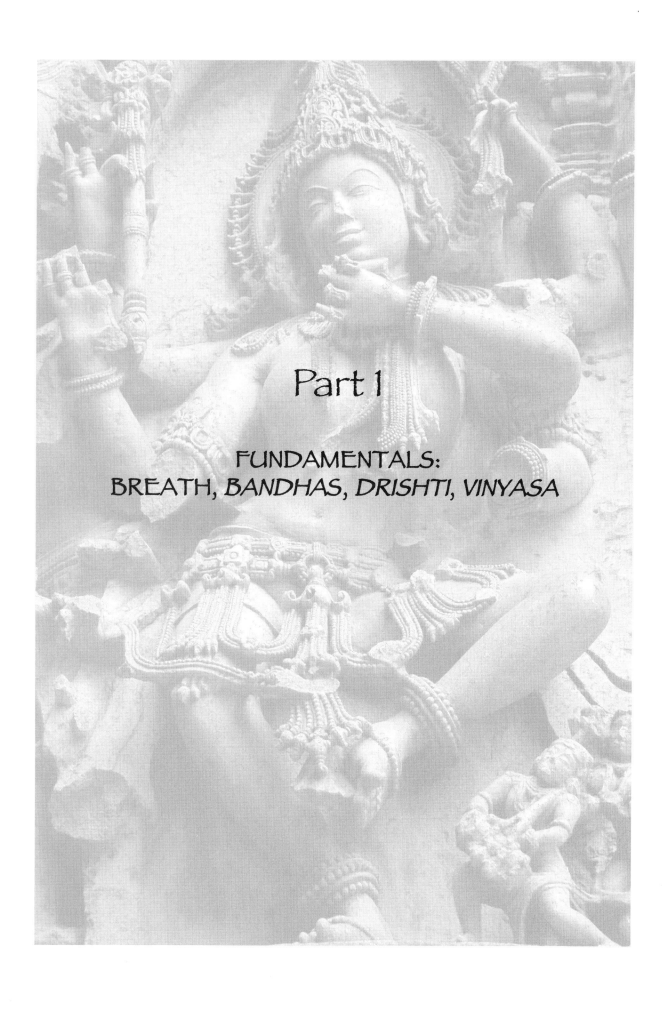

Part 1

FUNDAMENTALS:
BREATH, *BANDHAS*, *DRISHTI*, *VINYASA*

Breath

The most visible aspect of the Ashtanga Yoga system is the different yoga *asana*s (postures). More important, though, is the invisible content, which consists of three fundamental techniques. These techniques bind the postures together on a string so that they become a yoga *mala* or garland.[1]

In the Vinyasa Yoga system the body is used as a mantra, the postures represent beads, and the three fundamental techniques form the string that holds the beads together to create a garland of yoga postures. The system is designed to work as a movement meditation, where the transitions from each posture to the next are as important as the postures themselves.

For the beginner it is essential to learn these three fundamental techniques at the outset. Once they are mastered, the practice will happen almost effortlessly. Without them it can become hard work. The three techniques are *Ujjayi pranayama*, *Mula Bandha*, and *Uddiyana Bandha*. We now focus on the first of these.

Ujjayi pranayama means "victorious breath" or the victorious stretching of the breath. The term *pranayama* is a combination of two words, *prana* and *ayama*. *Ayama* means extending or stretching, while *prana* can have several meanings. It is usually taken to mean inner breath or life force, and as such it makes up part of the subtle anatomy of the body. Other elements of the subtle anatomy are *nadi*s (energy channels) and *chakra*s (energy centers). Sometimes, however, *prana* is used to refer to the outer or anatomical breath.[2] In this context *pranayama* means extension of breath: the adoption of a calm, peaceful, and steady breathing pattern. When the breath is calm, the mind is also calm.

1. The expression 'yoga *mala*' was coined by Shri K. Pattabhi Jois, and he is the author of a book with that title.
2. *Prana* has another meaning in the context of the principle of the ten individual currents within the life force, where it has reference to inhaling only.

Ujjayi pranayama is a process of stretching the breath, and in this way extending the life force. Practicing it requires a slight constriction of the glottis — the upper opening of the larynx — by partially closing it with the epiglottis. The epiglottis is a lid on the throat that is closed when we drink water and open when we breathe. By half closing the epiglottis we stretch the breath and create a gentle hissing sound, which we listen to throughout the entire practice. The sound produced seemingly comes from the center of the chest and not from the throat. The vocal cords are not engaged, as that would lead to strain: any humming that accompanies a sound like wind in the trees or waves on the shore should be eradicated.

Listening to the sound of your own breath has several implications. First and foremost it is a *pratyahara* technique. *Pratyahara*, the fifth limb of yoga, means "withdrawing the senses from the outer world" or, more simply, "going inside." This will be considered in detail later. For now it will suffice to say that listening to your own breath draws your attention inward and takes it away from external sounds. This is a meditation aid.

Furthermore the sound of the breath can teach us almost everything we need to learn about our attitude in the posture. At times the breath may sound strained, labored, short, aggressive, flat, shallow, or fast. By bringing it back to the ideal of a smooth, pleasant sound we begin to correct any negative or unhelpful attitudes.

To practice *Ujjayi*, sit in an upright but comfortable position. Start producing the *Ujjayi* sound steadily, with no breaks between breaths. Give the sound an even quality throughout the entire length of the breath, both inhaling and exhaling. Lengthen each breath and deepen it. Breathe evenly into the rib cage. Breathe simultaneously into the sides, the front, the back, and finally into the upper lobes of the lungs. The rib cage needs to have a gentle pulsating movement, which means the internal intercostals (the muscles between the ribs) relax on inhalation, allowing the rib cage to expand freely as we breathe.

Our culture tends to focus only on abdominal breathing, which leads not only to a slouching posture but also to rigidity of the rib cage. This is due to the intercostal muscles lacking exercise, which in turn blocks the flow of blood and life force in the thorax and opens the way to coronary disease and cardiopulmonary weakness. The slouching appearance in this area is due to a relaxation of the rectus abdominis muscle, commonly known as "the abs." This slouching makes the belly soft and promotes abdominal breathing.

Furthermore this relaxation of the rectus abdominis allows the pubic bone to drop, leading to an anterior (forward) tilt of the pelvis, which produces a hyperlordotic low back, commonly referred to as a sway back. This in turn lifts the origin of the erector spinae,[3] the main back extensor muscle. Thus shortened, the erector spinae loses its effectiveness in lifting the chest. The chest collapses, leading not only to a slouching appearance but also to a rigid, hard rib cage. This prevents the thoracic organs from getting massaged during breathing. The lack of massage and movement of heart and lungs lowers their resistance to disease. The compensatory pattern, leading to a sway back, an anteriorly tilted pelvis, and a collapsed chest, is one of the worst postural imbalances, and its main cause is favoring abdominal breathing and the resulting weakness of the abdominals.

In yoga we use both the abdomen and the thorax to breathe. The intercostals are exercised through actively breathing. The air is literally pumped out of the lungs until all that remains is the respiratory rest volume, the amount of air left after a full exhalation. The aim is to breathe more deeply so as to increase vitality. The way to achieve this is not by inhaling as much as possible but by first exhaling completely in order to create space for the new inhalation.

There are two vital reasons for wanting to increase breath volume. First, by increasing our inhalation we increase the amount of oxygen supplied.

Second, by increasing our exhalation we exhale more toxins.

These toxins fall into several categories:

• Mental toxins — examples include the thought of conflict toward another being or collective conflict like the wish to go to war with another nation for whatever reason.

• Emotional toxins — fear, anger, hatred, jealousy, attachment to suffering, and the like.

• Physical toxins — metabolic waste products that are not being excreted.

• Environmental toxins — lead, nicotine, carbon dioxide, sulfur dioxide, recreational drugs, and the like.

All of these toxins have a tendency to be held and stored in the body in "stale," "dead" areas where there is only a small amount of oxygen, often around the joints or in adipose tissue (fat). The buildup of these toxins — a literal energetic dying of certain body areas long before the death of the entire organism — can eventually lead to chronic disease. In fact the buildup of toxins and the simultaneous depletion of oxygen in certain tissues is the number-one cause of chronic disease.

By breathing deeply, exhaling accumulated toxins and inhaling oxygen, we take the first steps toward returning the body to its original state of health. More steps are required, and these will be covered later. Briefly they are storing energy (in the section that follows on *bandhas*) and awakening the whole body (Part 2, Asana).

The main reason for practicing *Ujjayi pranayama* is not, however, for its physical benefits, but rather in order to still the mind. Why should the mind be stilled? *Yoga Sutra* I.2 states, "Yoga is the stilling of the fluctuations of the mind." Sutra I.3 says, "Only then when the mind is still abides the seer in its true nature."

The mind can be likened to a lake. If thought waves (*vrtti*) appear, the surface of the lake is disturbed and ripples appear. Looking into the water you can see only a distorted representation of your appearance. This distortion is what we constantly see, and it is the reason we don't know our true selves. This leads to suffering (*duhkha*) and ignorance (*avidya*).

When the thought waves have subsided and

3. The origin of a muscle is the end that is closer to the center of the body, called the proximal end; its insertion is the end more distant from the center of the body, called the distal end.

the surface of the lake of the mind becomes still for the first time, we can see who we really are. The mind is completely clear and, as a result, we can achieve identity with the object it is directed at.[4] The notion of stilling the fluctuations of the mind is often referred to as the arresting of the mind or mind control in yogic literature. The term "mind control" is misleading and unfortunate, however. It was rigorously criticized by sages like Ramana Maharshi, who said that if you want to control the mind you need a second mind to control the first one, and a third to control the second. Aside from this infinite regression, having separate parts of your mind struggle for control over each other can lead to schizophrenia. In less extreme cases it can lead to becoming a "control freak," which makes for being a thoroughly unhappy person.

Ancient yogis found a solution to this problem when they realized that thinking (*vrtti*) and movement of life force (*prana*) happen together. According to the *Hatha Yoga Pradipika*, "Both the mind and the breath are united together like milk and water and both of them are equal in their activities. The mind begins its activities where there is the breath, and the *prana* begins its activities where there is the mind."[5]

We know now that mind and breath move together. Influencing the mind directly is regarded as difficult, but through directing the breath it can be achieved much more easily. The extension of the breath through the practice of *Ujjayi pranayama* smooths the flow of *prana*.

It is important always to breathe through the nose only. If we breathe through the mouth, heat and energy will be lost. It will also dry us out too much. According to Indian tradition, if the mouth is kept open demons will enter. Apparently demons become very jealous of the merit that a yogi accumulates. I will leave this view to individual evaluation.

Remember the connection between breath and movement: every movement comes out of breath. Rather than moving with and following the breath, the breath should initiate the movement. Practicing this way, we will be moved by the breath like the autumn wind picking up leaves.

4. *Yoga Sutra* I.41.
5. *Hatha Yoga Pradipika* IV.24, trans. Pancham Sinh, Sri Satguru Publications, Delhi, 1915, p. 50.

Bandhas

We have learned in the previous section about the importance of deep breathing. What is it exactly that makes yogic breathing so effective?

To answer this we have to look again at the idea of *prana*. As we already know, *prana* can refer to the anatomical breath, but it most often denotes life force, located in the subtle body. It is important to understand that the two are not identical. However, the movements of the life force that occur in the subtle or energetic body have some correlation to the movement of breath in the gross body. The flow of *prana* can be influenced by directing one's breath. It can even be accumulated and stored. Most of us have heard accounts of yogis who managed to survive without oxygen for extended periods of time. Although it is not the purpose of yoga to perform such feats, it is nevertheless possible using a set of exercises called *mudras*, *mudra* meaning "seal." They are a combination of posture, breath, and *bandha*, and they produce the sealing of *prana*. It is this process of gaining control of the life force that differentiates yogic exercise from mere gymnastics. Gymnastics and sport can make one fit, but they don't have the energy-preserving effect of yoga, because they do not use *mudra* and *bandha*. It is the combination of posture with *pranayama* and *bandha* that makes yoga so effective.

The term *bandha* is related to the English word "bonding." We bond breath, movement, and awareness together. The first *bandha* is called *Mula Bandha*, which translates as "root lock." The root referred to here is the root of the spine, the pelvic floor or, more precisely, the center of the pelvic floor, the perineum. The perineum is the muscular body between the anus and the genitals. By slightly contracting the pubo-coccygeal (PC) muscle, which goes from the pubic bone to the tailbone (coccyx), we create an energetic seal that locks *prana* into the body and so prevents it from leaking out at the base of the spine. *Mula Bandha* is said to move *prana* into the central channel, called *sushumna*, which is the subtle equivalent of the spine.

Locating the PC muscle might be difficult at first. It has been suggested that one should tighten the anus, or alternatively contract the muscle that one would use to stop urination, but these indications are not entirely accurate: *Mula Bandha* is neither of these two muscles but located right between them. These suggestions have their value, however, offering some guidance until we become more sensitive and are able to isolate the PC muscle more precisely. For females it is essential not to mistake *Mula Bandha* for a contraction of the cervix. This contraction tends to occur especially during strenuous activity. Should a woman do this on a daily basis when engaged in two hours of yoga practice, she could experience difficulty in giving birth.

In the beginning we employ mainly a gross muscular lock, which works mainly on the gross body. Through practice we shift to an energetic lock, which works more on the subtle or pranic body. When mastered, *Mula Bandha* becomes exclusively mental, and works on the causal body.

To become familiar with *Mula Bandha*, sit tall and upright in a comfortable position and focus on slightly contracting the perineum, which is the center of the pelvic floor. With the exhalation, visualize the breath beginning at the nostrils and slowly reaching down through the throat, the chest, and the abdomen until it eventually hooks into the pelvic floor, which contracts slightly. As the inhalation starts, there will be an automatic reaching upward. Since we keep the breath hooked into the pelvic floor through contracting the PC muscle, we create suction and an energetic lift upward through the entire core of the body. This is *Mula Bandha*. With this movement the first step is taken to arrest the downward flow of life force, which increases with age and invites death, disease, and decay like the withering of a plant, and convert it into an upward flow that promotes growth and further blossoming.

Mula Bandha is held throughout the entire breathing cycle and during the whole practice. Every posture needs to grow out of its root. This is only finally released during deep relaxation in complete surrender. The second *bandha* is *Uddiyana Bandha*. It is sometimes confused with *Uddiyana*, one of the *shat karmas* or six actions, also called *kriyas*, of Hatha Yoga. This *Uddiyana* is a preparation for *nauli*, the stomach roll. *Nauli* is practiced by sucking the entire abdominal content up into the thoracic cavity. It is done only during breath retention (*kumbhaka*), and it is very

different from the technique practiced in Vinyasa Yoga. The *Uddiyana Bandha* of Vinyasa Yoga is a much gentler exercise. It consists of lightly contracting the transverse abdominis muscle, which runs horizontally across the abdomen and is used to draw the abdominal contents in against the spine.

To successfully switch on *Uddiyana Bandha*, it is important to isolate the upper transverse abdominis muscle from the lower part and use only the part below the navel. Doing otherwise impinges on the free movement of the diaphragm. If the movement of the diaphragm is restricted for a long time, aggressive, boastful, egotistical, and macho tendencies can develop in the psyche. This is not endorsed by traditional teaching, however. Shankara and Patanjali provide us with the following explanations. True posture, according to Shankara, is that which leads effortlessly to meditation on Brahman and not to pain and self-torture. Patanjali says that *asana* is perfected when meditation on the infinite (*ananta*) is achieved through the releasing of excess effort.[6]

Some have claimed that Ashtanga Yoga is warrior yoga, and that warriors used it to psych themselves up for battle. This is a very sad misunderstanding. Those who have had a true experience of the practice will have come away feeling tired and happy — and definitely not psyched up for battle. Rather, one feels more like hugging one's enemy and, in complete surrender, handing them whatever they demand — perhaps even imparting genuine advice as to how to enjoy life and not waste it with such stupidities as aggression and warfare. There is no warrior yoga. War and yoga exclude each other because the first yogic commandment is *ahimsa* — nonviolence.

Richard Freeman says that *Uddiyana Bandha* is in fact only a slight suction inward just above the pubic bone. The more subtle *Uddiyana Bandha* becomes, the more blissful, peaceful, childlike, and innocent becomes the character of the practitioner. I suggest starting by firming the abdominal wall below the navel and then, as awareness increases with years of practice, allow *Uddiyana Bandha* to slide downward. Again, the more subtle it becomes, the more influence *Uddiyana Bandha* will have on the subtle body.

6. *Yoga Sutra* II.47.

As I have mentioned in the previous section, a lot of emphasis has been placed on abdominal breathing in our culture in the last forty years. This has its place in the performing arts — especially dance and theater — and for therapy. It is certainly helpful for singers and actors, and for someone undergoing psychotherapy. Abdominal breathing, with complete relaxation of the abdominal wall, is recommended as useful whenever we want to connect to our emotions and bring them to the fore. In the New Age movement in particular, emotions are seen as something sacred that one needs to follow and live out. Abdominal breathing is a good idea whenever one wants to intensify one's emotions.

In many other situations, though, it is not helpful to heighten one's emotions. After all, emotions are only a form of the mind. To be emotional means to react to a present situation according to a past conditioning. For example, if I am rejected in a certain situation that is new to me, I will feel hurt. If I find myself in a similar situation again, I will become emotional even before any new hurt has been inflicted. I will emote "hurt" before I actually feel it. An emotion is a conserved feeling that arises because the original feeling has left a subconscious imprint in the mind. Patanjali calls this imprint *samskara*. The theory that being emotional is being more authentic is flawed, since an emotional person is as much in the past as a person who is constantly "in his or her head."

Besides the fact that it makes one emotional, constant abdominal breathing also has negative physical repercussions. It leads to sagging, collapsing abdominal organs with enlarged, weak blood vessels and stagnant blood. Then follow a lack of oxygen supply, a decrease in vitality, and eventually the development of chronic disease.

If the lower abdominal wall is kept firm and the upper wall is relaxed, the diaphragm moves up and down freely and the whole abdomen functions like the combustion chamber of an engine, with the diaphragm as the piston. This produces a strong oscillation of intra-abdominal blood pressure, and it is exactly this mechanism that produces healthy abdominal organs. When the diaphragm moves down and the abdominal wall is held, the pressure in the combustion chamber will rise. When the diaphragm moves up, all the blood is sucked out of the abdomen and blood pressure drops. This strong oscillation of abdominal blood pressure constantly massages the internal organs and leads to strong, healthy tissue.[7]

We look now at the subtle mechanics of *Uddiyana Bandha*. *Uddiyana* means flying up. The *Hatha Yoga Pradipika* states that, because of *Uddiyana Bandha*, the great bird of *prana* flies up incessantly through the *sushumna*.[8] *Sushumna* is the central energy channel, which lies, albeit in the subtle body, roughly in front of the spine and originates at the perineum. It terminates within the head — some sources say at the highest point of the head, but more often it is described as ending where the head is joined to the spine. The *sushumna* is usually dormant. It is accompanied by two other *nadi*s (energy channels), which wind around it like the snakes of the caduceus. These are the lunar (*ida*) and solar (*pingala*) channels. There are certain parallels between solar and lunar energy channels on the one hand and the sympathetic and parasympathetic nervous systems on the other, but we cannot say that the one *is* the other.

The *Hatha Yoga Pradipika* explains that *prana* should be directed into *sushumna* by closing the *ida* and *pingala*.[9] The same text states that, by practicing *Mula Bandha*, *prana* will enter *sushumna*. In a later stanza of the text a great truth is revealed: time (which we perceive as the fluctuation of night and day) is produced by the sun and moon.[10] In other words, it is the illusion of time that prevents us from recognizing deep reality (Brahman), which is timeless and is fabricated by the moment of inner breath (*prana*) in the *pingala* (solar) and *ida* (lunar) energy channels.

The stanza goes on to reveal the key to all physical yoga, which is that the *sushumna* devours time. In other words, if *prana* is made to enter the central channel it will devour time, which is itself a creation of the fluctuating mind and which keeps us from abiding in deep reality, the timeless consciousness (Brahman). Time is the operating system of the

7. This process is described by Andre Van Lysbeth in his book *Die grosse Kraft des Atems*, which he wrote after he studied with K. Pattabhi Jois in the 1960s.
8. *Hatha Yoga Pradipika* III.56.
9. *Hatha Yoga Pradipika* III.73.
10. *Hatha Yoga Pradipika* IV.17.

human mind; to go beyond time is to go beyond mind. This is possible when the great bird of *prana* flies up in *sushumna*, and *sushumna* devours time. For this the use of *Mula* and *Uddiyana Bandha* is prescribed.

Even the great Shankara says that *Mula Bandha* should always be practiced, since it is fit for raja yogins. In other words, even raja yogins — those who practice mind suspension and who are sometimes disparaging about Hatha yogins and their preoccupation with their bodies — should take up the practice of *Mula Bandha*, since it leads to going beyond mind. If we remember now Patanjali's definition of yoga being the suspension of mind,[11] we begin to understand the importance of *Mula* and *Uddiyana Bandha*.

Drishti

We move on now to *drishti* or focal point. As we have seen, the fifth limb of yoga is sense withdrawal (*pratyahara*). The *Upanishads* explain that the senses deliver the fuel for the mind in the form of sense objects. The mind then develops desires, which are the source of suffering. The mind's basic concept is that we are lacking. This lack, according to the mind, can only be alleviated through a constant supply of stimulation from outside.

The concept of yoga, on the other hand, holds that we are always in the original and pristine state of bliss, which is consciousness. This original state is formless, however; and, since the mind has the tendency to attach itself to whatever comes along next, we forget our true nature. Sense withdrawal means to accept the fact that external stimuli can never truly fulfill us. Once that is accepted, we are free to realize that what we were desperately looking for on the outside was present inside all along. The *Upanishads* explain further that, as a fire dies down when the fuel is withheld, so the mind will return to its source when the fuel of the senses is withheld. The method — or rather the collection of methods — by which this can be brought about is sense withdrawal (*pratyahara*).

As has been explained, the withdrawal of the audio sense is brought about by listening to one's own breath rather than to external sounds. The withdrawal or turning in of the visual sense is practiced through *drishti*, the attachment of one's gaze to various focal points. These are:

- toward the nose
- toward the center of the forehead (third eye)
- toward the navel
- toward the hand
- toward the toes
- toward the side
- toward the thumb
- upward

By doing this, one prevents oneself from looking around, which would let the mind reach out. Following *drishti*, the practice becomes deeply internal and meditative.

Drishti is also a practice of concentration (*dharana*), the sixth of Patanjali's limbs of yoga. If we practice in a distracted way, we may find ourselves listening to the birds outside and gazing around the room. To perform all of the prescribed actions — *bandha*, *ujjayi*, *drishti*, and finding proper alignment — the mind needs to be fully concentrated; otherwise one of the elements will miss out. In this way the practice provides us with constant feedback about whether we are in *dharana*. In time *dharana* will lead to meditation (*dhyana*).

Drishti has also a significant energetic aspect. According to the *Yoga Yajnavalkya*, which contains the yoga teachings of the sage Yajnavalkya, "One must endeavour to retain all the *prana* through the mind, in the navel, the tip of the nose and the big toes. Focussing at the tip of the nose is the means to mastery over *prana*. By focussing on the navel all diseases are removed. The body attains lightness by focussing on the big toes."[12] According to A. G. Mohan, a student of T. Krishnamacharya and translator of the *Yoga Yajnavalkya*, the aim of yoga is to concentrate the *prana* in the body, whereas it is usually scattered. A scattered *prana* will correspond to a scattered state of mind.

The scattered state of mind is called *vikshipta* in the *Yoga Sutra*. *Prana* that is drawn inward and concentrated in the body corresponds to the single-

11. *Yoga Sutra* I.2.

12. *Yoga Yajnavalkya*, trans. A. G. Mohan, Ganesh & Co., Madras, pp. 81–82.

pointed (*ekagra*) and suspended (*nirodha*) states of mind, which lead to objective (*samprajnata*) and objectless (*asamprajnata*) *samadhi*. In the Ashtanga Vinyasa method, *drishti* is one of the vital techniques to draw the *prana* inward. Anyone who has practiced in front of a mirror may have noticed how looking into it draws awareness away from the core toward the surface. Exactly this happens to the flow of *prana*, which follows awareness. Practicing in front of a mirror might be helpful from time to time to check one's alignment if no teacher is present, but it is preferable to develop proprioceptive awareness — awareness that does not depend on visual clues. This type of awareness draws *prana* inward, which corresponds to what the *Upanishad*s call dissolving the mind into the heart. The permanent establishing of *prana* in the core of the body leads to *samadhi* or liberation.

As enthusiastic as some scriptures are about techniques like *drishti*, we have to remember we are still just operating within conditioned existence. The master Shankara reminds us: "Converting the ordinary vision into one of knowledge one should view the world as brahman (consciousness) itself. That is the noblest vision and not that which is directed to the tip of the nose."[13]

Vinyasa

Vinyasa Yoga is a system of yoga specifically designed for householders. The difference between a householder (*grihasta*) and a renunciate (*sannyasi*) is that the latter has no social duties and can therefore devote ten or more hours per day to practice. In fact, if individual techniques pertaining to all the eight limbs were practiced daily, one would easily spend more than ten hours practicing. For example a wonderful day could be had by practicing *asana* for two hours, *pranayama* for two hours, *mudra* and *japa* (repetition of mantra) each for one hour, reading of scripture one hour, chanting of scripture one hour, reflection and contemplation one hour, meditation one hour.

A householder — meaning someone who has a family and a job or a business to attend to — can never spend so much time on the practice. The idea

of completely turning your back on society is actually fairly recent, relatively speaking. It was introduced by Gautama Buddha and elaborated on by Shankara. The ancient vedic and upanishadic *rishi*s, although they spent considerable time in the forest, were not dropouts. *Rishi*s like Yajnavalkya, Vasishta, and Vishvamitra had wives and children, and held positions such as priest or royal counselor.

For a yoga practice to work for householders, it would be necessary to compress it into two hours and yet retain its benefits, and so the eight limbs would have to be practiced simultaneously and not sequentially. With this in mind Rishi Vamana created the Vinyasa Yoga. The *rishi* arranged the practice in sequences, such that the postures were potentiating their effects, and combined them with *mudra*, *pranayama*, and meditation so that a ten-hour practice could be effectively compressed into two hours.

One of Vinyasa Yoga's outstanding features is that postures are not held for a long time. One of the greatest traps in physical yoga is to get identified with postures and preoccupied with the body. One thinks, "Now I am sitting in *Padmasana*. This is yoga!" One couldn't be more wrong. To perceive the awareness that witnesses sitting in *Padmasana* — that is yoga.

The core idea of Vinyasa Yoga is to shift emphasis from posture to breath and therefore to realize that postures, like all forms, are impermanent. The formed — *asana*s, bodies of life-forms, structures, nations, planets, and so on — come and go. The quest of yoga is for the formless (consciousness) — for what was here before form arose and what will be here after form has subsided. For this reason it was necessary to organize the practice in such a way that nothing impermanent is held on to. Vinyasa Yoga is a meditation on impermanence.

The only thing permanent in the practice is the constant focus on the breath. According to the *Brahma Sutra*,[14] "ata eva pranah" — the breath verily is Brahman. The breath is here identified as a metaphor for Brahman (that is, deep reality, ultimate reality, infinite consciousness). This assertion is based on the authority of the *Chandogya Upanishad*, where the question is asked: Which is that divinity?[15]

13. *Aparokshanubhuti of Sri Shankaracharya*, trans. Sw. Vimuktananda, Advaita Ashrama, Kolkata, 1938, p. 63.

14. *Brahma Sutra* I.I.23.
15. *Chandogya Upanishad* I:II:5.

Answer: "Breath...Verily, indeed all beings enter (into life) with breath and depart (from life) with breath."[16] Through *vinyasa* the postures are linked to form a *mala*. A *mala* is commonly used to count mantras during mantra meditation, whereas in Vinyasa Yoga every *asana* becomes a bead on this *mala* of yoga postures. In this way the practice becomes a movement meditation.

The practice produces heat, which is needed to burn toxins. Not only physical toxins are meant here, but also the poison of ignorance and delusion. The full-*vinyasa* practice, which entails coming back to standing between postures, has a flushing effect through the constant forward bending. It can be recommended in cases of strong, persistent toxicity and for recuperation after disease. The half-*vinyasa* practice, in which one jumps back between performance of the right and left sides of sitting postures, is designed to create a balance between strength and flexibility and to increase heat.

If *asana* only is practiced, this might lead to excess flexibility, which can destabilize the body. The proper position of the bones in the body, and especially of the spine, is remembered by sustaining a certain core tension in the muscles. If the tension is insufficient, frequent visits to a chiropractor or osteopath may become necessary.

In the *vinyasa* method, this possibility is avoided by jumping back between sides, which gives us the strength to support the amount of flexibility that is gained. This concept is important to understand. Flexibility that cannot be supported by strength should not be aimed for.

The underlying principle here is that of simultaneous expansion into opposing directions. Whenever we expand into one direction, we at the same time need to counteract that by expanding into the opposite direction. In this way we are not caught into extremes of body and mind. Patanjali says, "Thus one is unassailed by the pair of opposites."[17] For this reason one needs to place the same importance on *vinyasa* as on *asana*. As Rishi Vamana put it, "Oh Yogi, don't practice *asana* without *vinyasa*."

16. G. C. Adams, Jr., trans. and comment, *Badarayana's Brahma Sutras*, Motilal Banarsidass, Delhi, 1993, p. 60.
17. *Yoga Sutra* II.48.

Vinyasa Count

In colloquial language today, the term *vinyasa* is taken to refer to the jumping back and jumping through between the sides of postures (half *vinyasa*) and the movement that brings us to standing between postures (full *vinyasa*).

In the ancient treatise *Yoga Korunta*, *vinyasa* refers to every counted movement, accompanied by breath and focal point. The *vinyasa* count is a format in which the Rishi Vamana recorded the Ashtanga practice in the *Yoga Korunta*.

Each movement that is needed to enter and exit a posture in the traditional way is counted. Since the postures differ greatly not only from each other but also in the way in which they are entered and exited, they also differ very much in regard to the number of sequential movements that are needed to perform them (their *vinyasa* counts). So *Padangushtasana* has only three *vinyasas* (counted movements) whereas *Supta Padangushtasana* has twenty-eight. All *vinyasas* are flowing movements. The only one that is held is the *vinyasa* where we are in the state of the *asana*. To be in the state of the *asana* means to be in and to hold a posture. For *Padangushtasana*, for example, this is *vinyasa* three. This *vinyasa* is held usually for five breaths, though for therapeutic purposes it may be held for twenty-five breaths or more. The fact that one *vinyasa* may consist of up to twenty-five breaths leads us to the understanding that *vinyasa* count and the number of breaths, the breath count, are not identical.

In the following section I describe the postures following the half-*vinyasa* count. That is the way I learned it in Mysore and it is the normal mode of practice today.

To make this text more accessible to beginners I have counted the *vinyasas* in English. The original *vinyasa* count is, however, in Sanskrit, and it is important to preserve this precious tradition. Accordingly, I use the Sanskrit count when I conduct a *vinyasa*-count class. For those who want to study the *vinyasa* count more closely, I recommend K. Pattabhi Jois's *Yoga Mala* and Lino Mieles's *Ashtanga Yoga*.

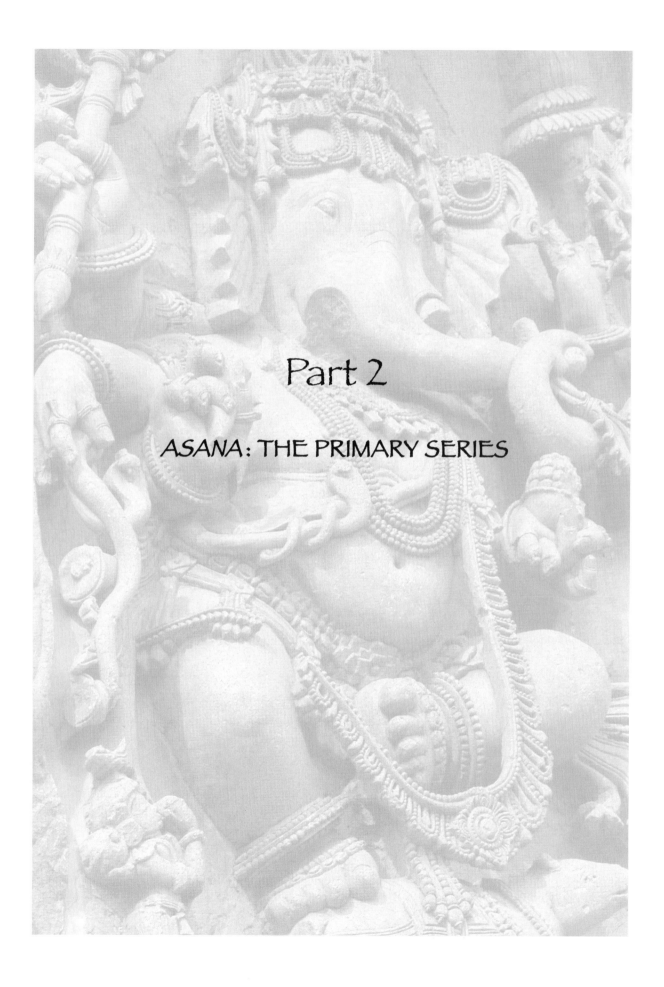

Part 2

ASANA: THE PRIMARY SERIES

Asana Names

Like the entire creation, the names of the *asana*s can be divided into four groups: lifeless forms, animal forms, human forms, and divine forms.

*Asana*s such as *Trikonasana* (Triangle Posture) and *Navasana* (Boat Posture), representing lifeless forms, occur predominantly in the Primary Series.

The Intermediate or Second Series is dominated by postures named after animals, for example *Shalabasana* (Locust Posture), *Kapotasana* (Pigeon Posture), and *Krounchasana* (Heron Posture).

The human race is represented by *asana*s dedicated to the ancient *rishi*s. Examples are *Marichyasana* (Posture of the Rishi Marichi), *Bharadvajasana* (Posture of the Rishi Bharadvaja), and *Durvasasana* (Posture of the Rishi Durvasa).

*Asana*s named after divine forms — such as *Natarajasana* (Lord of the Dance Posture), *Hanuman-asana* (Posture of Lord Hanuman), and *Skandasana* (Posture Dedicated to Lord Kartikeya) — occur, like those dedicated to *rishi*s, mainly in the Advanced A or Third Series.

The Yogic Approach

The Ashtanga Vinyasa Yoga practice is a movement meditation. The goal is that every breath taken becomes a conscious one. The set sequence, the consistent flow, the internal holding of the *bandha*s, the *drishti*, and listening to the sound of the *Ujjayi pranayama* are all techniques designed to withdraw the senses.

This facilitates focused concentration so that meditation becomes possible. Absence of the *Ujjayi* sound, shallow breathing, and fidgeting usually indicate that the mind has taken over and focus has been lost.

In the *Yoga Sutra*, Patanjali gives three stanzas on *asana*.[1] Their simplicity is profound.

1. *Yoga Sutra* II.46, 47, and 48.

Posture is steadiness and ease.
True posture is then when effort ceases and meditation on infinity occurs.
In *asana* there is no assault from the pairs of opposites.

Posture is steadiness and ease.

This stanza describes the qualities of posture. Steadiness implies effort and strength. Ease implies relaxation and release. These opposites are complementary. The effort required to build a strong body produces steadiness and gives ease of posture.

True posture is then when effort ceases and meditation on infinity occurs.

The ultimate aim of any limb of yoga is for us to experience our true nature. In practice, and in the following descriptions of how to perform each posture, sensitivity, awareness, and heightened concentration are demanded. Eventually, when the posture is known, we can drop the details and "be" in the posture. Effort ceases; the posture is expressed from within; meditation on infinity occurs. Infinity is a quality of our true nature.

In asana *there is no assault from the pairs of opposites.*

Steadiness and ease are themselves a pair of opposites, and yet, when in balance, each supports and allows the other to express itself fully. With excess effort the body becomes insensitive and the mind agitated. With excess ease the body becomes sluggish and the mind dull. Both aspects of this duality must be embraced. In his book *Awareness through Movement*, Moshe Feldenkrais points out that, if one lifts an iron bar and a fly alights on it, no difference can be noticed. If, however, you hold a feather you will notice if a fly lands on or takes off from it. With excess effort there is no room for improvement, as full effort has already been exerted. Sensitivity reserves the space to observe differences, to adapt the posture and to learn. In the space between the opposites, the mind falls still.

Action and Counteraction / Posture and Counterposture

These opposites also exist as fundamental differences between the actions that transport us into a posture and those that maintain it. As a rule of thumb, actions that take us into a posture need to be reversed when working in the posture itself. For example, while forward bending is performed by the hip flexors, once we are in the posture we use the hamstrings, which are hip extensors.[2] Back-bending is performed by the trunk extensors, but once in the posture we counteract these by engaging the abdominal muscles. To arrive in *Baddha Konasana* we use the external hip rotators; once in the posture we use the internal hip rotators.

The fact that every action performed in yoga does not continue endlessly means that we automatically perform the opposing action to counteract it and so reach a balanced state. As each posture is balanced by a counterposture, so each action within the posture is balanced by its counteraction until a neutral position is reached.

The neutral position is that in which the initial action has been balanced and correct alignment has been achieved. Alignment is correct when steadiness and lightness in the posture are achieved, holding it becomes effortless, and meditation is possible. This state is reached when all actions are balanced by opposing actions.

The posture remains alive and active as we continually play with balancing these opposites.

How to Stretch

There are three ways to stretch in a posture: passive, active, and dynamic/ballistic stretching. An example of passive stretching would be folding your torso forward from a standing position and then just hanging from your hip joints with your arms dangling down or your elbows clasped. Passive stretching is relatively ineffective, as it takes a long

time to produce results. A person with high muscle tension could hang in a passive stretch for half an hour without getting very far.

This type of stretching has the added disadvantage of not protecting the muscle stretched. For example, if in the posture previously described we reached for the toes and drew the torso down with our arms, the stretch would mainly be taken at the origin of the hamstring muscles, the ischial tuberosities, which are a part of the sit bones. This can result in tearing of muscle fibers, the so-called pulling of the hamstrings. Another downside of passive stretching is that it does not build strength to support the flexibility gained.

The technique employed in Ashtanga Yoga is active stretching. In this type of stretching we use an inherent reflex without which the body could not move. Whenever a muscle contracts, its antagonist (the muscle with the opposite function) releases. To understand this reflex one may look at the elbow joint. When the biceps (biceps brachii) contracts, the triceps (triceps brachii) releases, so that the elbow may be flexed. If the triceps also contracted, the elbow could not move. Likewise, when the triceps contracts, the nervous system simultaneously sends a signal to the biceps to release, and the elbow is extended.

A muscle that is being stretched will receive a signal to release when the opposing muscle is activated. In addition to gravity, it will also be stretched by the strength of the opposing muscle. At the same time, the opposing muscle will be exercised and increase in strength. With this method we will be able to close a joint — flex it — to about 85 percent. To access the remaining 15 percent, we will use a technique we call "active release," which is covered later.

The other form of stretching is dynamic stretching, mainly used in martial arts, rhythmic gymnastics, and calisthenics. Here one uses momentum to stretch. It is not often employed in yoga as it is considered too forceful. There are some exceptions in Vinyasa Yoga, such as *Supta Konasana* in the Primary Series and *Supta Vajrasana* in the Intermediate Series. Dropping into a backbend from standing, handstand drop-backs, and *Viparita Chakrasana* are other examples of dynamic stretching.

Apart from these exceptions, active stretching is used in the whole of the Ashtanga Yoga practice.

---

2. Flexion means bringing bones together; extension is the return from flexion. An exception is the movement of the humerus (the arm bone), where flexion is defined as raising the arm from its resting position forward and over the head. The flexors and extensors are respectively the muscles that bring these movements about.

Full *Vinyasa* versus Half *Vinyasa*

With the full-*vinyasa* system, one returns to *Samasthiti* (the basic standing posture) between each and every *asana*. The format I learned from Shri K. Pattabhi Jois in Mysore was the half-*vinyasa* system. This has one return to *Samasthiti* between different standing postures but transiting from one sitting posture to the next without coming to standing. This approach appears to be the more common one today.

It can be advisable to practice full *vinyasa* for some time to improve strength and stamina, for example after recovery from disease or to speed up metabolism. The full-*vinyasa* approach has an intensified flushing effect and can stimulate a sluggish liver. Although full *vinyasa* is more work, it also allows time for the practitioner "to come up for air" so to speak, and may actually de-intensify a practice. It certainly does eventually repay the energy expended. However, as a long-term practice it may be difficult to sustain.

Temperature

If you practice in a hot country, you will heat up quickly. This is especially true of males. Care needs to be taken not to overheat if one is engaging in strenuous practice in a hot environment. As with any type of engine, so also with the human body: overheating is not good. Sweating is healthy, but if sweat drips from the body it is a sign that the body is no longer able to cool itself adequately. Sweating to this degree on a daily basis literally drains life force from the body. A temperature of 68°F would be ideal for practice, with a range of 15° below and above that still possible, but practice speed needs to be adapted — faster when it's cold to increase heat and slower when it's hot to cool down. On a hot day, focus on the cooling quality of the breath.

Heating the yoga room to above 77° may produce more flexibility, but it decreases strength, stamina, and concentration. If yoga were only about flexibility, contortionists would be the greatest yogis. It is worth noting that extreme flexibility is often a result of biochemical imbalance. True posture is about the ability to focus deeply within.

The Ashtanga Vinyasa practice attempts to balance flexibility with strength. Real yoga "will walk the edge between opposing extremes."[3] Rather than desperately cranking ourselves into one particular direction in a posture, we expand simultaneously in all directions. The first pair of opposites that we discover in physical yoga is strength/flexibility. Excess flexibility is an obstacle because it means loss of strength and vice versa. We should never build up a degree of flexibility that is not matched by the necessary support strength. On the other hand, building up great strength without increasing one's flexibility restricts the range of joint movement.

A heated yoga room helps flexibility because it increases *vata* and *pitta*. A cold yoga room helps strength because it increases *kapha*.[4] A cold room also increases awareness and attention to detail. We have to study the posture more deeply to get to the same point in a cold room, but this pays off in terms of benefits. There is more learning if the temperature is low, and the body becomes sturdier due to the awakening of physical intelligence. We can avoid this process by turning up the thermostat, but everybody who has worked through a couple of winters with only moderate heating values the gain in refinement that it brings.

If temperatures are high, proper ventilation is necessary. The western fashion of keeping all windows closed in sweltering temperatures so that you can see puddles of sweat on the floor is surprising, considering that I have never seen a yoga room in India that even had closeable windows. The *Hatha Yoga Pradipika* warns in several places of the dangers of too much heat and too much heating, by staying too close to the fire for example, and also of excess physical exertion. Getting too cold, for instance by taking cold morning baths, is also not recommended. The idea here is moderation: staying away from the extremes and abiding in the center. Once a yogi is fully established, however, extremes will no longer be of concern.

---

3. *Yoga Sutra* II.48.

4. *Vata*, *pitta*, and *kapha* are the three humors, or constitution types, of the body. The terms are used in *Ayurveda*, the ancient Indian system of medicine. They have been translated as wind, bile, and phlegm, but, since the concepts behind them are complex, it is better to use the Sanskrit terms.

Samasthiti
EQUAL STANDING

Drishti Nose

Samasthiti is the basic standing posture. We stand with the base of our big toes touching and the heels slightly apart so that the feet are parallel. The straight line of the foot is from the second toe to the center of the heel. If we were to bring the heels together, the thighbones (femurs) would be outwardly rotated to a slight extent.

We start by establishing *Ujjayi* breathing with a smooth and even sound. The rib cage expands evenly in all four directions, and the *bandha*s are consciously engaged if they have not automatically been initiated with the breath. The inhalation reaches down in front of the spine and hooks into the pelvic floor, creating a lifting sensation from the center of the perineum (*Mula Bandha*). At the same time, the lower abdominal wall, between the navel and the pubic bone, gently draws in toward the spine. The natural up-and-down movement of the diaphragm and the accompanying movement of the upper abdomen or stomach area are unrestricted.

The toes spread as one would spread one's fingers, in order to completely awaken the feet. The weight of the body is placed above the ankles and equally distributes to all four corners of the feet — the bases of the large and little toes and the inside and outside edges of the heels. The body weight is also evenly distributed between the inner and outer arches of the foot, while the arches are lifted and active. The action of the toes influences the pubic bone while the heels relate to the tailbone (coccyx).

The fronts of the thighs are contracted, with the quadriceps pulling up the kneecaps. Quadriceps means four heads, referring to the four points of origin of this large muscle group. All four heads join into the common quadriceps tendon, which leads down to the shin. The kneecap (patella), a floating bone, is embedded within it.

Many students will have to tilt the pelvis posteriorly (backward), which reduces any excess curvature in the low back and makes one stand taller. This movement is achieved by engaging the abdominal muscles, which lifts the pubic bone as the coccyx drops. The strength of the legs creates a

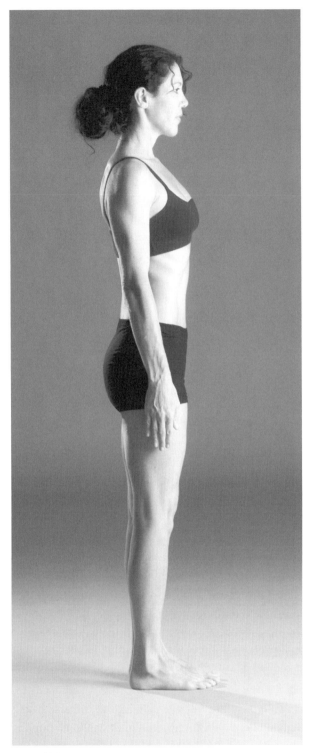

Samasthiti

vector of energy whose resonance is felt up the entire length of the body's core.

The front of the rib cage, the sternum, is lifted. (In common with many teachers, I will refer to this area as the heart.) One way of doing this pinches the shoulder blades (scapulae) together, which puffs the chest out as in a military posture of attention. This leads to a hardening and closing of the area behind the heart. Instead, as the heart is lifted, the area of the back behind the kidneys broadens and the shoulder blades widen and gently sink down the back. The shoulder blades flatten onto the back of

ANATOMICAL FOCUS
Inner Integrity

The bony vertebrae of the spine house the spinal cord, and its nerve ends exit between each vertebral body. The strong outer form of every posture supports the spine, enabling it to be fluid and extend freely. The nervous system remains unimpaired. This is the inner integrity that should be maintained within every posture.

Many chronic diseases, aches, and cultural ailments do not come from sick organs but from poor posture, which results in compression of the spine and impairment of the spinal nerves. Restoring the spine to its original state can alleviate these symptoms.

The spine becomes weak through lack of exercise and eventually loses its alignment due to weakness of the core muscles of the body. In many cases the spine actually shortens. The *vinyasa* method is an ideal tool to invigorate the spine and restore its natural elasticity. Any hardening, or any inability to extend the spine in a posture, is a sign of overexertion.

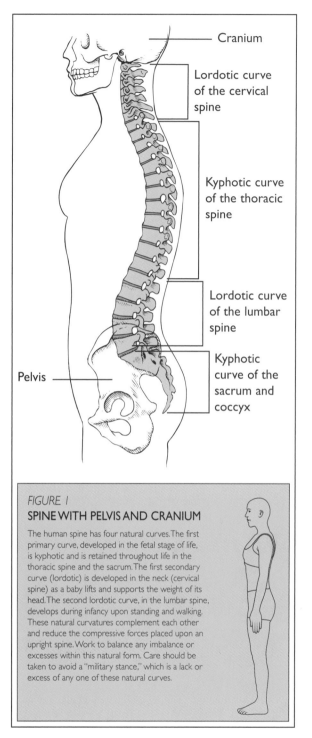

FIGURE 1
SPINE WITH PELVIS AND CRANIUM

The human spine has four natural curves. The first primary curve, developed in the fetal stage of life, is kyphotic and is retained throughout life in the thoracic spine and the sacrum. The first secondary curve (lordotic) is developed in the neck (cervical spine) as a baby lifts and supports the weight of its head. The second lordotic curve, in the lumbar spine, develops during infancy upon standing and walking. These natural curvatures complement each other and reduce the compressive forces placed upon an upright spine. Work to balance any imbalance or excesses within this natural form. Care should be taken to avoid a "military stance," which is a lack or excess of any one of these natural curves.

the chest and support the elevated and open position of the heart area. The lower ribs in the front of the chest soften back in toward the body. The arms may need to be "looped"[5] in the shoulder joint to reposition the head of the arm bone (humerus) so that it sits in the center of the shoulder joint. These actions leave the chest open and broad in all directions. The rib cage and lungs are free to expand, facilitating a full, free-flowing breath.

The chin drops slightly while the ears move back in line with the shoulders. Drawing the ears back in line with the shoulders corrects the

common postural condition of a forward head, where the ears are positioned in front of the shoulders when viewed from the side. In some cases this may measure more than four inches, which usually indicates that one's mind is racing ahead of one's actions. At the other extreme, those who remain in the past with their thoughts will often lean well back when they stand.

5. Looping means rolling back in a circular movement that is directed sequentially forward then upward, then backward and finally downward.

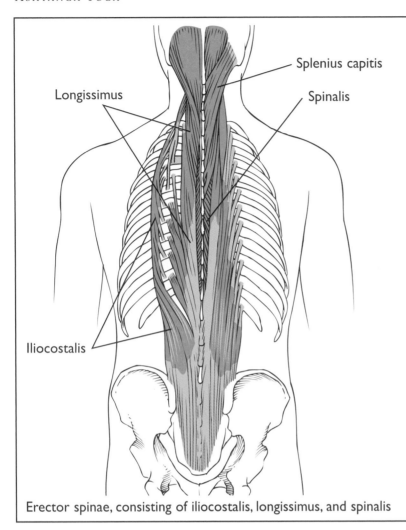

Longissimus

Splenius capitis

Spinalis

Iliocostalis

Erector spinae, consisting of iliocostalis, longissimus, and spinalis

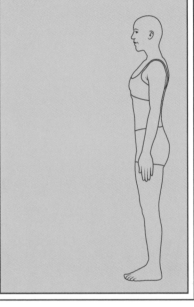

FIGURE 2 **ERECTOR SPINAE**

The erector spinae keeps the spine and thus the torso upright. Since it is situated posterior to the spine, it extends the spine (bends it backward) as it contracts. Its origin on the posterior crest of the ilium (hip bone) and the sacrum enables it to excessively curve the low back if it is permanently shortened.

The insertion of the erector spinae at the base of the skull enables it to take the head back. The many layers of the erector spinae also originate and insert at the transverse and spinous processes of most vertebrae and at the ribs, through which this complex muscle can maintain the integrity of the spine.

ANATOMICAL FOCUS

Postural Balance

Equal distribution of the weight of the body in the feet is imperative for balanced posture. When the body weight is placed too far forward in the feet, the low back (lumbar spine) hollows excessively (hyperlordosis) as the sacrum and coccyx lift. This puts excessive compressive forces onto the lumbar intervertebral discs and tightens the corresponding musculature (erector spinae and quadratus lumborum).

At the same time this positioning of the pelvis causes the abdominal muscles to release and weaken and the ribs to flare open. The area of the back behind the kidneys tightens and constricts, while the neck straightens, losing its natural lordotic curve, in an attempt to compensate for the excessive curvature produced in the lumbar spine and to bring the head back in line with the body's center of gravity.

On the other hand, if the weight is too far back in the feet, the hamstrings tighten and draw the pelvis and coccyx down in the back, while the pubic bone lifts at the front of the pelvis. As the body always strives toward equilibrium, this posture is usually accompanied by an increased curvature in the chest or thoracic spine (hyperkyphosis). The heart area collapses and the abdominals tighten. The shoulders round and the head shifts forward as the body compensates in an attempt to keep the center of gravity over the feet.

If too much weight is placed on the inside of the feet, the inner arches will collapse, placing stress on the medial menisci of the knees. This usually results in an anterior tilt of the pelvis, leading to excessive lumbar curvature.

To complete the picture, lift the highest point of the back of the head up toward the ceiling without losing the grounding of the feet. This action elongates and awakens the entire spine. Indian yogis have the exemplary tendency to humbly cast their gaze downward in *Samasthiti*. T. Krishnamacharya suggested that not to look down is to lose one's head.

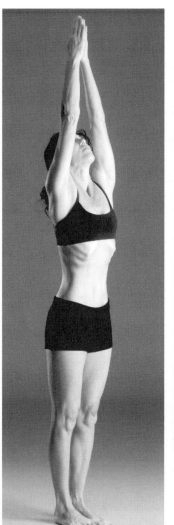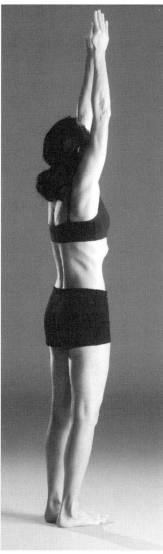

Surya Namaskara A, *vinyasa* one, correct shoulder position (left) and incorrect shoulder position (right)

The ideal alignment in *Samasthiti* is reached when all the major joints of the body — ankles, knees, hips, and shoulders — align one above the other, creating a vertical line that also passes through the ears. This establishes a posture with the least resistance to the forces of gravity, making effortless standing a possibility. *Samasthiti* is the blueprint for all other postures. Allow lightness and balance to be your guide.

Surya Namaskara A

SUN SALUTATION A

Drishti Thumbs, nose, navel

Surya Namaskara means Sun Salutation. It is traditionally done facing east, to greet the rising sun. Surya, the sun, is worshiped in many cultures as the giver of life; so too in India. The Sun Salutation is a warm-up exercise that is done a number of times to improve cardiovascular fitness. *Surya Namaskara* A is usually repeated five times, but more can be done on cold days, less in extreme heat — until the body feels awake and balanced. This sequence of *asanas* is also practiced to alleviate depression. It is said to bring health and vitality to the body and sunlight to the spirit.

Vinyasa One

At the beginning of the inhalation turn the palms out and reach far out to the sides and up, embracing as much space as possible until your palms are together above your head. The neck should always move as an extension of the spine, as indeed it is. The gaze lifts at the same pace as the lift of the arms. When the palms meet we are gazing up to the thumbs. The movement of the arms, the shifting of the gaze, and the movement of the breath should all be perfectly synchronized. This needs to be deeply understood, as it applies to the whole of the practice.

The lifting of the arms originates deep in the abdomen. This is done by hooking the breath into the abdomen and letting the power of the inhalation lift the arms. All lifting and upward movements are performed on the inhalation. The breath initiates each move and brings intelligence, grace, and ease to movement and posture.

When raising the arms, prevent hunching the shoulders up around the ears by actively drawing the shoulder blades down the back. This not only looks more elegant, but also prevents jamming of the neck (cervical) vertebrae and sets the correct pattern for arm balances and backbends. When looking up, do not throw the head back so that the face is parallel to the ceiling. This would be done either by collapsing the back of the neck or by overcontracting the trapezius muscle at the back of the neck.

Latissimus Dorsi

The action of the latissimus dorsi in drawing the shoulder blades toward the hips is anatomically called the depression of the shoulder girdle. Belonging to the outermost layer of muscles on the body, this muscle is difficult to overwork — in fact strengthening and toning of the latissimus dorsi relieves the burden usually placed on the trapezius and the other muscles that elevate the shoulder blades. The ideal approach is to commence training this muscle early.

Either way, it achieves no strength and offers no support to the neck. Instead, lift the chin to the ceiling, elongate the neck and the trapezius by engaging the latissimus dorsi muscle (the muscle that draws the shoulder blades down the back), and keep the back of the neck supported.

The head gently tilts on the atlas, the first of the neck vertebra. In Greek mythology, Atlas was the god who carried the world on his shoulders. This vertebra is also called C1, being the first of the seven cervical vertebrae.

Vinyasa Two

As we commence the exhalation, the pelvis begins to tip forward. On the way down, lead with the heart. The heart area remains lifted and open; do not collapse the chest. The arms are lowered at either side until eventually the hands are placed onto the floor, with the fingertips in line with the toes. Beginners and those with tight and shortened hamstring muscles should take care to keep the low back straight. As necessary, bend the knees when the pelvis no longer folds forward and the low back

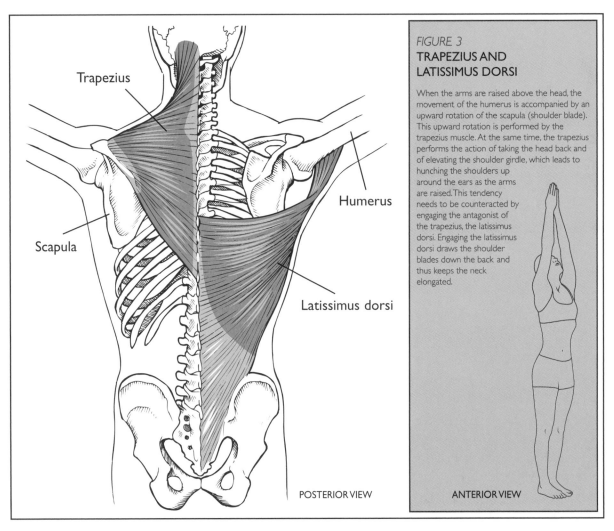

Trapezius

Scapula

Humerus

Latissimus dorsi

POSTERIOR VIEW

FIGURE 3
TRAPEZIUS AND LATISSIMUS DORSI

When the arms are raised above the head, the movement of the humerus is accompanied by an upward rotation of the scapula (shoulder blade). This upward rotation is performed by the trapezius muscle. At the same time, the trapezius performs the action of taking the head back and of elevating the shoulder girdle, which leads to hunching the shoulders up around the ears as the arms are raised. This tendency needs to be counteracted by engaging the antagonist of the trapezius, the latissimus dorsi. Engaging the latissimus dorsi draws the shoulder blades down the back and thus keeps the neck elongated.

ANTERIOR VIEW

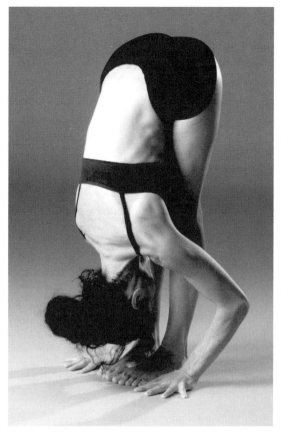

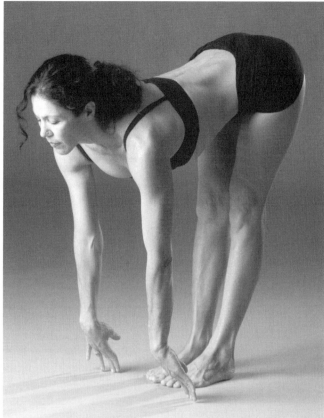

Surya Namaskara A, *vinyasa* two

Surya Namaskara A, *vinyasa* three

begins to round instead. Rounding of the low back places strain on the discs of the lumbar spine, eliminating the intended action of stretching the hamstring muscles. Even with the knees bent, one needs to feel a stretch in the hamstrings.

YOGIC CONTEXT
Breath Sense

All stretching needs to be done with sensitivity and awareness. In this way we work with, rather than against, the body. The breath is a great sensory tool that carries the natural intelligence of the body. It enables us to sensitize our awareness and thereby regulate the intensity of the stretch. As we inhale, we explore the new territory created and explored. This is the creative aspect of the posture. As we exhale, we release and relax into the new space gained. If you cannot breathe freely and extend the spine with your exhalation, you are trying too hard. All postures need to be worked with awareness, sensitivity and intelligence.

The abdominal muscles should be firm and supportive but not overcontracted, as this action would shorten the spine. At the end of the exhalation the crown of the head points down toward the floor. The neck is extended, with the head acting as a weight to lengthen the entire spine. Action is forever present in the feet, with the legs long, strong, and supportive. The groins are deep and soft (see *Padangushtasana*, page 37, for more details). The spine remains passive as it spills out of the hips, and only the shoulders are supported and lifted away from the ears.

Vinyasa Three

With the inhalation, lift the whole torso, attempting to concave or at least flatten out the low back while gazing up between the eyebrows. Unless one is extremely flexible, it is recommended to lift the hands off the floor and let only the fingertips keep contact with it. The legs work strongly, and the torso is buoyant, supported by the extensor muscles of the back. Keep the heart lifted, broaden the shoulders, draw the shoulder blades down the back, and press

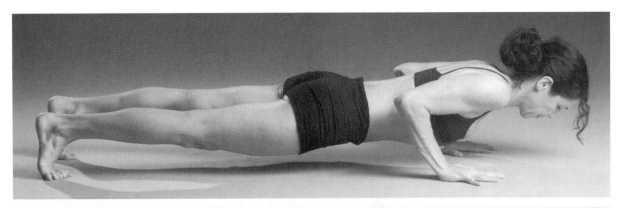

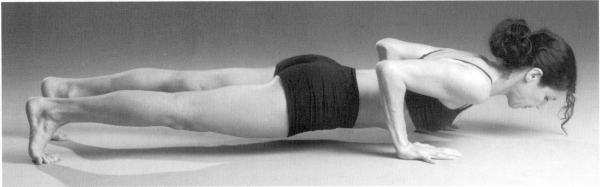

Surya Namaskara A, vinyasa four (Chaturanga Dandasana) — beginner's stance (above), final stance (below)

them on to the back. This positioning of the shoulders prepares them to take the weight of the body for the jump-back into *Chaturanga Dandasana*.

Vinyasa **Four** (*Chaturanga Dandasana*)

With the beginning of the exhalation, firmly ground your hands. The hands should be shoulder width apart, the middle fingers parallel to each other and the fingers spread. As the exhalation proceeds, move the feet back with a single hop so that the body forms

---

> **PRACTICAL TIP**
> *Stance for Beginners*
>
> As depicted in the top photo above, beginners may adopt a longer stance in *Chaturanga Dandasana* so that, on lowering down, the shoulders remain above the hands. Experienced students can work toward vertical forearms, tracking the elbows directly above the wrists on lowering the body. On moving into Upward Facing Dog, we aim toward positioning the shoulders above the wrists. Viewed from the side, the arms are perpendicular to the floor.

a straight line from the head to the feet. Land the feet so that they are hip width apart and flex them. Completing the exhalation, slowly bend the arms, lowering your body until you hover just above the floor. The elbows hug the body. Do not allow them to wander out to the sides: this stiffens the shoulders and tightens the pectoralis minor muscle. On the way down, the movement should be even, with the heart leading the way. Lift your face away from the floor to strengthen and support the back of the neck. By extending out through the heels, the coccyx drops, which lengthens the low back and positions the pelvis correctly for Upward Facing Dog, which follows. This action is balanced by an equal extension of the chest forward. The entire spine lengthens and the lower abdomen lifts away from the floor to support the lumbar spine.

Vinyasa **Five** (*Urdhva Mukha Shvanasana* — Upward Facing Dog)

Initiating the movement with an inhalation, straighten your arms and draw your chest forward, rolling the toes over until the feet point away from you. Press the tops of your feet down into the floor, using them as brakes to resist the forward-dragging action of the arms. Combined, these actions put the back in traction and elongate the spine.

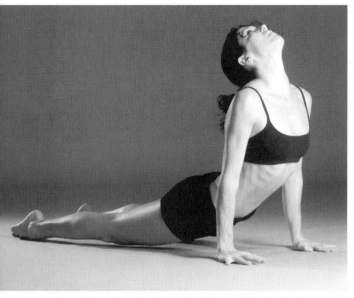

Surya Namaskara A, *vinyasa* five (Upward Facing Dog)

Rather than rolling the shoulders back (which pinches the shoulder blades together by contracting the rhomboid muscles and leads to a closing behind the heart), keep the shoulder blades wide (serratus anterior muscle) and draw them down the back (latissimus dorsi). Rolling the shoulders back will free up the chest to move forward and puff out proudly like that of a lion. Imagine the arms as the upright support of a swing, the shoulder joints as the fulcrum, and the chest as the seat of the swing. Slide the heart through the arms to gain length in the spine. The lowest ribs now move forward and lift upward.

Lifting the chin to the ceiling and keeping the back of the neck long, the head is taken back. Those with previous whiplash injuries should avoid this movement and keep the neck straight, gazing down toward the tip of the nose; this will prevent overcontraction of the back of the neck. Students who are in need of inducing more backbend can look up between the eyebrows. At the same time be careful not to limit the backbend to the neck only.

This posture is frequently confused with *Bhujangasana* (Cobra) from Hatha Yoga, and often hybrids between the two postures can be observed. Upward Facing Dog is distinctly different. As well

as the arms being straight, the legs are kept strong and straight, so much so that the knees remain off the floor. The strength in the legs provides support

> **ANATOMICAL FOCUS**
> *Spinal Junctions*
>
> The place where the spine meets the head (the cranium) is one of the important junctions of the spine. The others are the last cervical vertebra (C7) and the first thoracic vertebra (T1); the last thoracic vertebra (T12) and first lumbar vertebra (L1); and where the last lumbar vertebra (L5) articulates with the sacrum (S1-5). Laterally, the sacrum articulates with the pelvis, the sacroiliac (SI) joints. These are all areas where the spine encounters greater stresses. These areas have muscle attachments that work in opposing directions to equip us with a greater range of movement possibilities. It is therefore important to work these areas with awareness and respect in regard to their structural limitations and their vulnerability.
>
> At the same time, the rectus abdominis muscle (the six-pack muscle) must be engaged to anchor the lower ribs and prevent them flaring open. Flaring the lower ribs accentuates swaying of the low back. The rectus abdominis will also lift the pubic bone and allow the coccyx to drop. This will enable one to carry the spine long and tall in all postures.

for the lumbar spine. By keeping the legs straight, the stretch is taken in the front of the hip joint, lengthening the hip flexor muscles, which is imperative in all backbending postures. It is important to draw forward with the arms and lengthen the whole spine, rather than to collapse and dip into the low back. Incorrectly performed, this posture can easily lead to low-back pain. Performed correctly, it can relieve back pain caused by spending long hours sitting at a desk or in a driver's seat.

Urdhva Mukha Shvanasana is an extremely important posture in the sequence, as it is the only real preparation for backbending in the Primary Series. It should be deeply experienced every time it occurs in the series to awaken the spine for backbending.

Take your time, with long, conscious inhalations rather than a short breath, moving quickly into and out of this posture.

Vinyasa Six (*Adho Mukha Shvanasana* — Downward Facing Dog)

With the beginning of the exhalation, flex your feet and roll back onto the soles. Release the heels toward the floor. Raise your buttocks to the sky like a mountain as the hip flexors engage and the legs work toward straightening. At the same time, push the floor away with your hands to shift weight back toward the feet. Set your shoulders broad with the armpits facing downward. If the shoulders are hunched around the ears, the armpits will face out to the sides; performed this way the trapezius muscle is overcontracted and the posture will tighten the neck and the shoulders. The correct shoulder position needs to be learned here, as it builds upper-body strength and is needed later on in backbends and arm balances. If the armpits face out to the sides, the arm bones (humeri) need to be outwardly rotated until the desirable result is achieved.

PRACTICAL TIP

Stance Variations in the Dogs

The Upward and Downward Dog postures also have their intrinsic stances, which differ from person to person and may even change within one's practice life.

A person with a stiff backbend needs a longer stance in Upward Dog. If the stance is too short, the low back or neck muscles can spasm. A beginner will get more opening and be safer by choosing a longer stance. As the spine becomes more flexible in backbend, one can shorten the stance in Upward Dog.

Initiated by the feet, the legs work strongly in Downward Facing Dog. Attempt to ground the heels with weight equal to that which naturally falls into the balls of the feet. The strong action of the legs and hip flexors is used to tip the pelvis forward, tilting the sit bones so that they point up toward the ceiling. Those with a flexible forward bend must resist the tendency to sag in the low back by keeping

the junction of T12/L1 supported. The junction of T1/C7 is also supported, preventing the inside of the shoulders and the head from collapsing toward

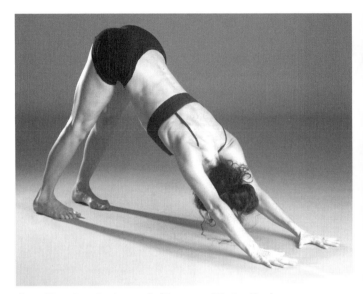

Surya Namaskara A, *vinyasa* six (Downward Facing Dog)

the floor. Instead, the top of the back of the head reaches forward toward the hands. Keep the chin dropped to the extent that there is no hardening in the front of the throat. The arms work as if you would try to lift your hands off the floor. The weight in the hands is cast forward so that only 40 percent is placed on the heels of the hands while the roots of the fingers carry 60 percent. Be sure that the bases of the little and ring fingers carry a load equal to that taken by the thumbs and pointing fingers.

The arms and legs act as strong supports so that the spine may be fully lengthened. The trunk flexors and trunk extensors are stretched, strengthened, and awakened, and carry the spine elongated.

Anyone who experiences stiffness in forward bending or who has short Achilles tendons needs a short stance in Downward Dog. If the heels are more than an inch or two off the floor, the angle of the legs to the floor does not enable the legs to be worked in such a way as to get sufficient stretch on the calves and Achilles tendons. In this case one needs to step the feet forward and shorten the stance. On the other hand, if the stance is too short the strengthening and lengthening effect on the spine and shoulders is reduced. To maximize this effect, ideally we would choose a long stance. For beginners, however, a long stance will place undue

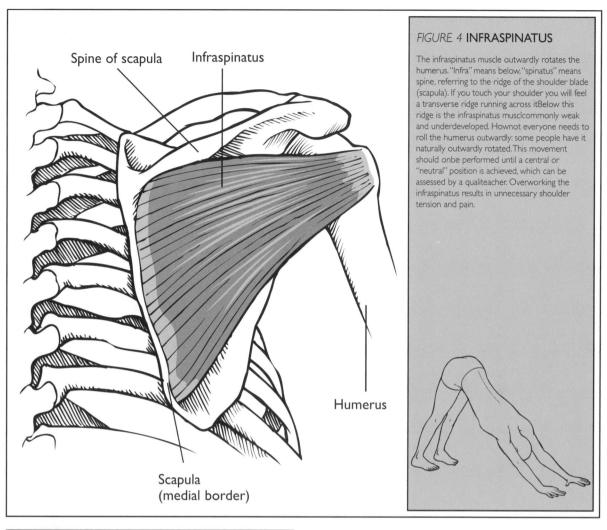

Spine of scapula   Infraspinatus

Humerus

Scapula
(medial border)

FIGURE 4 **INFRASPINATUS**

The infraspinatus muscle outwardly rotates the humerus. "Infra" means below, "spinatus" means spine, referring to the ridge of the shoulder blade (scapula). If you touch your shoulder you will feel a transverse ridge running across it Below this ridge is the infraspinatus muscl commonly weak and underdeveloped. How not everyone needs to roll the humerus outwardly: some people have it naturally outwardly rotated. This movement should on be performed until a central or "neutral" position is achieved, which can be assessed by a quali teacher. Overworking the infraspinatus results in unnecessary shoulder tension and pain.

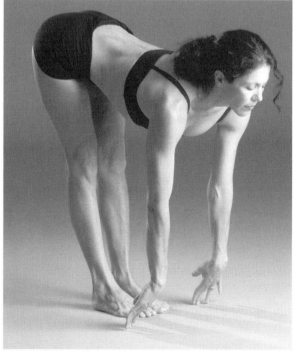

strain on the shoulders and wrists. Once the heels reach the floor, one should therefore lengthen the stance in Downward Dog. A competent teacher can assess the appropriate stance length.

Downward Dog is held for five breaths and, although the gaze would ideally be toward the navel, for most beginners this would lead to a collapsing of the shoulders and sacrificing the much-needed elongation of the spine. Gazing toward the feet or the knees is therefore recommended for beginners. It may take years to develop the flexibility and support strength to establish the final *drishti*, which is toward the navel. If a beginner starts with this gaze, it usually leads to compromising the inner integrity of this magnificent posture.

Similarly, the attempt to thrust the head down to the floor leads to a closing and hardening behind

Left, *Surya Namaskara* A, *vinyasa* seven (see next page)

the heart, to a splaying open of the lower ribs as the abdominal muscles are released, and to a collapsing around the junction of C7/T1. Downward Dog is like a handstand with the support of the legs and therefore needs a balance of trunk extension and trunk flexion. To go into either extreme misses the still point of balance.

Vinyasa **Seven**

With the end of the exhalation, the legs bend slightly, and with the inhalation the feet hop up between the hands. As the feet land they touch each other, and the torso lifts as the gaze is cast upward to the third eye *(Brumadhaya Drishti)*. This is a repetition of the third *vinyasa*.

Vinyasa **Eight**

The exhalation folds us forward, with the fingertips eventually coming into line with the toes. This is a repetition of the second *vinyasa*.

Vinyasa **Nine**

The inhalation lifts the heart so that the back remains straight as the torso lifts, with the arms reaching out to the side.

The next exhalation returns us to *Samasthiti*.

Surya Namaskara B

SUN SALUTATION B

Drishti Thumbs, nose, navel

Vinyasa **One**

Inhaling from *Samasthiti*, bend the knees deeply without the heels lifting off the floor. At the same time draw your arms up above the head, working them back toward the ears and bring the palms together. The gaze lifts upward beyond the folded palms. This is *Utkatasana*.

Utkatasana is a good example of the principle of simultaneous expansion in opposing directions (see figure 5, page 34). The ideal here would be to squat down until the thighs are parallel to the floor; then the trunk and arms lean forward as the body regains its center of gravity. This extreme gives the optimal effect in regard to strengthening the leg and buttock

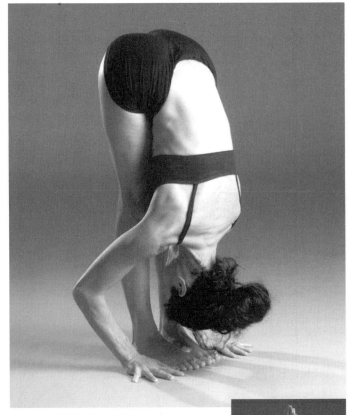

Above, *Surya Namaskara* A, *vinyasa* eight; right, *vinyasa* nine

muscles. The other extreme is to keep the back completely upright, without bending the legs enough. In this case we would compromise the powerful work of the legs and buttocks, which occurs only in a deep squat. The ideal is a balance between these two actions, working simultaneously in both directions.

Approach the limit of your flexibility slowly when squatting down, to give the ligaments time to lengthen and strengthen. While bending the knees do not tilt the pelvis forward or backward, but allow the pelvis to maintain its neutral position and the low back its natural curve. The knees remain together. Keep the arms drawing back into the shoulder joints to keep the shoulder blades down and the neck free of excess tension. If you have a tendency to whiplash symptoms, gaze straight ahead.

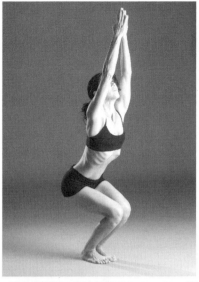
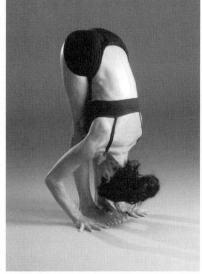
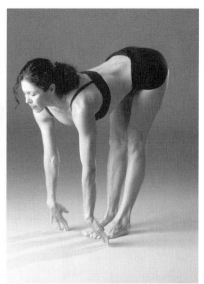
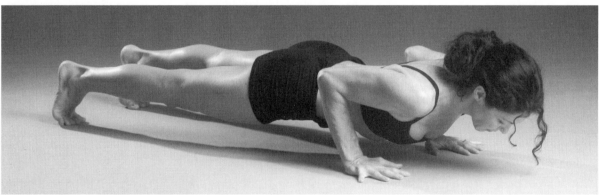

From left top, *Surya Namaskara* B, *vinyasa* one (*Utkatasana*), *vinyasa* two, *vinyasa* three; above, *vinyasa* four (*Chaturanga Dandasana*)

Beginners are advised to raise their arms straight out in front of them, drawing them from back to front. This action avoids hyperextending the low back. The more challenging option of raising the arms out to the side may be adopted when sufficient awareness and strength have been developed.

Vinyasa Two

With the exhalation draw your palms, folded into prayer position, to touch the chest (heart center) and, folding the torso forward as you straighten your legs, place the hands down on the floor on either side of the feet.

Vinyasa Three

Inhaling, lift the chest.

Vinyasa Four

Exhaling, hop the feet back and lower into *Chaturanga Dandasana*.

Vinyasa Five

Inhale into Upward Facing Dog.

Vinyasa Six

Exhale, draw back and up into Downward Facing Dog.

These last four *vinyasas* are the same as in *Surya Namaskara* A.

Vinyasa Seven (*Virabhadrasana* A)

At the beginning of the inhalation, turn your left foot on its ball and place the heel on an imagined center-line of the mat. The left foot becomes positioned at a 45° angle.

We now step the right foot forward, with a straight line going through the second toe, the heel of the right foot and the heel of the left foot. The placement of the right foot is crucial. Even when it is only

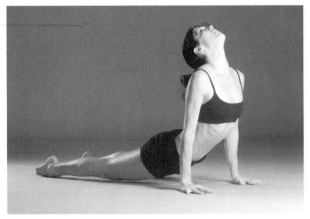 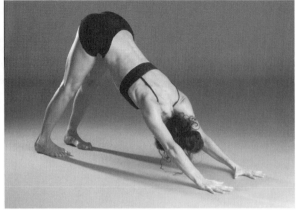

From left, Surya Namaskara B, *vinyasa* five (Upward Dog) and *vinyasa* six (Downward Dog)

slightly turned out, the tibia (shinbone) will externally rotate, disturbing the subtle balance of the posture. The front knee is bent and remains tracking directly above the ankle. To track the knee farther out beyond the ankle would promote forward travel of the femur (thighbone) on the tibia. Although this movement is prevented by the posterior cruciate ligament, it places undue strain on it and should be avoided. Likewise, to have the knee fall inward or outward of its position above the ankle, while it bears weight, places unnecessary stress on the inside (medial) and outside (lateral) collateral ligaments of the knee joint.

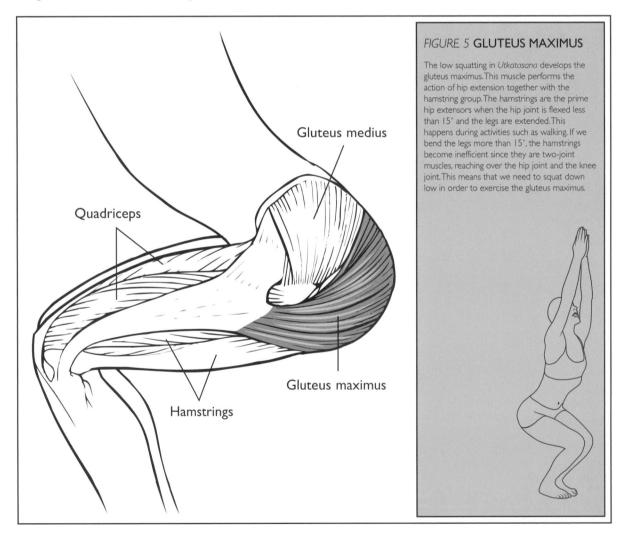

FIGURE 5 **GLUTEUS MAXIMUS**

The low squatting in *Utkatasana* develops the gluteus maximus. This muscle performs the action of hip extension together with the hamstring group. The hamstrings are the prime hip extensors when the hip joint is flexed less than 15° and the legs are extended. This happens during activities such as walking. If we bend the legs more than 15°, the hamstrings become inefficient since they are two-joint muscles, reaching over the hip joint and the knee joint. This means that we need to squat down low in order to exercise the gluteus maximus.

Gluteus medius

Quadriceps

Gluteus maximus

Hamstrings

Work your hips toward being completely square. This aids in stretching the hip flexor group of muscles, which run over the front of the hip joint. Bring the torso vertical so that the shoulders hover above the hips. Be sure to engage the abdominal muscles to draw the lower ribs in, as the back of the chest

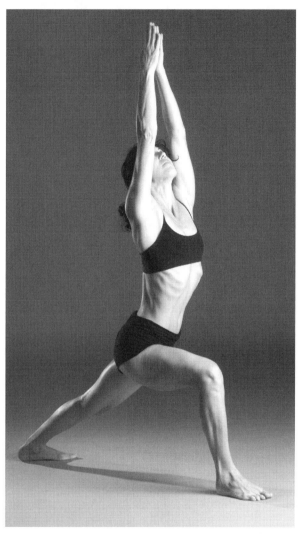

Surya Namaskara B, *vinyasa* seven (*Virabhadrasana* A, right side)

below the shoulder blades stays broad. The sit bones are heavy and sink toward the floor.

The strength of the back (extended) leg is important in supporting the softening needed to bend deeper into the front hip. This is achieved through totally awakening the back foot by spreading the base of the toes and keeping the outer arch of the foot grounded. Extending out through the heel of this foot will automatically position the foot at the perfect angle complementary to the direction of the knee of that leg. This also enhances the inward

(medial) spiraling required by the back leg in this posture. The bent leg spirals outward (laterally) to complement its partner, until a neutral position is reached — that is, when the hips are square. Although there is an obvious preponderance of weight distribution into the forward leg, maintain the action of

YOGIC CONTEXT
Importance of Correct Foot Position

All foot positions given in the standing postures mirror the direction of the knee at its final position in the posture. In *Virabhadrasana* A, we attempt to square the hips to the front foot. The knee will eventually face approximately 45° toward the front. If the back foot were, for example, placed at 90°, the knee would have to mediate between a thighbone (femur) that rolls in and a shinbone (tibia) that is turned out. In other words, the knee joint would do the rotation needed to accommodate the position of the foot. A 45° angle is therefore necessary on the back foot to work the hip into the required position. To place the foot so that it faces in the same direction as the knee protects the knee joint from excessive rotational force.

distributing weight back into the back foot by grounding the heel of that foot. This will create equilibrium between the flow of action in the legs. The strong support of the legs creates a vector of energy that supports the base of the spine and activates the *bandha*s, enabling the core of the body to rise.

While arriving in the final posture, the arms are simultaneously being raised above the head. Gaze upward beyond the folded hands.

Vinyasa **Eight**

With the exhalation, lift the left heel off the floor, lower the arms out to the side, drop the sit bones farther, and eventually place your hands down on either side of the front foot. When the hands touch down, step your right foot back to the left foot, feet hip width apart, and lower down into *Chaturanga Dandasana*.

Vinyasa **Nine**

Inhale into Upward Dog.

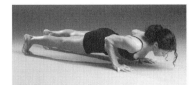

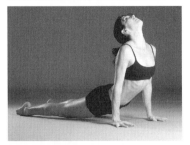

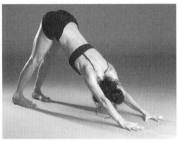

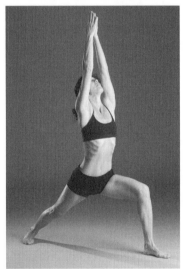

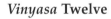

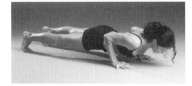

From the top, *Surya Namaskara* B, *vinyasa* eight (*Chaturanga Dandasana*), *vinyasa* nine (Upward Dog) , *vinyasa* ten (Downward Dog), *vinyasa* eleven (*Virabhadrasana*, left side), *vinyasa* twelve (*Chaturanga Dandasana*)

Vinyasa Ten

Exhale into Downward Dog.

Vinyasa Eleven (*Virabhadrasana* A)

Turn the right heel into the center, step the left foot forward, and repeat *Virabhadrasana* on the left side. The complex movement of stepping forward, lifting the torso, and raising the arms should all be completed on one inhalation without haste. It is a great tool for learning the extension of breath.

If you run out of breath on the way up, do not hold the breath. Beginners may need to commence by stepping the foot into position at the end of the exhalation in Downward Dog. Otherwise an additional short breath may be taken. You will soon be able to do the movement on one breath. In Ashtanga Yoga, movement is never done during *kumbhaka* (breath retention).

Vinyasa Twelve

With the exhalation, lift the right heel while placing the hands down, step the left foot back, and lower down. Again, this is a movement that requires us to extend the breath.

Vinyasa Thirteen

Inhale into Upward Dog.

Vinyasa Fourteen

Exhale into Downward Dog. This last Downward Dog is held for five breaths, while the other two are only transitional.

Vinyasa Fifteen

On the inhalation, hop forward, landing with the feet together, lift your chest, and gaze upward (identical to *vinyasa* three).

Vinyasa Sixteen

Exhaling, fold forward, straighten the legs, and place the fingertips in line with the toes (identical to *vinyasa* two).

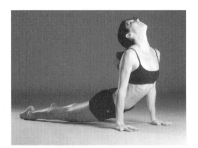

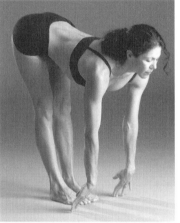

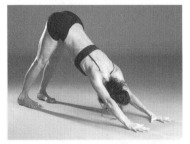

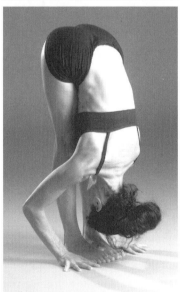

From the top, *vinyasa* thirteen (Upward Dog), *vinyasa* fourteen (Downward Dog), *vinyasa* fifteen, *vinyasa* sixteen

Vinyasa **Seventeen**

Inhale, bend your knees, draw your arms up above the head, and gaze up in *Utkatasana* (identical to *vinyasa* one).

Samasthiti

With an exhalation, straighten the legs, lower the arms, and gaze softly.

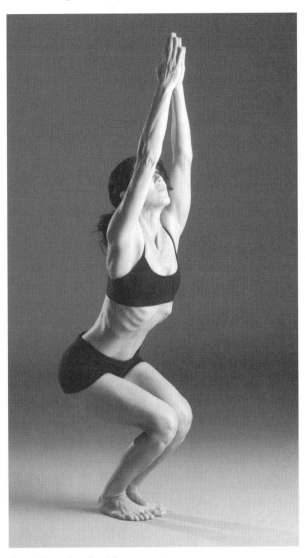

Surya Namaskara B, *vinyasa* seventeen

Do *Surya Namaskara* B until you start to perspire. Five rounds should be sufficient under average conditions, three in the tropics, and up to ten in colder regions.

> The standing postures teach us the basics of alignment and develop strength and poise.

Padangushtasana
HOLD-THE-BIG-TOE POSTURE

Drishti Nose

Vinyasa **One**

From *Samasthiti*, jump on inhalation and, exhaling, land with your feet parallel, hip width apart, placing hands on hips. "Hip width" means the ankle joints are positioned under the hip joints.

ANATOMICAL FOCUS
Disc Bulges

A disc bulge (see page 38) can occur when a weight is lifted off the floor with the spine flexed. Pressure on the discs between the vertebrae deforms them into a wedge shape and predisposes them to bulging. The intervertebral discs act as shock absorbers for the vertebrae. They consist of a fibrous band enclosing a fluid-filled nucleus. When this liquid-filled cushion is pushed beyond the boundary of the vertebrae, it is called a disc bulge. Often the disc will press against the spinal cord and cause considerable pain. The adjacent muscles spasm to arrest and thereby protect the spine, resulting in a complete inability to bend forward. A disc bulge usually corrects itself in a few weeks. A disc prolapse differs from this in that the fibrous nucleus of the disc is pushed beyond the boundary of the vertebrae. Allopathy[6] considers that this condition does not repair itself.

It is therefore important to avoid rounding the low back when bending forward, as in this position it bears the weight of the body. Instead, bend the knees while still maintaining some stretch in the hamstring muscles.

Inhaling, grow the legs tall and strong, and lift the torso up and out of the hips. Exhaling, fold forward at the hip joints, keeping the back straight and the heart lifted. Reach for the toes, hooking the big toes with the first and second fingers, palms facing inward, and closing the clasp of the fingers with the thumb. Students who cannot yet reach their toes may bend their legs. Bending of the low back to

6. The system of medicine based on Western science.

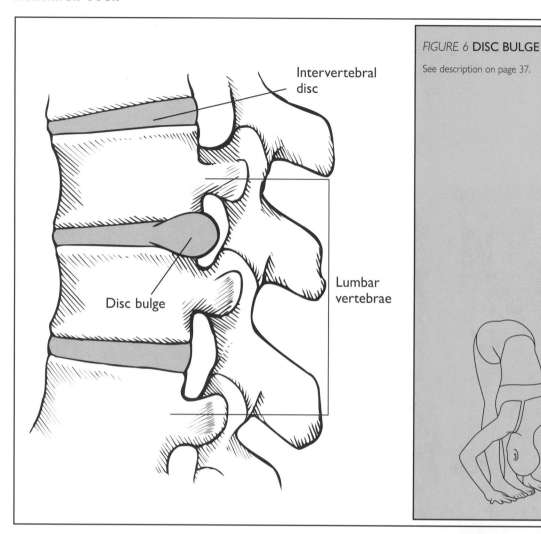

Intervertebral disc

Disc bulge

Lumbar vertebrae

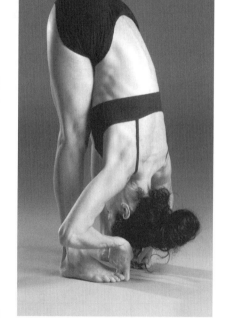

FIGURE 6 **DISC BULGE**

See description on page 37.

reach the toes is not recommended, as this places pressure on the lumbar discs, and may cause them to bulge.

On the next inhalation, keeping hold of the toes, lift the head and chest and cast the gaze up between the eyebrows.

Vinyasa **Two**

On exhalation, fold deeply forward, lifting the kneecaps. The lifting of the kneecaps is done by the quadriceps muscle, which is the antagonist to the hamstrings. Performed in this way, the stretch is active, which signals the hamstrings to lengthen. Deepen and soften your groins to lengthen the hip flexor muscles, and breathe into the hamstrings to release them.

The elbows draw out to the side, the shoulder blades move up toward the hips, and the crown of the head reaches to the floor. Let the weight of the head lengthen the spine and neck. As you support the posture with the action of the legs, the spine releases and is passive. The *drishti* is toward the tip of the nose. In this *vinyasa* we are in the state of *Padangushtasana*. Stay in the posture for five breaths.

Right, *Padangushtasana*

Vinyasa Three

Inhaling, lift your chest and gaze toward the tip of the nose. Exhaling, place the hands under the feet, stepping onto the fingertips and eventually the whole palm, with the toes touching the wrists.

Pada Hastasana
FEET-ON-HANDS POSTURE

Drishti Nose

Vinyasa One

From *vinyasa* three of *Padangushtasana*, inhaling, lift the head and chest and gaze upward. Attempt to concave the low back and keep the legs strong, keeping the hands under the feet.

> **YOGIC CONTEXT**
> *Active Balancing*
>
> Actively balancing the body in every posture means it is necessary to isolate those muscles that need to be contracted from the ones that need to be released and lengthened. Too often one sees students who contract their entire body. Active balancing strengthens the core muscles of the body as well as the superficial muscles. This creates a light carriage, as the skeletal structure is carried more efficiently. *Pada Hastasana* is a great posture to experience these principles at work.

Vinyasa Two

Exhaling, fold forward. You are now in the state of *Pada Hastasana*. Hold it for five breaths. As in the previous posture, keep the low back straight and, only when that is guaranteed, work at straightening the legs. The gaze is toward the nose. This posture is a more intense version of the previous one. You can make the stretch even more intense by shifting weight forward toward the toes.

The abdominal muscles — the term refers primarily to rectus abdominis — are engaged here to protect the low back. *Uddiyana Bandha* (the lower part of the transverse abdominis) prevents the breath from

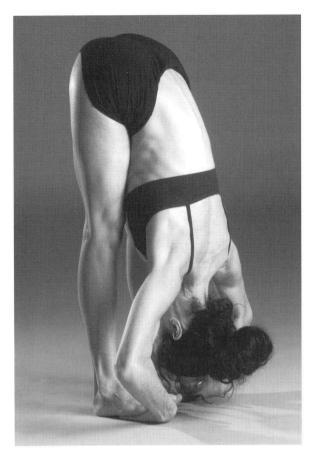

Pada Hastasana

distending the lower belly, which would destabilize the low back. Excess use of the abdominal muscles, however, would shorten the spine and lift the head away from the floor, as the abdominal muscles are primarily trunk flexors. Only a sensitive combination of leg work with trunk flexion and trunk extension will bring the desired result of elongating the spine. This is mainly felt at the waist. Subtle, intelligent work will increase the space between the lowest ribs and the pelvic crests, the upper rims of the hipbone. Both muscle groups of the trunk work isometrically (under tension but without shortening) and therefore both will be strengthened. This is active balancing.

Vinyasa Three

Inhaling, lift the head and chest as you straighten the arms. Exhaling, place the hands on the hips and return to *Samasthiti*.

Returning to *Samasthiti* on one breath is obviously a complex move. Beginners may break it down to retain the integrity of the movement.

39

Breath count for beginners: Exhale, place the hands on the hips, drop the tailbone, strengthen through the legs. Inhale and come up to standing, leading with the heart. Exhaling, hop back to *Samasthiti.*

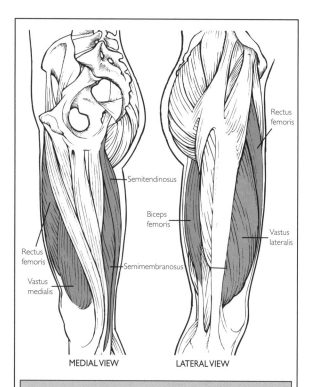

Rectus
femoris

Semitendinosus

Biceps
femoris

Vastus
lateralis

Rectus
femoris

Semimembranosus

Vastus
medialis

MEDIAL VIEW   LATERAL VIEW

FIGURE 7 HAMSTRINGS AND QUADRICEPS

Bending forward should involve flexing the hip joints and not the spine. The flexing of the hip joints is limited by the hamstring muscle group, which performs the action of hip extension and knee flexion. The hamstring group consists of three individual muscles. Of these the biceps femoris externally rotates the femur as it extends the hip, and the semitendinosus and semimembranosus internally rotate the femur as they extend the hip. We will encounter these muscles later in their secondary function as rotators of the femur.

If we passively hang in *Padangushtasana,* soreness can develop at the ischial tuberosities (sit bones), which is the origin of the hamstrings. To prevent this we need to engage the antagonists of the hamstrings, the quadriceps.

The quadriceps is engaged by pulling up on the kneecap (patella). The quadriceps consists of four separate muscles that jointly insert, via the patella tendon, at the tibia. The four heads of the quadriceps are the rectus femoris, vastus lateralis, vastus intermedius, and vastus medialis. The rectus femoris is the only two-joint muscle in the group. It originates at the front of the hip bone and can thus not only extend the leg at the knee but also flex the hip joint. The three vasti originate at the lateral, anterior, and medial surfaces of the femur respectively, and only perform extension of the knee joint.

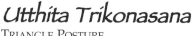

Utthita Trikonasana
TRIANGLE POSTURE

Drishti Raised hand

Vinyasa One

Inhaling, turn to the right and hop your feet about three feet apart and parallel. The arms extend out to the sides at shoulder level.

There is no "one stance fits all" here, but rather an ideal stance for every level of flexibility. This is of such importance that it should be assessed by the teacher on an individual basis. If the stance is too long, the inner integrity of the posture will be lost and its execution will bring little benefit. If it is too short, one will not gain spinal support, strength, and elongation. As flexibility increases over time and with practice, stances can be lengthened.

Vinyasa Two

Exhaling, turn your right foot out 90°. For the sake of precision, visualize a line going through the center of your mat lengthwise. Place the second toe of the right foot precisely along this line and check that the center of the heel is placed on the same line. A deviation of only 2° could be significant. Beginners often turn the foot out too much in order to gain stability, but this will result in a lateral (outward) rotation of the tibia, which is sometimes accompanied by a compensating inward rotation of the femur. This places stress on the knee. Dancers often prematurely wear out their knees through turning the feet out in this way.

Turn your left foot in approximately 5°, with the heel positioned on the same center-line on the mat. The 5° position will ensure that foot, shin, and thighbone all point in the same direction, again as the optimal position for the knee. To stay at 0°, or to turn the foot out, would place stress on the knee joint. On the other hand, if you turn the left foot in too far, say 30°, you will not achieve sufficient opening of the groins.

With the feet correctly positioned, let the right hip drop down (lateral tilt) as far as possible, bringing the pelvis toward being vertical to the floor. If the pelvis is left in a horizontal position, the spine has to flex laterally (sideways), which is not intended in

Opposite, Utthita Trikonasana

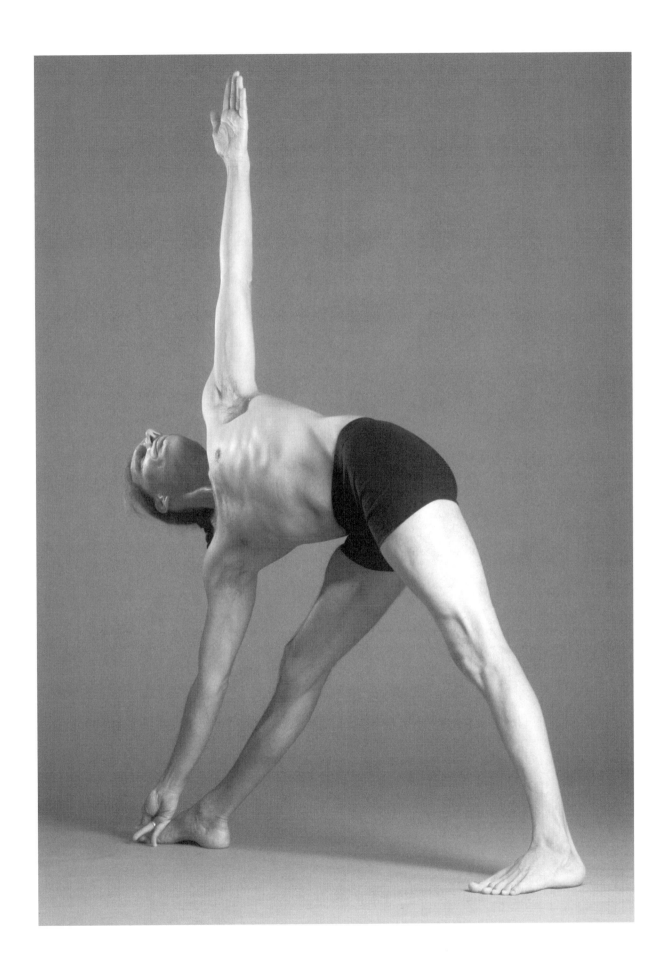

ANATOMICAL FOCUS
The Knee Joint

The knee is a modified hinge joint. A hinge joint can move in only one plane, but the knee does allow for some rotation. The action of straightening the leg is performed primarily by the quadriceps femoris muscle (front of the thigh), while the primary knee flexors, the hamstrings, draw the heel to the buttocks. But if we sit on a chair with the thighs held firm, we notice that we can swivel the feet left or right and the tibias will follow the movement.

The knee joint is complex, as the femur and tibia do not articulate well with each other. The lower end of the femur consists of two rounded protuberances called condyles, similar to two wheels, that roll — and also glide — over the upper end of the tibia. To cushion and secure this movement, two half-moon-shaped cartilages, the medial and lateral menisci, lie between the bones. Their function is similar to that of rail tracks for a train, the train being the femur and the wheels being the condyles. The difference is that the menisci actually follow the movement of the femur to allow for the roll and glide.

If the leg rapidly extends under pressure, the menisci may be unable to withdraw fast enough and are crushed. If we attempt to rotate the knee joint and at the same time straighten the leg against resistance, we can inflict serious damage, as often happens in some sports. The knee joint should never be rotated when under pressure or bearing weight.

Torn menisci heal very slowly, and medical doctors usually recommend surgery, but in many cases meniscus injuries can be healed with yoga in six to eighteen months. Cartilage has minimal blood vessels and therefore minimal nutrient supply, which is needed for the healing process. Yoga accelerates healing because the postures and transitions, when performed with precision, stimulate nutrient exchange. To heal a damaged knee will take much perseverance and patience, and especially careful precision. Whoever has worked with a meniscus injury knows that a change of only 2° in the positioning of the feet in standing postures can make the difference between comfort and healing and pain and aggravation.

Most knee problems, however, do not start with meniscus problems but with a strain of the cruciate ligaments. The posterior cruciate ligament prevents the femur from dislocating forward on the tibia, while the anterior cruciate ligament prevents backward dislocation. They are named after their points of insertion on the tibia, in the back and front respectively. Once the cruciate ligaments are strained, the knee becomes loose or unstable. Imprecise tracking of the femur on the tibia results, leading to wear on the menisci.

Strain of the cruciate ligaments comes about through hyperextension of the leg, in other words its extension beyond 180°. The anterior and posterior cruciate ligaments and the popliteus muscle restrict hyperextension, but it will occur if sufficient stress is applied. Continuous hyperextension of the leg will eventually weaken and strain the cruciate ligaments.

Hyperextension of the knee can often be observed in *Trikonasana*, students with low muscle tension being especially predisposed to it. Lifting the knee away from the floor and isometrically engaging the hamstrings counteracts this tendency. The engaging of the hamstrings can be achieved by attempting to draw or swipe the front foot over the floor toward the back foot. The foot will of course not move because it carries weight, but the muscles used to perform the action — the hamstrings — will engage. This important action needs to be performed in all postures where the front leg is straight.

If pain in the back of the knee persists, the knee needs to be bent slightly.

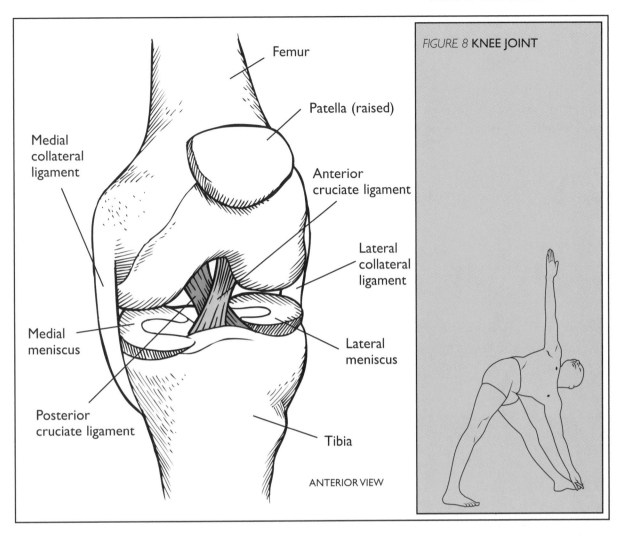

Femur

Patella (raised)

Medial collateral ligament

Anterior cruciate ligament

Lateral collateral ligament

Medial meniscus

Lateral meniscus

Posterior cruciate ligament

Tibia

FIGURE 8 **KNEE JOINT**

ANTERIOR VIEW

this posture. The left hip swings up and out to the left to allow the right hip to drop.

Reach out to the side and then down, imagining staying between two panes of glass that prevent any leaning of the torso out in front. The left shoulder remains on one plane above the right leg. The right hand eventually clasps the right big toe. If you are not able to reach the toe without compromising the posture (laterally flexing the spine), place your hand on the foot or shin. Do not lean into this leg, but keep both sides of the torso and neck lengthening and supported away from the floor. If it is comfortable, turn the head to gaze up to the thumb of the left hand, which hovers above the left shoulder. Keep the neck in a straight line with the rest of your spine without performing an unnecessary backbend in your neck. Otherwise gaze out to the side. Five breaths.

Getting into *Utthita Trikonasana* we externally rotated the right femur to turn the foot out. Once in

the posture, we inwardly rotate the femur until we reach the neutral position. The left thigh, which was medially (inwardly) rotated to take us into the posture, is laterally rotated once in the posture until the leg is again in the neutral position, with the four corners of the foot equally grounded. Check especially that both the outside of the left foot and the base of the right big toe are grounded. There needs to be a subtle balance between grounding the inner and outer arches of the front foot. This will lead to a subtle balance of inward and outward rotation of the thigh of the front leg, which is necessary for the hamstrings to lengthen evenly. Many beginners have a tendency to roll the thigh out to escape the stretching of the inner hamstrings — a tendency also common in *Padangushtasana* and *Pashimottanasana*, that needs to be counteracted if present. Keep the left hip lifted back over the right one as the right groin moves forward.

The underneath side of the torso reaches forward so that the right waist gets the same stretch as the left. Stay in the state of *Trikonasana* for five breaths.

Vinyasa Three

Inhaling, come up to the middle position: feet three feet apart and parallel; arms out to the side with hands positioned over the feet, looking straight ahead.

Vinyasa Four

Exhaling, repeat *Trikonasana* on the left side and hold for five breaths.

Vinyasa Five

The inhalation carries us back up to the middle position.

Parivrta Trikonasana

REVOLVED TRIANGLE POSTURE

Drishti Raised hand

Since we do not return to *Samasthiti* between *Utthita* and *Parivrta Trikonasana*, the first *vinyasa* of *Parivrta Trikonasana* remains uncounted and we start with *vinyasa* two.

Vinyasa Two

Ideally, we enter the posture on one exhalation. Beginners will need to break down the surprisingly complex entry movement into its constituents.

From the middle position, first shorten the stance by four to eight inches, unless you have really long hamstrings. Shortening the stance deducts the difference in distance between the hip joints from the intrinsic stance of *Utthita Trikonasana*, where the hips are parallel to the mat, to that in *Parivrta Trikonasana*, where they are square. Otherwise the position of the sacrum will be compromised — it should be parallel the floor — and the position of the spine will be compromised as a result. Students might think keeping the longer stance will produce a greater stretch, a more thrilling sensation, but in fact it impinges on the flow of *prana* up the *sushumna* (the central energy channel of the subtle body) and of cerebrospinal fluid in the gross body, which may or may not have some correlation.

Uninterrupted flow in these channels is a goal of yogic practice. If the underlying scientific principles of the practice are not understood, yoga may be of little use.

Having shortened the stance, turn the right foot out 90° and the left foot in approximately 45°. If the left foot is turned in farther than 90°, balance is easily lost, while if the left foot is not turned in sufficiently it is too difficult to square the hips — or if they are squared excess strain is placed on the left knee, since the tibia rotates outwardly and the femur rotates medially, following the movement of the pelvis. Now pin the right hip back by grounding the base of the right big toe, and draw the left hip forward by grounding the outside of the left foot, until the hips are square.

ANATOMICAL FOCUS
Spinal Movement

The lumbar spine is structurally unsuitable for twisting due to the orientation of its facet joints (L1–L5). Although twisting movements are limited in the lumbar spine, it has a great range of movement in flexion and extension (forward- and backbending respectively). In comparison, the orientation of the facet joints in the thoracic spine (T1–T11) allows ample rotation but limited extension. Extension is also limited here due to the direct attachment of the ribs onto the vertebral body and its transverse processes (twelve pairs of ribs attach to the twelve thoracic vertebrae).

With the left hand, reach far forward beyond your right foot. Exhaling, lower the hand and place it on the outside edge of the right foot, with the little finger next to the little toe. The fingers are spread and point in the same direction as the toes. Maintain the lift of the heart by not flexing but rather continuing to lengthen the trunk. Draw your shoulder blades down the back and bring your heart through from between the shoulders. If this is not possible with the hand on the floor, place it on your foot or shin. The left hand pushes the floor away. The right fingertips reach up to the ceiling, where the gaze is focused. Beginners may gaze down to the foot if looking up makes them lose their balance.

It is important to keep both hip joints at an even distance from the floor. To achieve this, avoid leaning into the front (right) foot. Instead, pin the right hip back by grounding the roots of the toes of the right foot and engaging the abductors of the hip on

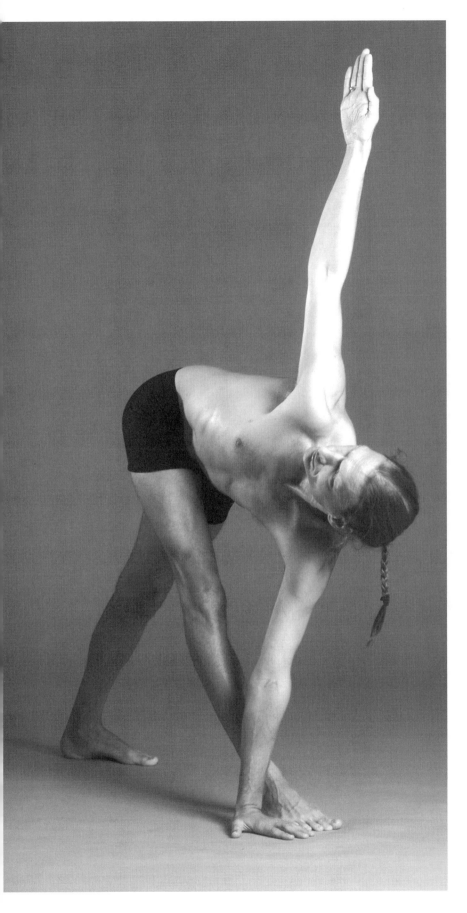

the right side. These actions prevent the left hip from sagging.

Position the head above the front foot and continue lengthening the spine and neck in this direction. Both hands and both shoulders are positioned on the same plumb line, this being achieved by rotating the thoracic spine 90°.

We stay in the posture for five breaths, working the legs strongly as support for the torso and spine. Extend out through the big toe and at the same time create a suction of the thigh back into the hip. Counteract the forward tendency in the posture by keeping the heel of the back foot heavy. Counteract the hip flexion on the front leg by drawing the front foot on the ground toward you. Ideally, as the feet ground downward there is a continuous line of energy flowing up the legs, over the hips, along the spine, and up through the crown of the head. In this way the posture is grounded and, simultaneously, energy is drawn upward.

Vinyasa Three

Inhaling, return back up to the middle position.

Vinyasa Four

Repeat *Parivrta Trikonasana* for five breaths on the left.

Vinyasa Five

Inhaling, return to the middle position. The next exhalation returns you to *Samasthiti*.

Parivrta Trikonasana

45

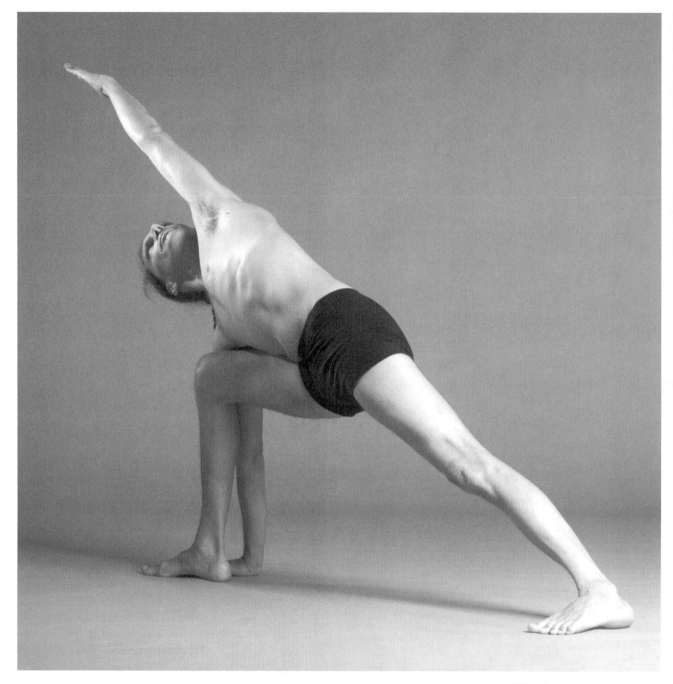

Utthita Parshvakonasana

Utthita Parshvakonasana

SIDE ANGLE POSTURE

Drishti Raised hand

Vinyasa One

Inhaling, turn to the right, hopping into a long stance (the longest of all the standing postures).

Vinyasa Two

Exhaling, open the right foot to 90° and turn the left foot in 5° only. Bend the right leg until the knee is positioned exactly above the ankle, which brings the tibia perpendicular to the floor (see *Virabhadrasana* A in *Surya Namaskara* B, page 33). It is not a defining factor of the posture to have the femur parallel to the floor: this is achieved when the strength necessary to support such flexibility is developed. Place the right hand on the floor alongside the outside edge of the foot, with fingers pointing in the same direction as the toes. Keeping the base of the big toe grounded, the right knee presses against the right shoulder. This action engages the abductors of the right hip

posture is neutralized. Keep tension between the bent knee and the opposite hip to work the groins open. The palm faces down to the floor and the left armpit faces out to the side (and not up to the ceiling). This is achieved by engaging the infraspinatus muscle, which laterally rotates the humerus (arm

---

MYTHOLOGICAL BACKGROUND

Perfect World

Lord Subramaniam, second son of Lord Shiva, also known as Skanda the fierce lord of war, once went to visit Lord Shiva and complained that the current world, which was created by Lord Brahma, was imperfect — full of corruption, crime, and injustice. Shiva suggested that he create a better world. Subramaniam then defeated and incarcerated Brahma, and destroyed his world. Then he created his own, better world.

After some time Lord Shiva visited Subramaniam and looked at his perfect world. In it nothing moved or lived or changed, as everything was arrested, frozen in the static state of perfection. There were not even sentient beings, as their essential nature is to strive for perfection and, if perfection is reached, life has come to an end. Liberated beings are not reborn. The Buddha, after reaching Mahaparinirvana, never came back. That is why *bodhisattvas* avoid perfection: they are thus able to continue to serve others. According to Indian thought, the state of perfection exists only as consciousness, called *purusha* or *atman*, which is the seat of awareness. What changes is the transitory world of manifestation, which includes body, mind, egoity, and all objects made up of the gross elements and subtle elementary particles.

Shiva pointed out to Subramaniam that this world was not a world at all, but only a frozen image of perfection. The purpose of a manifest world is to supply beings with the right cocktail of pleasure and pain, which eventually leads to self-knowledge. For this purpose it has to be in constant flux, and hence imperfect. Seeing the flaw in his world, Subramaniam freed Brahma to reinstall his old, imperfect world.

---

joint. At the same time, take the left arm over the head to form a diagonal line from the left foot all the way up to the left hand. Beginners may need to increase their stance at this point to achieve this line.

In this posture it is important not to collapse into the hips but to keep them supported. There should be a feeling of buoyancy in the hips and legs away from the floor. Ground the outer arch of the left foot and use it as an anchor to establish an outward rotation in the left thigh, which will lift the left hip back over the right. The right hip joint makes an attempt to dive through under the left one to stretch the right adductor group (see figure 17, page 101) in anticipation of the half-lotus and lotus postures to come.[7] The right thigh rotates inward until the lateral rotation that brought us into the

bone). This movement does not need to be performed by people whose arm is naturally in this position, which can be assessed by a qualified teacher. Indiscriminate outward rotation may lead to inflammation of the rotator cuff and an infraspinatus that is chronically in spasm.

Keep the shoulders down, away from the ears, by depressing the shoulder girdle using the latissimus dorsi muscle. The shoulder is kept up off the neck by abducting the shoulder blades with the serratus anterior muscle (see figure 9, page 48). Stay in the state of *Utthita Parshvakonasana* for five breaths.

7. The Latin prefix *ad-* means "toward" and *ab-* means "away." Adductors are muscles that draw bones toward the midline of the body, whereas abductors draw them away from the midline.

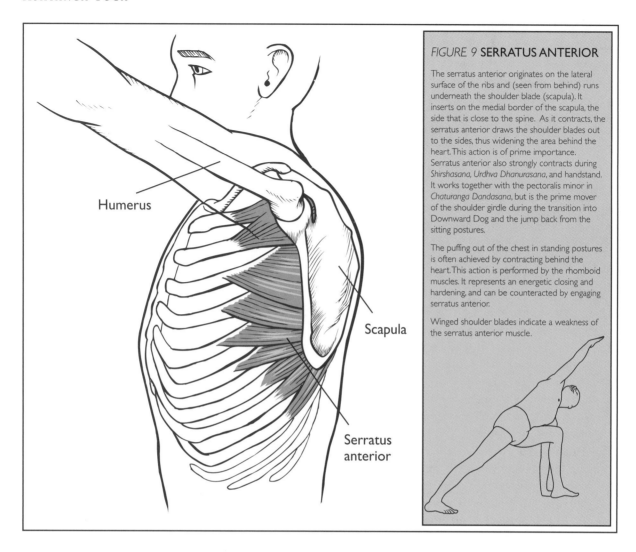

FIGURE 9 SERRATUS ANTERIOR

The serratus anterior originates on the lateral surface of the ribs and (seen from behind) runs underneath the shoulder blade (scapula). It inserts on the medial border of the scapula, the side that is close to the spine. As it contracts, the serratus anterior draws the shoulder blades out to the sides, thus widening the area behind the heart. This action is of prime importance. Serratus anterior also strongly contracts during *Shirshasana, Urdhva Dhanurasana,* and handstand. It works together with the pectoralis minor in *Chaturanga Dandasana,* but is the prime mover of the shoulder girdle during the transition into Downward Dog and the jump back from the sitting postures.

The puffing out of the chest in standing postures is often achieved by contracting behind the heart. This action is performed by the rhomboid muscles. It represents an energetic closing and hardening, and can be counteracted by engaging serratus anterior.

Winged shoulder blades indicate a weakness of the serratus anterior muscle.

Humerus

Scapula

Serratus anterior

The head turns to face the raised arm, looking along the arm to gaze at the palm of the hand without contorting the neck. If all instructions so far have been followed precisely, the face will show an expression of serene bliss. If we are pulling a face of strain, effort, or ambition, the chances are that we have become lost in some extreme of the posture, and it is time to pull back.

If we have achieved the subtle balance between all muscles involved, freedom, lightness, and inner silence will result. This is yoga.

Parshvakonasana is a beautiful teacher for learning the balancing and embracing of opposites, as are many other postures. The complexity of the standing postures especially calls for simultaneous awareness in all directions. As Shankara says,

"True posture is that which leads to spontaneous meditation on Brahman."

Only after the effort that moved us into the correct posture (and not the perfect posture, since everything that is perfect is static and therefore dead) has been recognized as empty in nature can this moment of silence and lightness, which is true posture, be experienced.

Vinyasa **Three**

The inhalation carries us back up into the middle position.

Vinyasa **Four**

Exhaling, we repeat the posture on the left side.

Vinyasa **Five**

Inhaling, we come back to the middle.

Parivrta Parshvakonasana

REVOLVED SIDE ANGLE POSTURE

Drishti Raised hand

Parivrta Parshvakonasana is not really a posture for beginners, but it can be added in after some proficiency has been gained in *Marichyasana* C (see page 86). Since we do not return to *Samasthiti* between *Utthita* and *Parivrta Parshvakonasana*, the first *vinyasa* of *Parivrta Parshvakonasana* is uncounted.

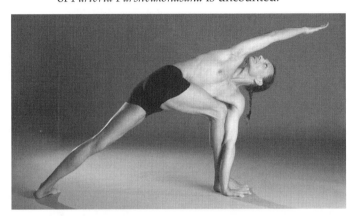

Parivrta Parshvakonasana

Vinyasa Two

Exhaling, shorten the stance slightly and turn the back foot in 45°, as we do in all standing postures where the hips are squared. The right foot is turned out 90°. Keeping the back leg straight, again track the right knee over the right ankle. Squaring the hips, hook the left shoulder outside the right knee (the emptier the lungs are the easier this is). You can assist yourself by pressing the right thigh toward the center with your right hand. Press the left hand into the floor outside the foot, spreading the fingers.

Now take the right arm overhead to form a diagonal line from the left foot to the right hand. The palm faces downward, the face is turned toward the right arm, and the gaze is up toward the palm. Spread the base of the toes of the back foot to encourage the leg to be straight and strong. Strong abduction of the right knee, countered by the left arm, will inspire the spine to spiral.

Do not fake the spinal twist by letting your right hip sag toward the floor, but work the hips toward being level and square. Lift the shoulder blade off the neck and draw it down away from the ear.

Keep the lower abdomen firm and use deep breathing into the chest to elongate the spine. Create space between the left shoulder and right hip. Extend out simultaneously through your sit bones and through the crown of the head. Hold *Parivrta Parshvakonasana* for five breaths.

> **YOGIC CONTEXT**
> ## *Intelligent Action*
>
> Any movement in a posture can be over-exercised, and at any stage one should be able to initiate its countermovement, which is to retract the action. This is intelligent action.
>
> Most muscles have more than one action. For example, latissimus dorsi primarily extends the humerus.[8] It also medially rotates the humerus. The first of the two actions indirectly causes the arm to bend at the elbow. This is counteracted by the deltoid, which flexes the humerus (raises the arm above the head). The medial rotation of the humerus calls the infraspinatus into play. One action is played against its opposite to reach the desired balanced posture.

For beginners who cannot enter the posture in one breath, it may be approached in phases:

• Turn to face the right leg and place the left knee on the floor. Keeping the leg bent, hook the left shoulder outside the right knee and press the left hand into the floor.

• Keeping the knee over the ankle and the shoulder hooked outside the knee, lift the back knee off the floor and straighten the leg.

• Maintaining all of the above, work the left heel down, placing the foot at a 45° angle.

• Raise the right arm and gaze at the palm.

Stay at any of these phases for as long as necessary until the stage is attained. In this way your integrity in the posture is not sacrificed. Once you can do the complete posture, attempt to enter into it on one breath.

Vinyasa Three

Inhaling, come back up to the middle position.

---

8. Extension is defined as returning from flexion, and flexion of the humerus is raising the arm out to the front.

Vinyasa Four

Exhaling, repeat the posture on the left side.

Vinyasa Five

Inhaling, come back up and, on exhalation, return to *Samasthiti*.

Prasarita Padottanasana A
WIDE STANCE FORWARD BEND A

Drishti Nose

Vinyasa One

Inhaling and turning to the right, jump to land in a medium-width stance. The exact width of the stance will be determined by the ratio between the spine length and leg length of each individual practitioner.

The outside edges of the feet need to be parallel to track the knees, as the thighs tend to roll forward when folding forward. Recheck that the feet have not turned out after each of the four versions of this posture. The hands are placed firmly on the hips. As the hips sink toward the floor, lift the entire spine, including the sacrum, out of the hips. The heart lifts and leads the forward folding of the trunk.

Vinyasa Two

Exhaling, fold at the hip joints and place the hands on the floor. Spread the fingers and work toward having the fingertips in line with the toes. Position the hands shoulder width apart.

Inhaling, lift the chest, straighten the arms, and concave the low back. The legs work strongly to support the passive lengthening of the spine. Gaze toward the nose.

Vinyasa Three

Exhaling, fold forward. Counteract the medial roll of the thighs by drawing them back out to the side. Position the torso between the thighs, then "close the door" with the thighs by returning to medial rotation until the knees face straight ahead. Flexible students can rest the crown of the head (the highest point) on the floor. Students with long torsos compared to the length of their legs may have to bring the feet closer together to keep their necks elongating,

while students with relatively short torsos may have to widen their stance to get the same effect.

If the crown of the head is rested on the floor, a flushing effect of the cerebral glands (hypophysis, epiphyses) will ensue.

To enhance this purificatory effect, four versions of the posture are given. This is a subtle posture. Initially one thinks that contracting the abdominals and hip flexors as much as possible will get one deeper into it, but both rectus abdominis, the main abdominal muscle, and the psoas, the main hip flexor, shorten the torso and therefore draw the head away from the floor.

See *Padangushtasana* (page 37) and *Pada Hastasana* (page 39) for the subtleties of forward bending. We assist with the hands in bringing the torso between the legs, while the shoulder blades draw up to the ceiling. Hold the *asana* for five breaths.

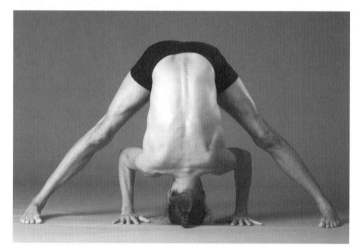

Prasarita Padottanasana A

Contraindications: If there is pain in the outer ankle, ground the inside of the feet. With pain in the inner ankle, ground the outside of the foot. A tendency of the hip abductors to spasm in these postures (pain on the outside of the hip above the greater trochanter) indicates an underdevelopment of these muscles. In this case, shorten the stance.

Vinyasa Four

Inhaling, lift your head and straighten your arms. Exhaling, return the hands to the hips.

Vinyasa Five

Inhaling, come to upright and exhale.

Prasarita Padottanasana B
WIDE STANCE FORWARD BEND B

Drishti Nose

Vinyasa One

Inhaling, raise your arms out to shoulder height, and broaden the chest and shoulders.

Vinyasa Two

Exhaling, place the hands back on the hips. Inhaling, lift the heart high and lengthen through the waist.

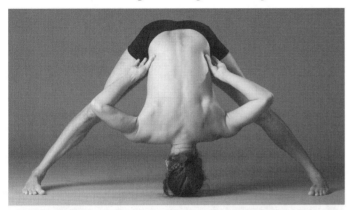

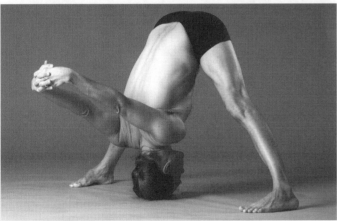

Prasarita Padottanasana B (top) and C

Vinyasa Three

Exhaling, fold forward at the hip joints, keeping the hands on the hips with fingers lightly pressing onto the abdomen to keep *Uddiyana Bandha* alive. Keep the groins deep and the psoas long to maintain the lengthening of the torso gained in *vinyasa* two. Hold this posture for five breaths.

Vinyasa Four

Inhaling, raise the trunk back up and exhale.

Prasarita Padottanasana C
WIDE STANCE FORWARD BEND C

Drishti Nose

Vinyasa One

Inhaling, extend the arms out to the sides.

Vinyasa Two

Exhaling, draw the arms behind your back and interlock the fingers. It is important here to roll the arms back in the shoulder joint and work the arms straight. If the arms sit forward in the joint, it is both uncomfortable and impossible to open the shoulder joint. Inhale and lift the heart.

Vinyasa Three

Exhaling, fold forward, dropping the head.

There are two hand positions for this posture. The first is where the palms face each other and the thumbs point down when one stands upright. This is the same hand position as in *Halasana* (page 118) and *Karnapidasana* (page 119). Pressing the heels of the hands together to intensify the stretch is contraindicated in students who have hyperextended elbows. If this condition is present, the teacher should not apply weight to the student's hands to get them deeper into the posture, as it may exaggerate the condition.

Once the first hand position is mastered, one can switch to the second, which is more challenging. Here we medially rotate the humeri (arm bones). In the forward bend the palms will face away from you with the thumbs pointing down to the floor. Apart from the arm position, the instructions for *Prasarita Padottanasana* C are the same as for B, with the added weight of the arms opening the shoulder joints and bringing more gravitational force into play in the stretching of the hamstrings. Hold this posture for five breaths.

Vinyasa Four

Inhaling, come upright.
Exhaling, place the hands on the hips.

Prasarita Padottanasana D

WIDE STANCE FORWARD BEND D

Drishti Nose

Vinyasa **One**

Inhaling, lift the front of the chest, keeping the hands on the hips.

Vinyasa **Two**

Exhaling, fold forward and clasp the big toes as in *Padangushtasana*.

Inhaling, lift the heart, gaze up softly, and straighten the arms.

Vinyasa **Three**

Exhaling, fold forward, placing the torso between the thighs and, if possible, the crown of the head down onto the floor. Shift the weight forward toward the toes to intensify the stretch. Keep spreading the toes.

The wrists and elbows draw out to the sides. The shoulder blades and the sit bones reach up to the ceiling. The crown of the head and the heart reach down to the floor. Hold for five breaths.

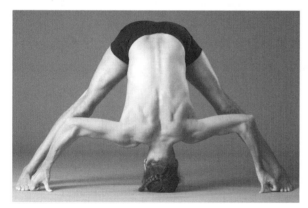

Prasarita Padottanasana D

Vinyasa **Four**

Inhaling, lift the torso to straighten the arms and look up.

Exhaling, place the hands back on your hips.

Vinyasa **Five**

Inhaling, come upright.

Exhaling, return to *Samasthiti*.

Parshvottanasana

INTENSE SIDE STRETCH

Drishti Nose

Vinyasa **One**

Inhaling, turn to the right and jump into a short stance. This is a square-hip position as in *Parivrta Trikonasana*. The *vinyasa* count encourages us to turn toward the right foot and place the hands in prayer on our back, all on the same inhalation.

For the sake of precision, beginners may break down these movements. To do so, turn out to the right on exhalation, to face the back of your mat. The left foot needs to be turned in 45°. Place the palms together behind the back and bring them up as high as possible between the shoulder blades. On

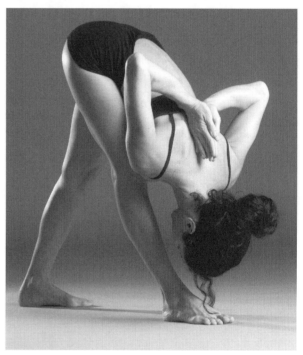

Parshvottanasana

the next inhalation spread the toes and lift the chest high, wrapping it back over your folded hands.

Vinyasa **Two**

Exhaling, fold forward over the straight front leg. The subtle alignment of the front foot is here probably more important than in any other standing posture. There needs to be a straight line going through the second toe and the center of the tibia and femur, with both bones in neutral rotation. The common tendency is to turn the front foot out too much, which rotates the tibia and femur away from each other. Pin the right hip back by grounding the right big toe. The entire thigh of the front leg is sucked back into the hip by engaging the quadriceps and the hamstrings. Without lifting the heel of the foot off the floor, point the toes. This action also engages the hamstrings, which serves to protect them in this intense stretch.

There is a strong tendency here to lean into the front foot, which causes the left hip to sag down to the floor. This avoids the stretch of the right hamstrings. Counteract this tendency by casting weight back into the left foot, spiking down the back heel. Keep the hips square and at an even distance from the floor. The back leg is straight and active, with an emphasis on grounding the outer arch of the foot. Gentle inward rolling of the thigh supports the squaring of the hips. All rotational movements need to be individually assessed by a teacher with knowledge of anatomy, as they can easily be overdone.

The elbows and shoulders have a tendency to droop forward and are lifted by the action of the rhomboid muscles, which lie between the shoulder blades. The palms, especially the roots of the fingers, press together. The entire trunk still performs *Samasthiti*, with the spine, neck, and back of the head in line as if standing upright. Allow neither the forehead to collapse to the shin nor the chin to jut forward to meet the shin. Instead, encourage the crown of the head and the heart to reach forward toward the front big toe, while the shoulder blades and sit bones draw backward, thereby putting the entire spine into traction. Hold for five breaths.

Vinyasa Three

Inhaling, come up and turn to the left.

Vinyasa Four

Exhaling, duplicate the posture on the left.

Vinyasa Five

Inhaling, come up and enjoy stretching the arms as the shoulders release.

The exhalation carries us back to *Samasthiti*.

Utthita Hasta Padangushtasana
UPRIGHT HAND-TO-BIG-TOE POSTURE

Drishti Toes, out to the side

Vinyasa One

From *Samasthiti*, inhaling, shift your entire weight into the left foot and draw the right knee up to the chest with both hands. This intermediate position is an opportunity to "set up" for the posture. It lengthens the hamstrings over the hip joint — here check that the right hip has not been lifted with the leg and deepen the groin by releasing the psoas.

> **ANATOMICAL FOCUS**
> *Strengthening the Feet*
>
> Beginners often develop cramps in their feet, especially if they have fallen arches. This should not be discouraging. Cramping indicates a weakness of the foot, but this will quickly be corrected through this posture if it is performed correctly. This is important, as fallen arches stress the medial meniscus and eventually weaken the knee joint. To correct this we have to lift the inner and transverse arches away from the floor. The anatomical names for these actions are plantar flexion (pointing the foot) and inversion of the foot (turning the sole of the foot upward) respectively. We will return to this action again and again, as it is the same one that protects the knee on entering into the half and full lotus postures. The muscles that perform both actions are tibialis posterior, flexor digitorum longus, and flexor hallucis longus. All three originate on the tibia and fibula and insert on the underside of the foot.

Establish the support of the standing leg by grounding the base of its big toe. The subtle medial spiraling achieved in the leg indicates the awakening of the abductor muscles. When you are standing on one leg, these muscles are vital in supporting the suspended hip and leg.

The right hand reaches down the outside of the knee and "binds" the right big toe, that is, wraps two fingers around it. Place the left hand on the left hip.

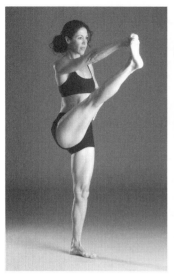 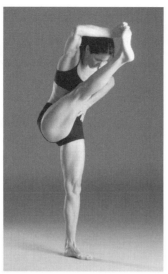 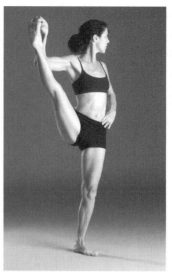 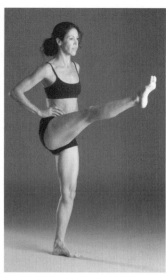

Utthita Hasta Padangushtasana, vinyasa one (left), *vinyasa* two, *vinyasa* four, and *vinyasa* seven

Now straighten the right leg, but only to a point where the back can be held upright. Sacrificing the alignment of the spine defies yogic principles. With

YOGIC CONTEXT
Outer Structure and Inner Freedom

Yoga Sutra II.47 says that the posture is correctly performed when the effort to perform it develops a quality of emptiness.

What does this mean? Initially effort is necessary. Otherwise the gross body, which is tamasic by nature,[9] will never become vibrant and alive in every aspect of the posture. Once the outer frame of the posture is achieved, we need to meditate on the inner nature of effort. When this is witnessed, it is recognized as the deep nature of all phenomena: *shunya* — emptiness.

There is effort at the surface and silence in the heart; form at the surface, formlessness at the core; structure outside, freedom inside.

Needless to say, this method does not work without first putting in the effort. Both aspects of this duality must be embraced; both need to be experienced. As Patanjali says, "abhyasa vairagyabhyam tannirodhah"[10] — the thought waves cease through application of the dual means of practice and letting go.

the leg straight, lift it high and lengthen out through the inseam[11] of both legs. If the right shoulder has been pulled forward by the weight of the leg, draw it back until the shoulders are again square.

Check that both hips are an even distance from the floor. The hip is often pulled up to escape the hamstring stretch. Check that the standing leg is still straight. Grow tall and elongate the spine up to the ceiling as the sit bones descend to the floor. The spine has the tendency to compress from carrying the additional weight of the lifted leg.

Vinyasa Two

When you have managed to fulfill all the above instructions you can lean forward on the exhalation. Place the torso squarely along the front leg, without altering its position.

Initially this position may feel awkward, but it is a powerful tool for gaining access to *Uddiyana Bandha*. It is, however, only effective if the alignment has been closely studied and the necessary flexibility gained. Hold this *vinyasa* for five breaths.

Vinyasa Three

Inhaling, come back upright, raising the torso.

Vinyasa Four

Exhaling, take the leg out to the right side while shifting the gaze to the left. It is important to do this

9. *tamas* = inertia, dormancy, mass.
10. *Yoga Sutra* I.12.

11. An imaginary line roughly corresponding to the inner seam of a pair of trousers.

movement without raising the right hip. Beginners can achieve this by first laterally rotating the thigh, which encourages the hip to drop but lifts the right heel into the center.

Once the leg is out to the side, the thigh can be rotated medially to turn the heel back down. The foot is taken out to the side as far as possible and the right hip joint worked open. The aim is to bring both hip joints and the right foot into one plane, which provides a maximum stretch for the right adductor muscle group (see figure 17, page 101). This is a perfect preparatory warm-up for the next posture, *Ardha Baddha Padmottanasana*. The stretching of the adductors is a safety precaution for the knees, necessary for all lotus and half-lotus postures. Hold this *vinyasa* also for five breaths.

Vinyasa **Five**

Inhaling, bring the leg back to center.

Vinyasa **Six**

Exhaling, fold forward again onto the right leg.

Vinyasa **Seven**

Inhale and come upright. Let go of the foot and hold the leg up away from the floor. This is an important exercise for strengthening the psoas muscle (see figure 12, page 67). This action is initiated by the psoas and completed by the rectus femoris (hip flexor). Due to its origin (anterior superior iliac spine), it tends to tilt the pelvis anteriorly (forward). A tight/weak psoas also has the tendency to exaggerate the lordosis of the low back (swayback). Both of these tendencies need to be counteracted by the rectus abdominis muscle (see figure 16, page 89), which pulls the pubic bone up in front and tilts the pelvis posteriorly.

If the abdominal muscles do not work, the leg cannot be lifted very high. *Utthita Hasta Padangushtasana*

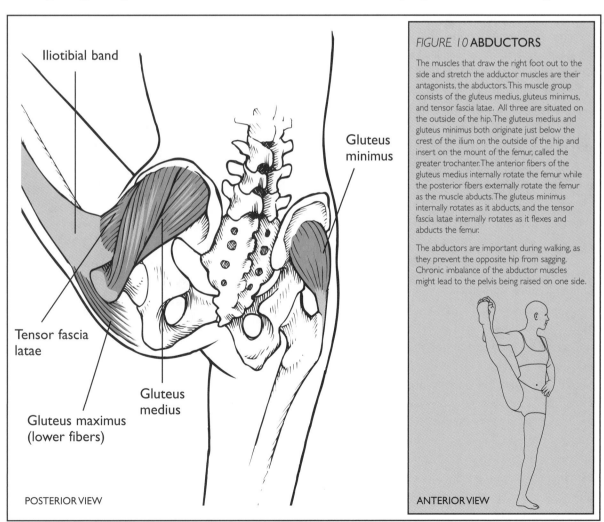

Iliotibial band

Gluteus minimus

Tensor fascia latae

Gluteus medius

Gluteus maximus (lower fibers)

POSTERIOR VIEW

FIGURE 10 **ABDUCTORS**

The muscles that draw the right foot out to the side and stretch the adductor muscles are their antagonists, the abductors. This muscle group consists of the gluteus medius, gluteus minimus, and tensor fascia latae. All three are situated on the outside of the hip. The gluteus medius and gluteus minimus both originate just below the crest of the ilium on the outside of the hip and insert on the mount of the femur, called the greater trochanter. The anterior fibers of the gluteus medius internally rotate the femur while the posterior fibers externally rotate the femur as the muscle abducts. The gluteus minimus internally rotates as it abducts, and the tensor fascia latae internally rotates as it flexes and abducts the femur.

The abductors are important during walking, as they prevent the opposite hip from sagging. Chronic imbalance of the abductor muscles might lead to the pelvis being raised on one side.

ANTERIOR VIEW

is an optimal exercise for both the hip flexors and the abdominal muscles.

Exhaling, lower the right leg.

Vinyasas Eight to Fourteen

Repeat for the left leg.

Ardha Baddha Padmottanasana

INTENSE BOUND HALF LOTUS

Drishti Nose

Vinyasa One

Since this is a surprisingly complex posture, we will break it down into phases. Beginners should study these phases closely.

PHASE 1

Inhaling, lift the right knee to the height of the chest and draw the heel to the right sit bone. To do the posture safely, we have to be able to touch the sit bone with the heel. This means that we have completely closed the gap between femur and tibia. Only then can the two bones move as a unity in the posture, which avoids any strain on the knee joint. If you cannot perform this movement, you should not attempt to go all the way into the posture, but concentrate instead on preparation. If you cannot completely close the knee joint you need to lengthen the quadriceps. Long quadriceps are also of great advantage in backbending.

PHASE 2

Pick up the right foot and, cradling it in both hands, point and invert it. Now direct the knee far out to the side. Gently draw the foot up into the *right* groin, with the knee still out to the side. This educates the hip to perform lateral rotation. The main prerequisite for the lotus and half-lotus postures is the ability to rotate the femur in the hip joint, and resistance may be encountered here. It is important to realize that the half-lotus and lotus postures belong to a group that involve hip rotation and not knee rotation. If we do not open the hip joints (which are ball-and-socket joints and move in all directions), the "opening" will go into the knee joints. These are, however, hinge joints, designed to

move in only one direction. The "opening" will be nothing but a destabilization.

The ancient yogis had no problems in this area: they always sat on the floor, which keeps the hip joints mobile and flexible. In our society we sit in chairs off the floor and with the hip joints flexed. We therefore need to invest extra time into postures that prepare us for the Primary Series.

PHASE 3

From having the knee pointed far out to the right and the right heel in the right groin, we now lift the heel toward the navel, keeping foot and knee the same distance from the floor.

If you closed the gap between tibia and femur, both bones will now move as a unity, preventing any strain on the knee joint. I like to refer to this knee position as "sealed." It ensures that the rotation happens between the femur and its hip socket (acetabulum) and not between the femur and the tibia (knee joint). When you have acquired the necessary hip rotation, you will be able to touch your heel to your navel.

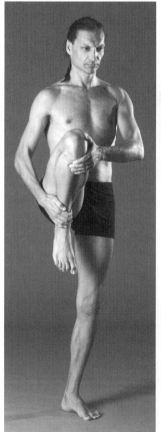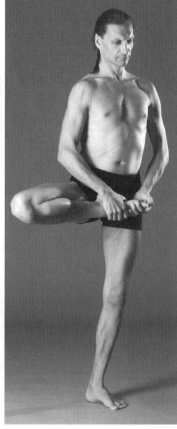

PHASE 4

Keeping the heel in line with the navel, let the knee slide down toward the floor. Ideally at this point we would medially rotate the femur to an extent that the previous lateral rotation is annulled, and the sole of the foot faces forward instead of upward. Lift the right foot into the opposite groin, making sure the heel stays in line with the navel. Keep hold of the foot with the left hand while the right hand reaches around your back for the left elbow. Bind the elbow or if possible the big toe of the right foot. Check that there is no limitation here from failing to lift the shoulder as the arm reaches back. Now draw the shoulder blade down the back.

Only when you have managed to bind the big toe with the opposite hand can you safely proceed to fold forward. The ability to bind indicates that the knee is in a safe position to fold forward. If the toe cannot be bound, the foot is probably not high enough in the groin but rather somewhere on the opposite thigh. This means that the knee joint is not flexed completely and the ligamentous structures and cartilage will be subject to stress.

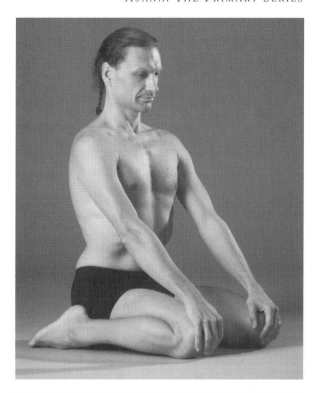

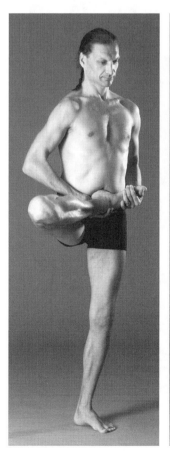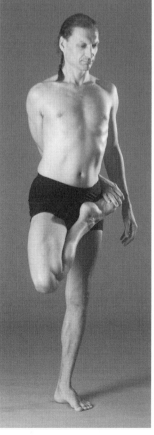

PRACTICAL TIP
Lengthening the Quadriceps

The easiest way to lengthen the quadriceps is to spend fifteen minutes or longer each day engaged in *Virasana* and, later, *Supta Virasana*. Do this outside of your *vinyasa* practice.

In the beginning you may sit on blankets or pillows. As flexibility increases, slowly reduce the height of your seat. After *Virasana* has become easy, practice *Supta Virasana*.

It is beneficial to use a belt in this posture. Without a belt the knees will have the tendency to come apart. Actively drawing the knees together every day for an extended period will shorten the adductor muscles.

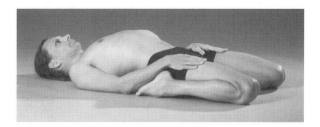

From opposite page, left to right, going into *Ardha Baddha Padmottanasana* phase 1, phase 2, phase 3; *vinyasa* one
Top, *Virasana*; above, *Supta Virasana*

Opening the Hip Joints

To open the hip joints, we need to spend as much time as possible sitting in *Ardha Siddhasana*.

Practice this posture after *Virasana*. Again, blankets can be used and slowly decreased in height as your flexibility increases. Keep the knees as wide apart as possible. You can eat, write, or watch TV in this posture. If one spends an hour in it daily, the hip joints will quickly open. After you have gained some flexibility, progress on to *Siddhasana*.

Vinyasa Two

Exhaling, bend forward, keeping the big toe bound, and place the left hand on the floor alongside the left foot. Spread the fingers and point them forward. Spread the base of the toes of the standing leg. Gently shift a little more weight than that held in the heels forward into the base of the toes. Lift the inner arch of the foot away from the floor to protect the knee. Release the hip flexors and the buttocks (gluteus maximus) but work the supporting leg strongly (vastus group), eventually placing the chest squarely down on the leg. The crown of the head points downward toward the floor. The shoulder blades are drawn up to the ceiling to keep the neck long.

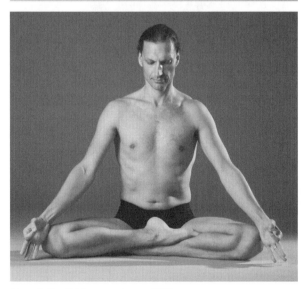

Top, *Ardha Siddhasana*; above, *Siddhasana*

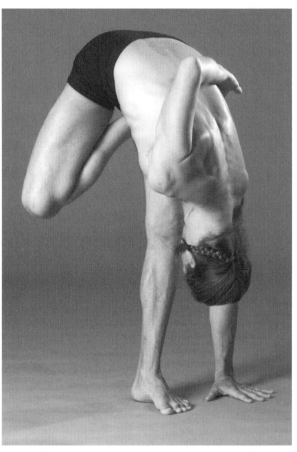

Ardha Baddha Padmottanasana, vinyasa two

The folded knee gently works toward the back end of the mat with a light medial rotation of the femur. To prevent the hip of the bent leg from sagging, keep this foot and leg active so there is an even tone in both legs. The angle between the two femurs should be 35° to 45°, depending on the ratio of tibia to femur length. (People with a long shinbone need

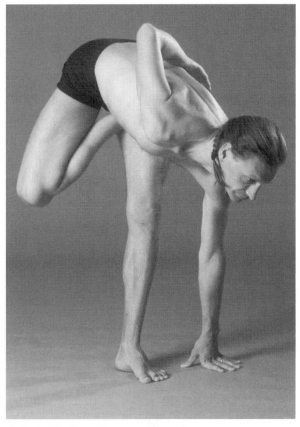

Ardha Baddha Padmottanasana, vinyasa three

to have the knee lifted farther out to the side to level the hips.) This action is performed by the abductor muscle group, especially the gluteus medius and gluteus minimus.

They are two very interesting muscles, as they are often the cause of a twisted pelvis if there is an imbalance between the two sides.

Stay in the state of *Ardha Baddha Padmottanasana* for five breaths.

PRACTICAL TIP

Bending the Leg in Transit

A trick for beginners to gain confidence is to bend the standing leg a little to reach the hand to the floor. When you have the hand securely on the floor, straighten the standing leg.

The same method can be used on the way up. The bent leg will help the other foot to slide deeper into the groin, with the bent leg more forgiving as you develop your sense of balance.

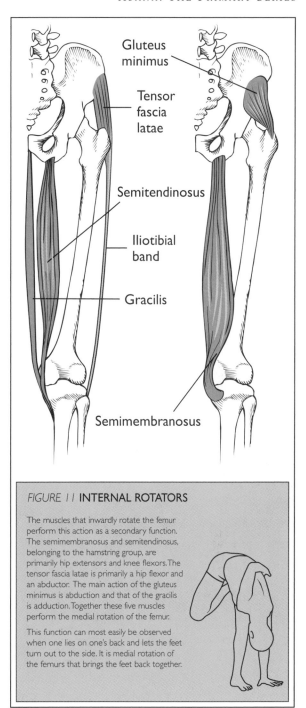

FIGURE 11 **INTERNAL ROTATORS**

The muscles that inwardly rotate the femur perform this action as a secondary function. The semimembranosus and semitendinosus, belonging to the hamstring group, are primarily hip extensors and knee flexors. The tensor fascia latae is primarily a hip flexor and an abductor. The main action of the gluteus minimus is abduction and that of the gracilis is adduction. Together these five muscles perform the medial rotation of the femur.

This function can most easily be observed when one lies on one's back and lets the feet turn out to the side. It is medial rotation of the femurs that brings the feet back together.

Vinyasa **Three**

Inhaling, lift the torso and head and, maintaining the posture, exhale.

Vinyasa **Four**

Inhaling, come up, but keep the half lotus bound until you are completely upright. This will draw the foot farther up into the groin and increase the opening effect on the hip joint.

Vinyasa Five

Exhaling, release the big toe, carefully take the foot out of position using both hands, and stand in *Samasthiti*.

*Vinyasa*s Six to Nine

Repeat on the left side.

Caution: If you experience pain in your knee at any point, go back and attentively study the previous steps. If you are starting out with very stiff hip joints, it could take the better part of a decade to open them. It is well worth the work.

Utkatasana
POWER POSTURE

Drishti Upward

The following three postures build strength and stamina. They are the only standing postures that are woven together with full *vinyasa*. The sequence concludes with a *vinyasa* to sitting.

Vinyasa **One**	Inhale, raise arms.
Vinyasa **Two**	Exhale, fold forward.
Vinyasa **Three**	Inhale, lift chest.
Vinyasa **Four**	Exhale, *Chaturanga Dandasana*.
Vinyasa **Five**	Inhale, Upward Dog.
Vinyasa **Six**	Exhale, Downward Dog.

Vinyasa **Seven**

Inhaling, hop your feet to your hands, big toes together. Bend the knees and, keeping the heels grounded, lower your sit bones toward the floor. Raise the arms, bring the palms together, and gaze up past your hands to the ceiling. Balance between the two poles of keeping the torso and arms upright and deepening the squat (see *Surya Namaskara* B, *vinyasa* one, page 32). Keep the lower abdomen firm and allow the rib cage to pulsate with the breath. Hold the state of *Utkatasana* for five breaths.

Vinyasa **Eight**

Exhaling, place the hands on the floor and, with the inhalation, hop up into an arm balance. The knees are bent. Attempt to hover here for the duration of

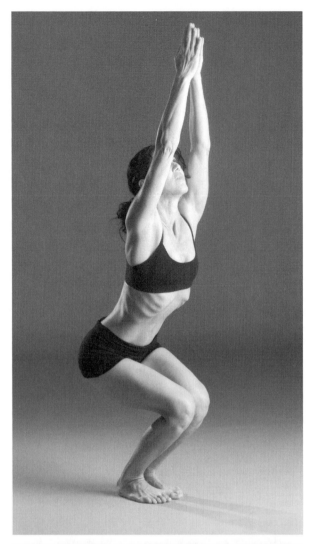

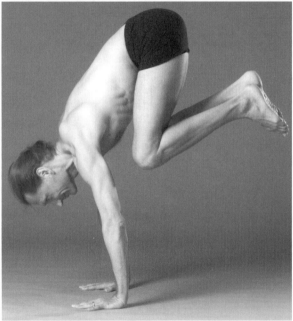

Top, *Utkatasana*, *vinyasa* seven; above, *vinyasa* eight

the inhalation. Keeping the legs bent will develop greater strength, whereas straightening the legs into a full handstand enables us to rely more on our sense of balance.

Balancing on the arms develops core strength. The body must draw all forces together and work as one unit. This is an important aspect, especially necessary for those whose bodies are naturally soft and flexible. There is a tendency for students who swiftly gain flexibility to progress more and more in that direction. Flexibility, however, often accompanies low muscle tone. Low muscle tone is the ability to lengthen

---

YOGIC CONTEXT
Asana — The Seat

In some contemporary forms of yoga the lotus and half-lotus postures are neglected. If the student practices out of ambition, and the underlying technical principles are not understood, these postures can in fact be detrimental. This is a great shame, as the hip rotations are arguably the most important yoga postures, with *Siddhasana* and *Padmasana* (lotus posture) high in their ranks. The *Hatha Yoga Pradipika* calls *Siddhasana* "the principal *asana*" and claims it to be "the gate to freedom." About *Padmasana* it says, "It opens the path to liberation." The *Gheranda Samhita* says about *Siddhasana*, "It leads to freedom" and about *Padmasana*, "It wards off all diseases."

Shiva Samhita recommends that *Siddhasana* should be adopted if quick success in yoga is desired, and agrees with the *Gheranda Samhita* that *Padmasana* "protects from all diseases." The *Yoga Yajnavalkya* says that, "*Padmasana* is esteemed by all."

There is enough evidence to deem the hip rotations as the most important category of yoga postures, with all other postures preparing us to stay for a longer time in *asana*s such as *Padmasana* and *Siddhasana*.

---

muscles with a relative inability to contract them. This tendency needs to be counteracted by focusing on building strength rather than more flexibility.

This exercise might initially seem daunting, but a sincere effort every day will take you a long way in a year.

Vinyasa **Nine**	Exhale, *Chaturanga Dandasana*.
Vinyasa **Ten**	Inhale, Upward Dog.
Vinyasa **Eleven**	Exhale, Downward Dog.

Virabhadrasana A
WARRIOR POSTURE A

Drishti Upward

Since we follow in this text the half-*vinyasa* system, which is the common practice in India, every posture from now on will commence from *vinyasa* seven. In other words, from Downward Dog in the previous posture we enter the following posture. To start every posture with the first *vinyasa* would mean returning to *Samasthiti* between every *asana*, which is the full-*vinyasa* practice.

Vinyasa **Seven**

Inhaling, turn the left heel into the center of your mat so that the foot is placed at 45° to the center-line of the mat. Step the right foot up and place it between the hands (check that the hips are square and the left foot correctly positioned).

Continuing the inhalation, bring the torso upright and raise your arms. Bring the palms together and gaze upward. Draw the shoulder blades down and out to the side to prevent the shoulders from hunching around the ears. The outer arch of the back foot grounds, and the thigh rolls medially to aid the left hip in remaining forward. The sit bones are heavy and sink downward. Without losing the squareness of the hips, track your right knee out over the right ankle, bringing the shin perpendicular to the floor.

If we sacrifice the squareness of the hips here, we forsake the best opportunity in the Primary Series to stretch the psoas and quadriceps muscles. For this stretch to occur, it is necessary to keep the pelvis upright.

The tendency will be to tilt the pelvis anteriorly and collapse into the low back. Apart from avoiding the lengthening of psoas and quadriceps, we will also weaken where we need to be strong: in the low back.

To protect this vulnerable area we need to bring the abdominal muscles into play. Engaging rectus

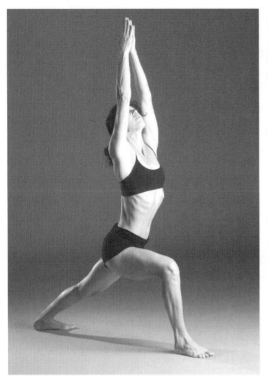

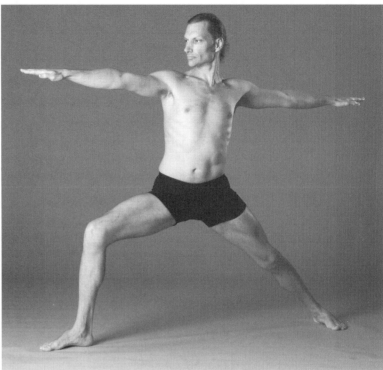

Virabhadrasana A

Virabhadrasana B

abdominis lifts the pubic bone and tips the pelvis posteriorly, allowing us to stretch those important muscles. Hold *Virabhadrasana* A for five breaths.

Vinyasa Eight

Exhaling, lower the gaze to the horizon and, keeping the arms up, turn to the left and repeat *Virabhadrasana* A on the left side. Once fully into the posture, lift the gaze upward.

Virabhadrasana B
WARRIOR POSTURE B

Drishti Hand

Vinyasa Nine

Exhaling, draw the right hip back until the pelvis is parallel with the long edge of the mat. At the same time lower the arms until the hands hover above your feet. Open the right foot to 5° to accommodate the opening of the groins (technically, "groin" here refers mainly to the adductors). You will need to

elongate the stance up to ten inches, the distance gained from opening the hip position. The gaze reaches out to the right hand. Hold for five breaths.

The outer arch of the right foot grounds and the right leg rolls laterally to open both groins. Note that the rotation of the thigh of the back leg, which is determined by the turn-out of the foot, is different from that of *Virabhadrasana* A. Sink the hips down as low as possible until you get the feeling of being suspended between two rubber straps. Resist the tendency to lean the torso toward the front leg by positioning the shoulders squarely above the hips. For the working of the legs see *Utthita Parshvakonasana* (page 46), which is identical.

Vinyasa Ten

Exhaling, turn and imitate the posture on the right side. The gaze shifts to the right hand. Five breaths.

Vinyasa Eleven

Exhaling, place both hands down at the front end of the mat and, inhaling, lift up and hover for the

> In the *Mahabharata*, Arjuna is frequently addressed as "Oh mighty armed one." With regular training, *vinyasa* eleven will give us a chance to replicate Arjuna's strength.

Vinyasa **Twelve**

Exhaling, lower into *Chaturanga Dandasana*.

Vinyasa **Thirteen**

Inhaling, arch into Upward Dog.

length of the inhalation in an arm balance, with the left leg straight and the right leg bent. This is again an opportunity to balance flexibility with strength.

Vinyasa **Fourteen**

Exhaling, draw back into Downward Dog. We are now ready to jump through to sitting.

MYTHOLOGICAL BACKGROUND

Shiva's Wrath

Virabhadra was a fierce warrior of Lord Shiva's army. The head priest, Daksha, was an orthodox rule-maker and preserver of traditional society. Against his consent, his beautiful daughter Sati married Lord Shiva. Shiva destroys the world at the end of each world age, and he also destroys the ego. He is therefore the Lord of Mystery.

For various reasons Daksha considered Shiva impure. Shiva had peculiar habits such as meditating in burial grounds smeared with the ashes of the dead, and meditating on mountaintops for long periods, rather than participating in society. But the main reason for Daksha's disdain was that Shiva always carried a skull with him. The story behind this was that, to punish him for his vanity, Shiva had once cut off one of the five heads of Lord Brahma, whereupon Brahma laid a curse on Shiva: that the skull would stick to his hand. To this day some worshipers of Shiva always carry with them a skull.

At one time Daksha organized a great ceremony to which he invited all deities and dignitaries with the exception of Shiva and Sati. Against Shiva's advice, Sati attended her father's ceremony. Before the thousands of guests she asked her father why he had not invited her husband. Daksha responded by exclaiming that Shiva was a despicable character, an outcast who did not know the conventions of society.

With this insult to her husband, Sati's anger was so aroused that she burst into flames and was reduced to ashes. When Shiva, in his solitude, heard of Sati's death he became terribly angry, jumped up and danced the dance of destruction.

Eventually he tore out one of his *jatar*s (dreadlocks) and smashed it to the ground. From the impact the terrible warriors Virabhadra and Bhadrakali arose. Shiva ordered them to proceed to Daksha's festival, destroy the hall, kill everybody one by one, behead Daksha, drink his blood, and throw his head into the fire.

The story continues, but as far as our posture is concerned we can leave it there. *Virabhadrasana* is dedicated to this terrible warrior.

Pashimottanasana

INTENSE WESTERN STRETCH[12]

Drishti Toes

As with all following *asana*s (excluding the finishing postures), here we pick up the *vinyasa* count at seven.

Vinyasa Seven

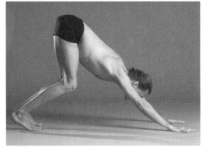
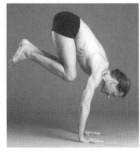
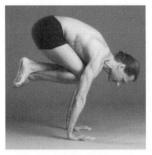
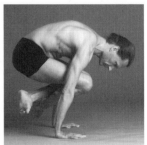

Inhaling, jump through to a seated position.

At first you may execute this movement using momentum. With increased proficiency you will be able to jump through with little or no momentum while still clearing the floor. The key to effortless performance here is to connect the breath to the *bandha*s. As long as we are airborne in the jump, we must continue to inhale, as the inhalation has a lifting and carrying effect. Once the lift-through is complete we initiate the exhalation to lower down.

To learn this movement it should be divided into two clearly distinguishable separate phases. Phase 1 is hopping forward into an arm balance with the shoulders over the wrists, and the hips and folded legs lifted high. Phase 2 consists of letting the torso and legs slowly swing through the arms, using the shoulders as an axis. As you swing through, suck the feet up into the abdomen and the knees into the chest to clear the floor. With the last of the inhalation, straighten the legs into *Dandasana*, still suspended in the air. With the exhalation, slowly lower down like a helicopter. Performing the movement in this way will establish a firm connection between breath and *bandha*s. It will also strengthen the abdomen and the low back, preparing for the challenging backbends and leg-behind-head postures in the later sequences.

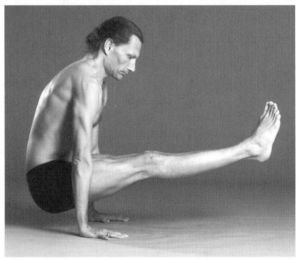

Sit in *Dandasana* for five breaths. *Dandasana* has no *vinyasa* count of its own: rather, the seventh *vinyasa* of *Pashimottanasana* is the state of *Dandasana*. Nevertheless *Dandasana* is the basic sitting posture. We will usually transit through *Dandasana* before and after each half *vinyasa*.

Dandasana is like *Samasthiti* seated. The sit bones ground and the spine lengthens with the attempt to reproduce its natural curvature. The heart is lifted and buoyant, open in the front and broad and open

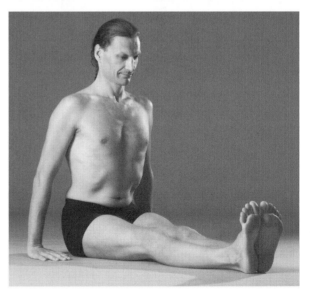

12. Referring to the back of the body, which traditionally faced away from the rising sun and therefore toward the west.

Left to right, top to bottom, jump through to *Dandasana*

in the back. The armpits lift in the front as the tops of the arm bones (humerus) are positioned in the center of the shoulder joints. Extend the arms and place the hands on the floor with the fingers pointing toward the feet. If your arms are longer than your torso, place the hands slightly behind the hips. The

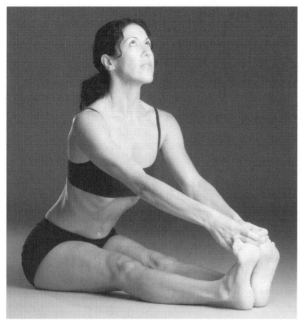

Pashimottanasana, vinyasa eight

kneecaps are pulled up. Lengthen out through the base of the toes and spike the heels down into the floor to awaken the hamstrings. The gaze is toward the nose.

Vinyasa **Eight**

Exhaling, reach for the big toes. The low back must be kept flat. To round the back in a seated forward bend is the equivalent of bending down from a standing position to lift a heavy object off the floor while rounding the back and keeping the legs straight. To avoid the danger of disc bulge and prolapse (see page 37, and figure 6, page 38) it is necessary to keep the low back straight in any weight-bearing situation. This includes all forward bending postures and also leg-behind-head postures like *Ekapada Shirshasana*. In postures where gravity is the only load, such as *Karnapidasana* and *Bujapidasana*, the spine can be safely flexed.

Without resorting to bending your back and/or using a strap, you have two options if you are too stiff to reach the big toes in *Pashimottanasana*. One is

to bend the knees and take the toes. This enables the pelvis to tilt forward, which is the imperative first stage of a forward bend. Keeping the iliac crests (upper front of the hip bones) in close proximity to the thighs, work on slowly straightening out the legs. Press out through the base of the feet and, at the same time, reach the sit bones away from the feet. The pubic bone slips down between the thighs. The other option is to take hold of the shins, ankles, or whatever you can reach. With a firm grip, slowly work your way forward as the hamstrings lengthen.

Some students will find their hamstrings so stiff that the pelvis tilts posteriorly when sitting on the floor with legs straight. This means that gravity is working against you. In this case, it is advisable to

> **YOGIC CONTEXT**
> *The Use of Props*
>
> All *asana*s are designed to form energetic cycles — especially postures like *Pashimottanasana* and *Baddha Padmasana*, where the hands are connected to the feet. The earth, being receptive, draws out our energy. These bound postures recycle energy that is otherwise lost. Yogis often meditate on a seat that consists of consecutive layers of *kusha* grass, deer or tiger skin, and cotton to insulate them from the earth. These energy cycles are thought to have a profound influence on the pranic sheath (*pranamaya kosha*), which is reduced when the energy flow is interrupted through belts and straps.
>
> The use of a strap or belt might seem like an easy solution for students with stiff hamstrings who find it difficult to reach their toes with their back straight. However, as Shri K. Pattabhi Jois has pointed out, the use of props interrupts the energy cycle of the posture.

elevate the sit bones by sitting on a folded blanket. This helps to bring the pelvis upright, enabling proper alignment of the spine. Whichever approach you choose, with the inhalation lift the chest and straighten the arms.

Look up between your eyebrows as you pull up on your kneecaps, and draw your shoulder blades down your back. Lengthen your waist, letting the

Psoas — The Seat of the Soul

The hip flexor muscle group includes the rectus femoris of the quadriceps, the sartorius, the tensor fascia latae, and the deeply internal psoas muscle. Continuing to contract the rectus femoris after it has tilted the hips in a forward bend causes it to bunch up in the front of the hip and prevent one from working deeper into the posture. The psoas muscle originates from the sides of the body of T12 (the last thoracic vertebra), where it touches the diaphragm and all five lumbar vertebrae. It runs along the back of the abdominal cavity (the front of the spine) through the pelvis and inserts at a mount on the inside of the thighbone (femur), the lesser trochanter. It flexes the hip joint and laterally rotates the femur in the process.

When the thigh is fixed, as in standing and seated postures, the psoas is flexed. Ida Rolf states that a healthy psoas should elongate during flexion and fall back toward the spine.[13] It is necessary to release and lengthen the psoas, once the hips are tilted forward, in order to deepen any forward-bending postures.

The superficial muscles of the body relax completely after they have been worked, but the deep muscles always retain a certain tension, even at rest. This is especially true of muscles that originate on the spine, like the psoas. They are therefore prone to spasm if worked intensely. The conscious relaxing of these muscles is as important as exercising them.

The psoas is the deepest muscle in the body. Its importance is such that it has been described by some as the "seat of the soul." To see the psoas in action one has to imagine the graceful gait of African or Indian women carrying large water containers on their heads. To do this, the head has to maintain a continuous forward motion without any sudden jerks. The movement is only possible with a strong but relaxed psoas muscle. The psoas swings the pelvis forward and backward like a cradle. This swinging action initiates the movement of the legs with the rectus femoris (the large hip flexor at the front of the thigh) only coming into action well after the psoas. The

swinging of the pelvis creates a wavelike motion up the spine, which keeps the spine healthy and vibrant, and the mind centered in the heart. If you have ever tried to walk with a large object balancing on your head you know how difficult this makes it to follow the tangents of the mind. Connecting with the core of the body (the psoas) shifts the attention from the mind to the heart — this is why the psoas is regarded as the seat of the soul.

The other extreme can be observed when we watch an army march. Soldiers are required to keep the psoas hardened. Being constantly shortened, the muscle spasms and is weakened. In the military attention posture, when the chest is swelled, one naturally dips into the low back, which also weakens the psoas muscle. When marching, the pelvis is arrested and the thighs are aggressively thrust upward and forward. This movement only uses the rectus femoris. The spine is frozen, and this keeps the soldiers' attention in their minds. In this state the mind can more easily be convinced to be noncompassionate to fellow human beings, who are instead labeled as the enemy.

If we all walked with our psoas active and our spines caressed with the wavelike motion this produces, our minds would possibly arrive at a state of silence. We would then see every human being as part of the same consciousness that animates us all. One of the reasons our Western culture has conquered much of the world with its arms is that we have abandoned natural awareness and have fallen under the tyranny of the mind. Yoga calls for restoring this awareness, which draws us to naturally abide in nonviolence. Nonviolence becomes a nonimposed ethical law.

As one starts practicing yoga it is very important to abandon the Western aggressive conquering attitude of wanting to derive an advantage out of yoga, but rather to approach the postures from a deep surrender into what is already here. All forward bends inspire this attitude. If, rather than developing yet another wish — such as to lengthen the hamstrings, which actually shorten and contract with greed — we let go into the knowledge that everything we may ask for is already here, the hamstrings will release by themselves. Ambition shortens hamstrings.

13. Rolf, I.P., *Rolfing: The Integration of Human Structures*, Santa Monica, Dennis-Landman, 1977, p. 112.

lower ribs reach away from your hip bones by releasing the psoas muscle. The psoas is the only muscle that connects the lower extremities to the spine, which makes it an integral stabilizing core muscle.

we can conclude that *Uddiyana Bandha* is not engaged sufficiently. Let these movements be motivated from deep within, working the posture from the core out toward the periphery.

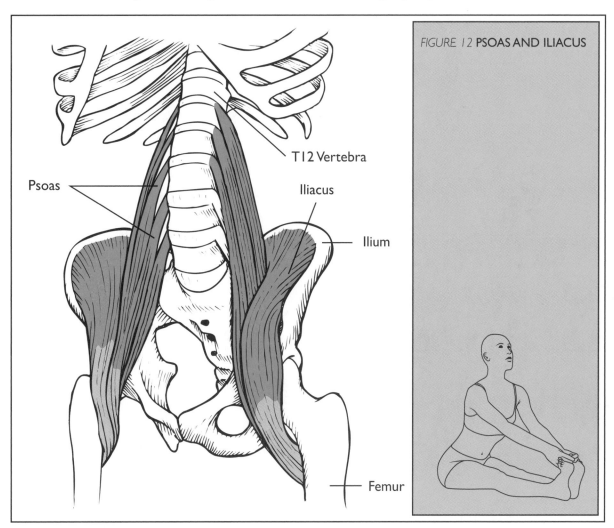

FIGURE 12 **PSOAS AND ILIACUS**

Psoas

T12 Vertebra

Iliacus

Ilium

Femur

Vinyasa Nine

Exhaling, fold forward at the hip joints, maintaining the lift created in *vinyasa* eight. Rather then collapsing the head down toward the knees, lift the heart forward toward the toes.

The work of *Uddiyana Bandha* is important here to support the low back. Do not breathe excessively into the belly, as is often done in forward bending, but encourage the rib cage to participate in the breathing process.

The inhalation is used to reach the heart forward, whereas the exhalation is used by surrendering deeper into the posture. If this instruction leads to the student "bouncing" up and down in the posture,

The kneecaps are permanently lifted in all forward-bending postures. As explained in *Padangushtasana* (page 37), the antagonist of each muscle to be stretched needs to be engaged. The muscle group being stretched here is the hamstrings; their antagonist is the quadriceps. For beginners it is often impossible to keep the kneecaps pulled up due to an inability to access the quadriceps. It may seem as if we need to grow a new nerve connection to this muscle. This learned coordination is possible through concentration and perseverance. The teacher may gently press the thumbs into both thighs to "awaken" the quadriceps.

In all forward bends it is important to release

and spread the buttocks. The buttocks are often tightened in a fear response to the stretch felt. Tightening the buttocks, however, draws us up out of the forward bend since the gluteus maximus muscle is a hip extensor. The ligaments of the sacroiliac joints (sacrum / pelvis joints) can also be

around the ears and blocks the flow of energy to the cervical spine. Excessive contracting of the neck muscles can lead to a red face in forward or back bending, which indicates a constriction of the blood flow to the head. Use the anchoring of the hands to counteract this, by drawing the shoulder blades

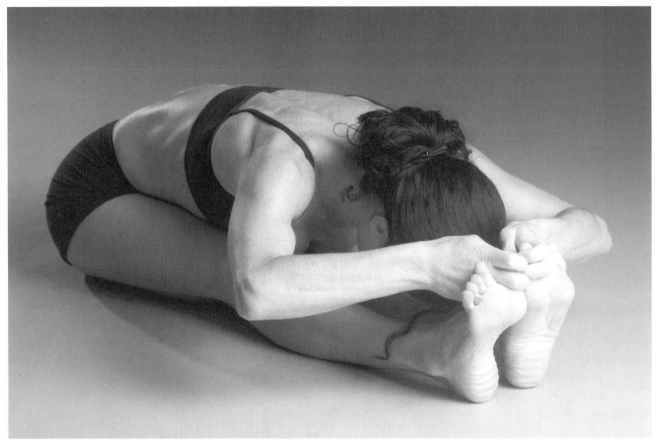

Pashimottanasana A (the state of the *asana*)

strained. Focus on releasing the buttocks, allowing them to spread, and lengthen through the low back. This is eccentric lengthening of the quadratus lumborum muscle. Eccentric lengthening means that the muscle is active, as we need it to keep the back straight, but at the same time it becomes longer as we elongate the waist. In other words the muscles lengthen against resistance. It is important to create additional space between the hipbone and the lowest rib because a shortened, contracted waist is an obstacle in all forward bending, backbending, and leg-behind-head postures.

The shoulders move away from the ears in *Pashimottanasana*. Contracting the trapezius and levator scapulae muscles hunches the shoulders

down the back, which is called depressing the shoulder girdle (latissimus dorsi), and by drawing them out to the sides, called abduction of the scapulae (serratus anterior).

Pashimottanasana is another great posture to demonstrate the principle of simultaneous expansion in opposing directions. The feet, the heart, and the crown of the head are reaching forward to elongate the spine. The shoulder blades, the sit bones, and the heads of the femurs are extending backward. The elbows and the shoulder blades reach out wide to the sides. The muscles hug the body, compressing *prana* into the core. The core remains open, receptive, and bright. Its luminescence permeates the whole of the posture and shines forth.

Surrender is most important in *Pashimottanasana*. This posture is not about conquering the hamstrings but about letting go. To breathe into and release the hamstrings can be very upsetting. We store many powerful emotions, such as suppressed anger, competitiveness, and fear of inadequacy, in our hamstring muscles. All suppressed emotions are potentially

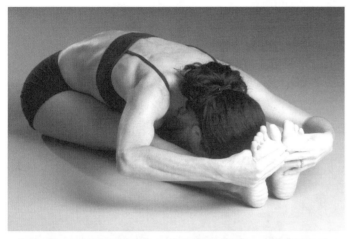

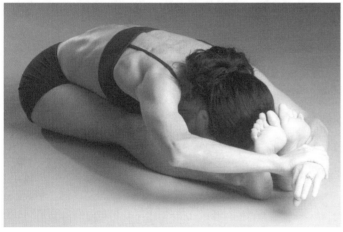

Pashimottanasana B (top) and C

crippling to our health: they are toxic and have an impact on our personality. It is essential that, if strong emotions do arise when we breathe awareness into the hamstrings, we acknowledge whatever we feel and then let go of these emotions. Breathing through a posture requires that the stretch be kept at a manageable intensity. If the stretch is too strong we will harden and numb ourselves further. One needs to stretch with compassion and intelligence. Otherwise, instead of letting go of our old unconscious conditioning, we will superimpose yet another layer of abuse. Stay in the state of *Pashimottanasana* A for five breaths.

Vinyasa Ten

Inhaling, lift the torso away from the legs, straightening the arms. Exhaling, take the outsides of the feet.

The next three *vinyasas* reflect *Pashimottanasana* B, and the three *vinyasas* after that reflect *Pashimottanasana* C.

Vinyasa Eight

Inhaling, lift the heart and the entire front of the torso.

Vinyasa Nine

Exhaling, *Pashimottanasana* B, five breaths.

Vinyasa Ten

Inhaling, lift the torso away from the legs, straightening the arms. Exhaling, reach around the feet to lock the wrists.

Vinyasa Eight

Inhaling, lift the torso, straightening the arms.

Vinyasa Nine

Exhaling, fold forward, *Pashimottanasana* C, five breaths.

These three variations of *Pashimottanasana* stretch the inside, outside, and center of the hamstrings, which coincide with the three separate muscles of the group: semitendinosus, semimembranosus, and biceps femoris (see figure 7, page 40).

Vinyasa Ten

Inhaling, lift the torso, straightening the arms. Exhaling, place your hands to the floor.

Vinyasa Eleven

Inhaling, lift up and move the feet back with a single hop so the body forms a straight line from the head to the feet.

The inhalation has a natural upward lifting function; the exhalation has a grounding and rooting function. Imagine the autumn wind playing with leaves and effortlessly lifting them off the floor. The same power is used in the *vinyasa* movement. The inhalation inspires the lift, with the shoulder and arm muscles providing the structural support. This is only possible with *Mula* and *Uddiyana Bandha* engaged. The

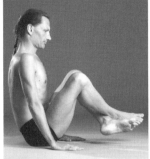
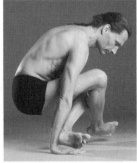
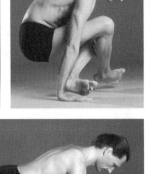
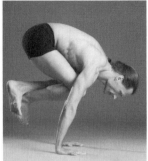
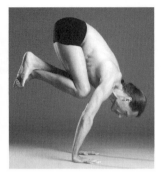

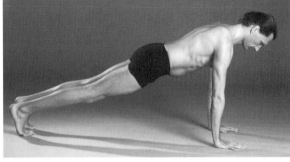

Above from left, *vinyasa* eleven jump back, in phases
Left, start of *vinyasa* twelve

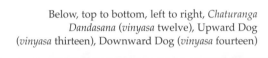

Below, top to bottom, left to right, *Chaturanga Dandasana* (*vinyasa* twelve), Upward Dog (*vinyasa* thirteen), Downward Dog (*vinyasa* fourteen)

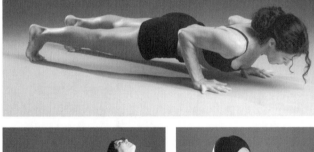

inhalation reaches down, hooks into the *bandha*s, and lifts the body up like an elevator. Movement must follow the breath. If the breath is connected to the *bandha*s, it will move the body effortlessly and one will feel light and rejuvenated after the practice. If the *bandha*s are not firmly established, one might feel drained and exhausted after practice because energy has been lost. Feel how the inhalation reaches down and attaches itself to the engaged pelvic floor and lower abdominal wall. Continue to inhale, creating a suction that lifts your trunk off the floor. Support this lift with the frame and action of your arms and shoulders.

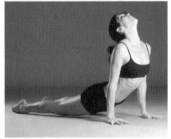
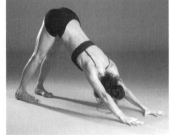

Left, *Lollasana*

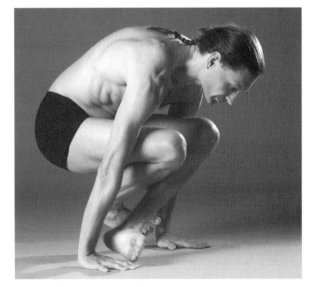

> **PRACTICAL TIP**
> *Lollasana*
>
> If your arms and shoulders are weak, do the following exercise. Sitting on your heels, cross your ankles, point your feet backward, and lift your knees and feet off the floor. Hold *Lollasana* for as long as you can. Add on one breath every day until you can hold it for ten breaths. Then gently begin to swing back and forth without dragging your feet over the floor. Eventually insert this movement into your *vinyasa*.

Vinyasa Twelve

Exhale into *Chaturanga Dandasana*, the fourth position of *Surya Namaskara* A.

Vinyasa Thirteen

Inhale into Upward Dog.

Vinyasa Fourteen

Exhale into Downward Dog.

We are now ready to jump through to sitting for the next posture.

PRACTICAL TIP

Different Foot Positions in Forward Bending

There are three different foot positions for forward bends. In the first, the foot is flexed (dorsal flexed), which means that the upper side of the foot is drawn toward the shin. This position can be used for the less intense type of forward bends — for postures where the hamstrings do not bear the weight of the torso, such as *Dandasana* and *Marichyasana* C.[14]

The second foot position, the one used in *Pashimottanasana*, is between pointing and flexing. To achieve this, first extend out through the heels and then through the bases of all the toes. Keeping the feet flexed in *Pashimottanasana* is one of the main sources of hamstring injuries. This second foot position is also chosen in other semi-intense forward bends like *Ardha Baddha Padma Pashimottanasana*, *Triang Mukha Ekapada Pashimottanasana*, *Janushirshasana*, and, very important, in *Upavishta Konasana*.

The third foot position is to have the feet pointed (called plantar flexion, which means that the surface of the foot draws away from the shin). Pointing the feet gives maximum protection to the hamstrings. This position is employed in the most intense group of forward bends, which includes *Hanumanasana*, *Trivikramasana*, *Tittibhasana*, and *Vasishtasana*.

---

14. For the purpose of this explanation we can look at *Marichyasana* C as a forward bend. In this asana the hip flexors of the straight leg (the muscles that fold the trunk forward) are engaged to stay upright. This is also the case in *Dandasana*.

Purvottanasana

INTENSE EASTERN STRETCH[15]

Drishti Nose or third eye

Purvottanasana is the counter and complementary posture to the *Pashimottanasana* series.

Vinyasa Seven

Inhaling, jump through to sitting. Place the hands shoulder width apart on the floor with a hand's-length space between your fingertips and your buttocks. The fingers are spread and pointing forward, toward the feet.

Vinyasa Eight

Inhaling, broaden the shoulders and draw the shoulder blades down the back. Straighten the arms and free up the chest. Lift the heart high and tip the chin toward the chest.

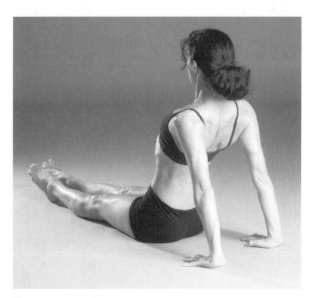

Purvottanasana, vinyasa seven

The legs are straight and strong. Point the feet. Drop the coccyx toward the heels and dig the back of the heels down into the floor. This engages the hamstrings and the gluteus maximus. Lift the pelvis and uncoil the spine. Work the toes toward the floor until the soles of the feet cup the floor. Once up in the posture, the hamstrings can take over and you can release the buttocks; to go on contracting them

---

15. Referring to the front of the body, which traditionally faced the rising sun.

would place a strain on the sacroiliac joints. Keep lifting the chest and continue to open it by positioning the shoulder blades broad and drawing them down the back, and by arching the upper back (erector spinae).

The head is the last to go back. Release the front of the throat and allow the head to hang back, relaxed. Gaze to the tip of the nose to keep the back of the neck elongated. This head position should not be adopted, however, if the student has neck

Vinyasa **Nine**

Exhaling, exit the posture by first replacing the buttocks on the floor, then bringing the head back upright. Finally, the hands come forward.

Vinyasa **Ten**

Inhaling, lift the feet between the hands.

Vinyasa **Eleven**

Exhaling, jump back into *Chaturanga Dandasana*.

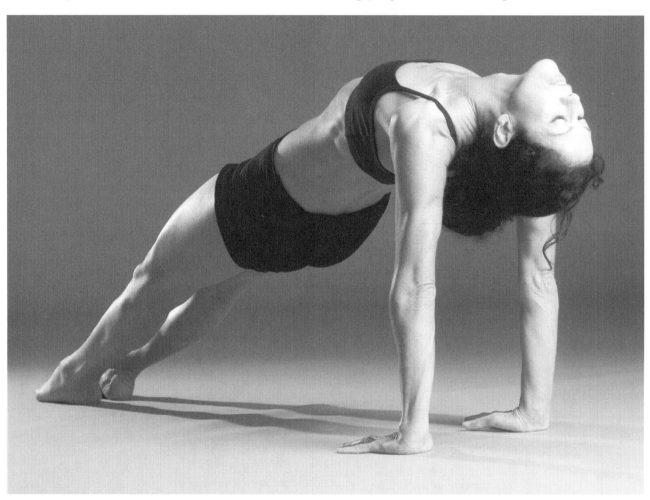

Purvottanasana, vinyasa eight

problems or has suffered whiplash. The old pattern of a whiplash injury could be set off in the transitions in and out of this posture.

Instead, one can gently place the chin on the sternum and keep it there throughout the posture. Gaze toward the feet. The head should be lifted only when one has come back down to sitting. Done in this way, the neck muscles are not provoked into a spasm reflex. Hold *Purvottanasana* for five breaths.

Vinyasa **Twelve**

Inhale into Upward Dog.

Vinyasa **Thirteen**

Exhale into Downward Dog.

Ardha Baddha Padma Pashimottanasana

BOUND HALF LOTUS FORWARD BEND

Drishti Toes

Ardha Baddha Padma Pashimottanasana starts a new cycle of postures that combine forward bending with hip rotation. The Primary Series mainly consists of these two themes.

The postures are grounding and rooting, and they form the basis of the more exhilarating themes of backbending, leg-behind-head, and arm balances, which form the subject of the Intermediate and Advanced Series. From a yogic point of view the foundation must be properly prepared before we advance to a more complex practice.

Rotation Pattern

The next five postures establish the rotation pattern of the femur for the Primary Series. Sown here, this seed can eventually fructify in the performance of such complex postures as *Mulabandhasana* (the most extreme medial rotation) and *Kandasana* (the most extreme lateral rotation). The rotation pattern is as follows:

• *Ardha Baddha Padma Pashimottanasana* — medial rotation

• *Triang Mukha Ekapada Pashimottanasana* — lateral rotation

• *Janushirshasana* A — medial rotation

• *Janushirshasana* B — lateral rotation

• *Janushirshasana* C — medial rotation

ANATOMICAL FOCUS

The Paradox of Active Release

This is an important understanding that needs to be grasped in order to master the art of working deeply and harmoniously in all postures. Active release derives its effectiveness from the following principle: To enter a posture we use prime muscle groups that perform particular actions. Once in the posture, we must release those muscle groups and engage their antagonists to work harmoniously and more deeply into the posture.

For example, to go into a backbend we engage the trunk extensors (erector spinae, quadratus lumborum). Ultimately, however, these muscles limit backbending. They shorten the back and pinch the spinous processes of the vertebrae together. Once we have arrived in a backbend we need to release the trunk extensors and instead engage the trunk flexors (abdominal muscles). This lengthens the back, creates space between the spinous processes, and deepens the backbend.

The same principle is applied in hip rotations such as *Ardha Baddha Padma Pashimottanasana* and *Baddha Konasana*. We laterally rotate the femur to go into hip rotations, but when in the posture we release the lateral rotators by medially rotating the femur. This action takes us much deeper into the posture. In all forward bends such as *Pashimottanasana* we engage the hip flexors, particularly the psoas and rectus femoris, to

go into the posture. Once the hip joint is flexed to about 160° we won't be able to close the joint any farther because the bulging hip flexors are in the way. To illustrate, try out the following: Standing, bend the knee joint by merely contracting the hamstrings and the calf muscles. You will not be able to close the joint completely because the very muscles that perform the action also prevent its completion. Now use your hand to draw your heel to your buttock. At the same time resist your hand by gently attempting to straighten your leg. This slight leg extension, performed by the antagonists of the prime movers, will release and flatten out the leg flexors so that the joint can now be completely closed.

In the case of *Pashimottanasana* the principle of active release is applied by drawing the heels down into the floor. This engages the hamstrings and enables the psoas and rectus femoris to release. Once they are released the front of the hip joint can be fully closed and the forward bend completed.

This action does not mean the kneecaps will be released. The quadriceps, which pulls up the kneecaps, has four heads, rectus femoris being only one of them. If rectus femoris (the only two-joint muscle in the group) is released, the other three heads (vastus lateralis, medialis, and intermedius) can still pull up the kneecap and work to extend the leg.

These femur rotations refer to the action performed after one has arrived in the posture. To get into the posture the action is the opposite. When the rotation pattern is performed in this way, the more challenging postures in the series, such as *Marichyasana* D and *Baddha Konasana*, become easily accessible.

Vinyasa Seven

Inhaling, jump through to sitting and straighten the legs. An experienced practitioner would go into the posture in one breath. For the sake of precision and safety we will break this rather complex movement down into various phases, identical to the standing half lotus (*Ardha Baddha Padmottanasana*).

PHASE 1

Sitting in *Dandasana*, flex the right knee joint completely until your right heel touches the right buttock. If this is not possible, resort to daily practice of *Virasana* and *Supta Virasana*. (See "*Lengthening the Quadriceps*," page 57.)

PHASE 2

From here abduct the right thigh until the right knee touches the floor. Establish a 90° angle between the thighs. Pointing and inverting the right foot, draw the right heel into the *right* groin, or as close to it as possible. You are now in the position for *Janushirshasana* A (page 79). Transiting through this posture on the way into half lotus prepares the adductor muscle group. Keeping the foot pointed and inverted, draw the knee far out to the right to further stretch the adductors. Tight adductors constitute the main obstacle to lotus and half-lotus postures. This method gives beginners maximum opening. It is not recommended that beginners pull the foot into position without first releasing the adductors. This movement can be repeated several times to produce the desired effect.

PHASE 3

Draw the heel in toward the navel. Transiting via the navel on the way into half lotus will ensure that the knee joint remains sealed.

PHASE 4

Now draw the right foot across to the left groin. Reach your right arm around your back to bind the right big toe. The palm faces downward. The palm

facing up would lead to excessive inward rotation of the humerus and, with it, hunching of the shoulder. An inability to bind is often due to stiffness in the right shoulder because of a short pectoralis minor muscle (see figure 13, page 76). In this case reach the right arm far up and out to the right side. Spin the

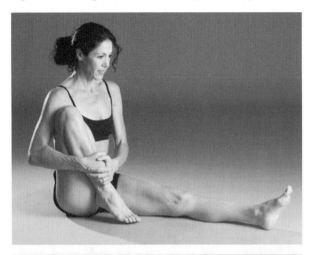

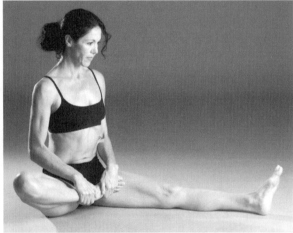

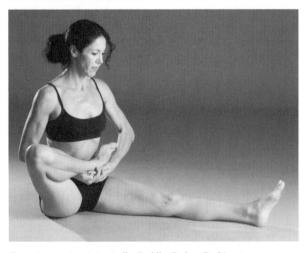

From top, going into *Ardha Baddha Padma Pashimottanasana*, phases 1, 2, and 3

arm inward so that the palm faces backward. Reach far behind, lowering the hand. Abduct and depress the shoulder girdle to avoid jutting the shoulder forward. As you proceed, release the muscle that draws the shoulder forward (pectoralis minor). If you still cannot reach the toe, work intelligently in *Parshvottanasana*, *Prasarita Padottanasana* C, *Urdhva Dhanurasana*, and Upward and Downward Dog. These postures reduce tightness in the shoulders.

If you are unable to bind your big toe, you are not ready to fold forward in this posture. If the foot is situated on the thigh rather than in the groin, bending forward can strain ligaments and/or damage cartilage.

outward (lateral) rotation of the thigh. To work in the posture, we now medially rotate the thigh. To aid medial rotation, keep the right foot pointed and inverted. The muscles that inwardly rotate — two hamstrings (semimembranous, semitendinous) an adductor (gracilis), an abductor (gluteus minimus), and a hip flexor cum abductor (tensor fascia latae) — all have the tendency to suck the thigh into the hip. This can lead to a build-up of tension in the knee. To counteract this, let the femur reach outward and away from the hip. This action releases the adductors, and its importance cannot be overemphasized.

Continue to gently draw the knee down to the floor and out to the side. The ideal angle between the

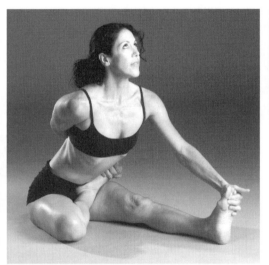

Ardha Baddha Padma Pashimottanasana, vinyasa seven

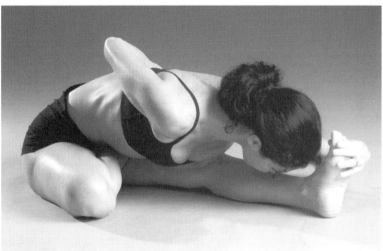

Ardha Baddha Padma Pashimottanasana, vinyasa eight

Instead, continue to work on opening the hips. Sit upright and keep drawing the foot upward with the left hand while you work the extended left leg. Be patient. Many of the other postures will aid the loosening of your hip joints and adductors. Then you will be able to perform the posture safely.

If you managed to bind the right foot, gently place the knee out to the side and down toward the floor. The left hand reaches forward and takes the outside of the left foot. Inhaling, lift the chest and straighten the left arm. Square your hips and shoulders to the straight leg.

two thighs is around 40°, depending on the ratio between tibia and femur length of each individual. The heel of the foot sits in the navel during the entire posture. Only then can the purpose of this posture, the purification of liver and spleen, be fulfilled.

Square your shoulders to the front leg and keep them at an even distance from the floor. Draw your elbows out to the sides, away from each other.

The sit bones ground; the buttocks spread. The crown of the head reaches toward the feet while the shoulder blades draw toward the hips. Hold for five breaths.

Vinyasa Eight

Exhaling, fold forward. The straight left leg works in the same way as the legs in *Pashimottanasana*. To place the right foot into the left groin we performed

Vinyasa Nine

Inhaling, lift the chest and straighten the left arm. Exhaling, take the leg out of half lotus and place the hands on the floor.

Vinyasa **Ten**   Inhaling, lift up.

Vinyasa **Eleven**   Exhale, *Chaturanga Dandasana*.

Vinyasa **Twelve**   Inhale into Upward Dog.

Vinyasa **Thirteen**   Exhale into Downward Dog.

*Vinyasa*s Fourteen to Twenty

Repeat the posture on the left.

Triang Mukha Ekapada Pashimottanasana

ONE-LEGGED FORWARD BEND WITH
THREE LIMBS FACING FORWARD

Drishti   Toes

Vinyasa Seven

Inhaling, jump through to sitting. Bend up the right leg and fold it back so that the right foot is placed outside the right buttock, with the sole and heel facing upward. Eventually, one can work toward jumping through and folding the right leg back in mid-air to land seated, with the left leg straight and the right foot pointing backward.

If necessary, lift the right thigh off the calf muscle and use your hand to roll the calf muscle out of the way. Now draw the right sit bone down to the floor. Adjust the rotation of the femur to make sure the front edge of the tibia points straight down to the floor. Most students will have to laterally rotate the femur in this posture. Medial rotation is necessary to get into the posture. If you experience discomfort or pain in your knee as you attempt to get your right sit bone down, proceed with compassion toward yourself. Inability to ground the right sit bone is due to stiff and short quadriceps. This prevents complete flexion of the knee joint.

To give the quadriceps time to lengthen, sit on

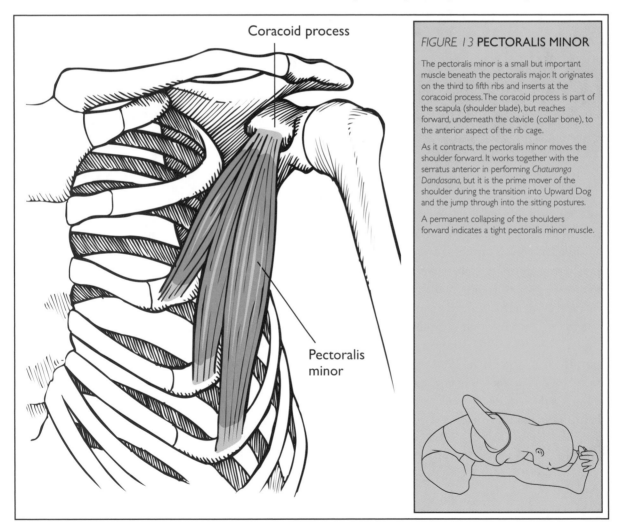

Coracoid process

Pectoralis minor

FIGURE 13 **PECTORALIS MINOR**

The pectoralis minor is a small but important muscle beneath the pectoralis major. It originates on the third to fifth ribs and inserts at the coracoid process. The coracoid process is part of the scapula (shoulder blade), but reaches forward, underneath the clavicle (collar bone), to the anterior aspect of the rib cage.

As it contracts, the pectoralis minor moves the shoulder forward. It works together with the serratus anterior in performing *Chaturanga Dandasana*, but it is the prime mover of the shoulder during the transition into Upward Dog and the jump through into the sitting postures.

A permanent collapsing of the shoulders forward indicates a tight pectoralis minor muscle.

a folded blanket. The blanket should be under your sit bones and the foot down on the floor. This tips the pelvis forward, returning the lordotic curve to the low back, enabling you to sit upright with ease. A tight quadriceps is often the cause of knee problems. Sit in *Virasana* whenever possible to lengthen it (see *"Lengthening the Quadriceps,"* page 57, which includes a photograph of *Virasana*). This posture

work of both legs to stay upright. Both thighs have to rotate to the right, which means that the left thigh needs to rotate medially and the right thigh laterally. The abdominals, lengthening eccentrically, draw the right sit bone down. If you are still in danger of keeling over, elevate the blanket on which you are sitting.

Inhaling, straighten the arms and lift the chest while still holding the foot.

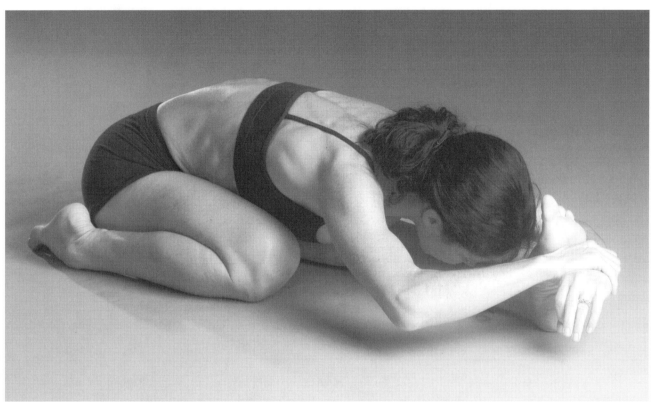

Triang Mukha Ekapada Pashimottanasana

consists of two *Triang Mukha Ekapada*s combined. Performed outside of *vinyasa* practice, this posture is even more effective. Then residual stiffness in the cold muscle is targeted — stiffness that may not be apparent when the muscles are warmed up. Spend as long as possible in *Virasana* and the quadriceps will quickly lengthen. As in *Triang Mukha*, it is essential that the foot does not turn out to the side and that the heel faces upward.

Ground both sit bones. Now reach forward with both hands to take the left foot or shin. Initially there may be a tendency for the right sit bone to lift off the floor and the body to lean over to the left side. This can be counteracted by using your right arm as a support, but it is more therapeutic to use the combined effort of the core muscles of the trunk and the

Vinyasa **Eight**

Exhaling, fold forward. Keep both buttocks evenly grounded and your shoulders at an even distance from the floor. In the beginning one often makes the mistake of focusing too much on the forward-bending aspect of the posture. It is much more important to ground the right buttock, which works directly on the hip and develops abdominal strength. Apart from jumping through and back, *Triang Mukha Ekapada Pashimottanasana*, *Marichyasana* A, and *Navasana* are the three main producers of abdominal strength in the series. This abdominal strength is much needed, later in the series, for *Supta Kurmasana*. Allocate at least 50 percent of your effort to the hip work in this posture — grounding the sit bone and stretching the quadriceps — and the

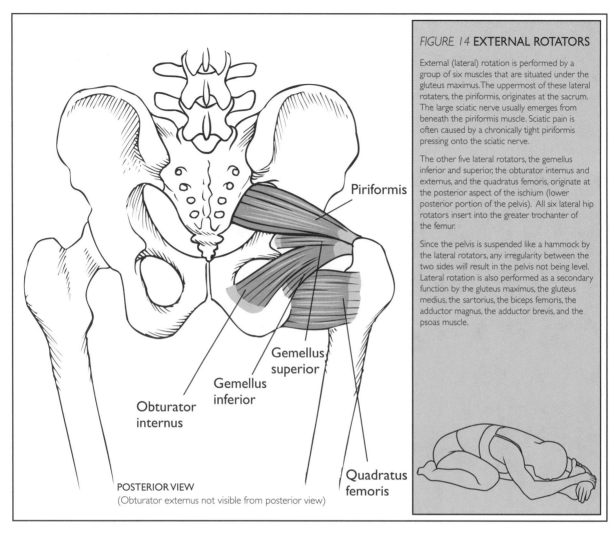

FIGURE 14 **EXTERNAL ROTATORS**

Piriformis

External (lateral) rotation is performed by a group of six muscles that are situated under the gluteus maximus. The uppermost of these lateral rotaters, the piriformis, originates at the sacrum. The large sciatic nerve usually emerges from beneath the piriformis muscle. Sciatic pain is often caused by a chronically tight piriformis pressing onto the sciatic nerve.

The other five lateral rotators, the gemellus inferior and superior, the obturator internus and externus, and the quadratus femoris, originate at the posterior aspect of the ischium (lower posterior portion of the pelvis). All six lateral hip rotators insert into the greater trochanter of the femur.

Since the pelvis is suspended like a hammock by the lateral rotators, any irregularity between the two sides will result in the pelvis not being level. Lateral rotation is also performed as a secondary function by the gluteus maximus, the gluteus medius, the sartorius, the biceps femoris, the adductor magnus, the adductor brevis, and the psoas muscle.

Gemellus superior

Gemellus inferior

Obturator internus

Quadratus femoris

POSTERIOR VIEW
(Obturator externus not visible from posterior view)

rest to the forward bend. With its stretching of the quadriceps and creation of abdominal strength, this humble posture is one of the most underestimated in the framework of the Primary Series.

Extend out through the heel and the bases of all toes of the left foot. Folding forward, make sure that you lift the heart toward the foot and keep the low back flat. Lengthen through the low back and let the buttocks spread. Do not hunch the shoulders. Lengthen the back of the neck. Practicing in this way, you might look stiffer, but also more elegant. Maintaining the inner integrity of the postures makes the practice far more effective. Hold this *vinyasa*, which constitutes the state of the *asana*, for five breaths.

Vinyasa Nine

Inhaling, lift the chest, still holding the foot. Exhaling, place your hands down. There are two ways to jump back:

• At count ten, lift the left leg up off the floor and hop back. This version demands a little more flexibility, but, as one can assist the jump back by pushing the floor away with the right foot, strengthwise it is not as taxing.

• Bring the right leg forward to *Dandasana* and jump back from there.

This makes for a cleaner lift and generates greater strength. It is therefore the preferred method to commence with.

Vinyasa **Ten**   Inhaling, lift up.
Vinyasa **Eleven**   Exhale, *Chaturanga Dandasana*.
Vinyasa **Twelve**   Inhale into Upward Dog.
Vinyasa **Thirteen** Exhale into Downward Dog.

Vinyasas Fourteen to Twenty

Repeat the posture on the left.

Janushirshasana A

HEAD-BEYOND-THE-KNEE POSTURE A

Drishti Toes

Janushirshasana A, like no other posture, combines the two main themes of the Primary Series — forward bending and hip rotation. *Pashimottanasana* and *Baddha Konasana* are the cardinal postures of these two actions. *Janushirshasana* A is in fact identical to performing *Pashimottanasana* on one leg and *Baddha Konasana* with the other. There may be more exhilarating postures in the sequence, but it is *Janushirshasana* A that most lets us experience the underlying principles of the first series.

Vinyasa Seven

Inhaling, jump through to *Dandasana*. Bend the knee and take the right thigh back, working toward creating a 90° angle between the thigh bones. This action, called abduction, hip flexion, and lateral

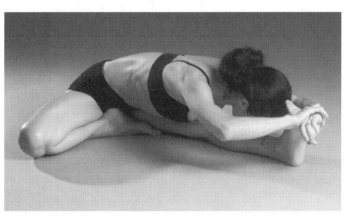

Janushirshasana A

rotation of the femur, is primarily performed by the sartorius muscle. Point and invert the right foot, as this aids subsequent medial rotation of the femur. Draw the right heel into the right groin, thus completely sealing the knee joint. Ideally the right heel would touch the right groin, but beginners may take some time to cultivate the necessary length in the quadriceps. This length needs to be gained in the previous posture, *Triang Mukha Ekapada Pashimottanasana*. We can now move the entire folded leg as a unity, minimizing friction in the knee joint.

As you reach forward to take the left foot, the right thigh begins its countermovement, rolling forward (medial rotation). If possible, the left hand binds the right wrist. Inhaling, lift your heart and square your shoulders to the left foot. Lift through the entire front of the body while the shoulder blades flow down the back and the sit bones ground down.

ANATOMICAL FOCUS
The Buddha's Lotus

Pointing the foot while executing *Janushirshasana* A allows the tibia to track the medial rotation of the femur until its front edge (it is a triangular bone) points down to the earth and the heel up to the sky. This fundamental movement can be applied in all lotus postures. It will lead to sitting in lotus posture with the heels and the soles of the feet facing upward, as in depictions of the Buddha. This is the anatomically correct position. The position adopted by many Westerners, in which the heels and soles face toward the abdomen, places undue strain on the knee joints.

To invert the foot at the same time as pointing it deepens the medial spiraling of the thigh, thereby deepening the lotus position. Combining these actions, create a vector of energy out from the groin. This counteracts the tendency for beginners to suck the thigh back into the hip, which shortens the adductors and creates an obstacle to opening the hips. All hip rotations require that the adductors are released and lengthened.

Lengthening along the insides of the thighs in *Janushirshasana* A loosens the adductors and reduces pressure on the knee. The knee gently draws down and back (abduction of the femur), increasing the length of the adductors.

Habitually short adductors (see figure 17, page 101) are observed in many Westerners. Our culture trains us to govern and to subdue nature; we place ourselves above nature. This is reflected in our habit of sitting on chairs — above the earth and removed from it. Asians and those of many other civilizations sat on the ground. This corresponded to a view in which humans are a part of nature and not its lord. And sitting on the ground leaves the hip joints open.

Vinyasa **Eight**

Exhaling, fold forward squarely over the inseam of the straight leg. The left leg and the torso follow the instructions for *Pashimottanasana*. The right foot points and inverts. The thigh rolls forward (rotates medially) and reaches back until a state of equilibrium is achieved. Every movement needs to contain its countermovement. In the present case the inward rotation of the thigh is terminated by a corresponding outward rotation, when the neutral state is reached. To prevent the excessive performance of a movement, receptivity is necessary to recognize the neutral state. Work for five breaths in the posture. Both shoulders are kept at an even distance from the floor.

Janushirshasana A beautifully lengthens the quadratus lumborum, a small back extensor muscle in the low back. Lengthen the low back, attempting to square the whole of the chest to the straight leg. Keep the back of the neck long. Jutting the chin forward in an ambitious attempt to touch it to the shin impairs the blood and nerve supplies to the brain, and the contracted neck muscles have the strength to subluxate cervical vertebrae. This action cultivates an aggressive go-getter attitude and a decrease of compassion.

It often helps if the teacher places a finger on a particular vertebra and encourages the student to lift it upward, C7 being one vertebra frequently in need of support. Students who have a tendency to whiplash or who carry a whiplash pattern should maintain a straight line from the spine along the neck and across the back of the head. Do not look up to the foot until your neck is cured. Hold *Janushirshasana* A for five breaths.

Vinyasa **Nine**

Inhaling, hold on to the foot, lift the torso, and straighten the arms. Exhaling, place the hands down, ready to lift up.

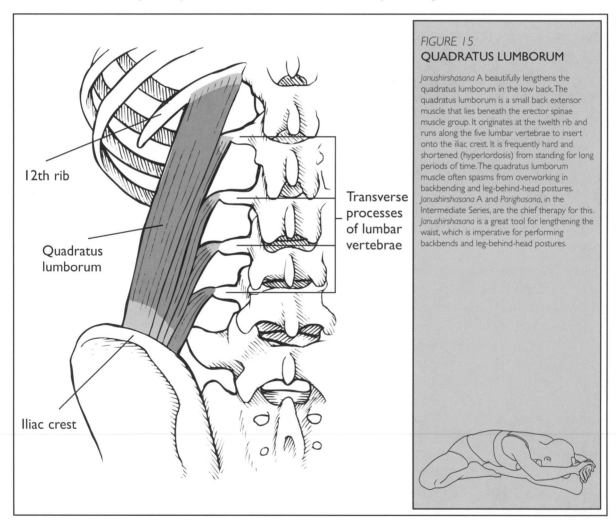

12th rib

Quadratus lumborum

Iliac crest

Transverse processes of lumbar vertebrae

FIGURE 15
QUADRATUS LUMBORUM

Janushirshasana A beautifully lengthens the quadratus lumborum in the low back. The quadratus lumborum is a small back extensor muscle that lies beneath the erector spinae muscle group. It originates at the twelfth rib and runs along the five lumbar vertebrae to insert onto the iliac crest. It is frequently hard and shortened (hyperlordosis) from standing for long periods of time. The quadratus lumborum muscle often spasms from overworking in backbending and leg-behind-head postures. *Janushirshasana* A and *Parighasana*, in the Intermediate Series, are the chief therapy for this. *Janushirshasana* is a great tool for lengthening the waist, which is imperative for performing backbends and leg-behind-head postures.

Vinyasa **Ten**   Inhaling, lift up.

Vinyasa **Eleven**   Exhale, *Chaturanga Dandasana*.

Vinyasa **Twelve**   Inhale into Upward Dog.

Vinyasa **Thirteen**   Exhale into Downward Dog.

Vinyasas Fourteen to Twenty

Repeat the posture on the left.

Janushirshasana B

HEAD-BEYOND-THE-KNEE POSTURE B

Drishti Toes

Vinyasa Seven

Inhaling, jump through and fold the right leg back to a maximum of 85°. Place the sole of the flexed (dorsally flexed) right foot against the left inner thigh. Without changing the position of the right foot, place the hands down and lift the buttocks off the floor. Shift your weight forward by letting the left heel glide forward over the floor, and sit down on the inside of the right foot (rather than on the heel only). The toes of the right foot still point forward to the left foot.

In *Janushirshasana* B the right foot is flexed and the right thigh rotates laterally, as opposed to

Right, going into *Janushirshasana* B; below, *Janushirshasana* B

Janushirshasana A, where the foot is pointed and the thigh rotates medially. Both these thigh movements are crucial to opening the hip joints for the more advanced postures.

Those whose tibias are short compared to the length of their femurs will have to bring the knee farther forward than 85° in order to find a comfortable seat on the foot. Both sit bones are off the floor. Square the chest to the left leg and reach forward to clasp the left foot.

Flexible students can reach around the foot to clasp the right wrist with the left hand. Inhaling, lift the chest and straighten the arms.

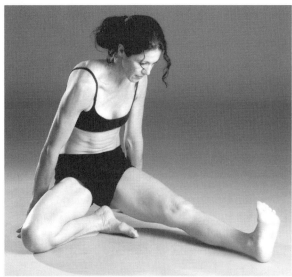

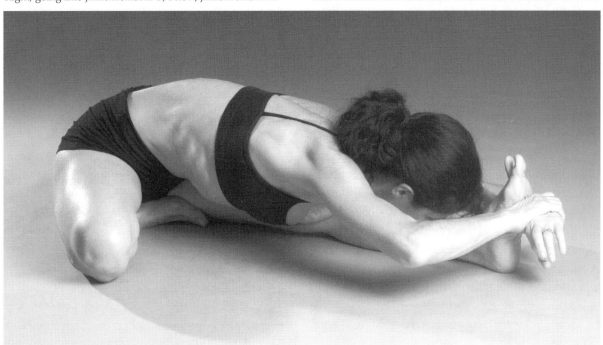

Vinyasa Eight

Exhaling, fold forward, keeping the spine and neck extended in a straight line. The right kidney area reaches forward to the left foot in an attempt to flatten out the back. The shoulders are at an even distance from the floor.

Draw the shoulder blades toward the buttocks. The lower abdomen and the pelvic floor are firm. The buttocks release, and the sit bones reach backward without touching the floor. The right knee grounds down while the right thigh rolls laterally until neutral. The heart and the crown of the head reach toward the left foot. Hold *Janushirshasana* B for five breaths.

Vinyasa Nine

Inhaling, still holding the foot, lift the chest and straighten your arms.

Exhaling, take the leg out of position and place the hands down.

Vinyasa **Ten**	Inhaling, lift up.
Vinyasa **Eleven**	Exhale, *Chaturanga Dandasana*.
Vinyasa **Twelve**	Inhale into Upward Dog.
Vinyasa **Thirteen**	Exhale into Downward Dog.

Vinyasas Fourteen to Twenty

Repeat the posture on the left.

Janushirshasana C

HEAD-BEYOND-THE-KNEE POSTURE C

Drishti Toes

Vinyasa Seven

Inhaling, jump through. Fold the right leg as if you were placing it into half lotus, but with the foot flexed. Now thread your right arm between the inner thigh and the underneath side of the calf. Hold the front of the foot, pulling the toes back toward the shin. Keeping the foot and toes flexed, draw the heel toward the navel. Let the right thigh roll medially, until you can place the base of the toes down on the floor, running along the inside of the left thigh.

Ideally, your foot would be vertical to the floor, with the heel directly above the toes and pointing

upward. If this is not yet the case, place your hands down on the floor, lift your sit bones, and gently slide forward to bring the foot more upright. Continue to rotate the thigh medially.

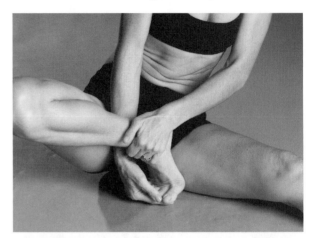

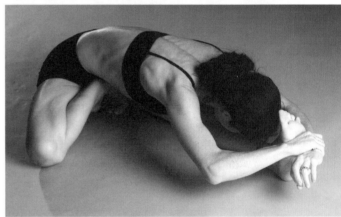

Top, going into *Janushirshasana* C; above, *Janushirshasana* C

Square the hips and allow the right knee to find its position. This will depend on the end position of the heel: the more upright the heel, the farther forward will be the knee. With the heel sitting directly above the toes, the knee will rest at 45° to the left leg. Draw the knee down to the floor. It may be necessary to lift the left buttock off the floor to bring the knee down. With the aid of gravity, the lifted buttock will in time meet the floor. To reach the knee to the floor with muscular action would require contracting the hamstrings, which is contraindicated in this posture as it sucks the thigh back into the hip joint.

Take your time with this posture. If necessary stay weeks or months in any of the phases described above. Done correctly, the posture is very therapeutic for the knees, and it can cure chronic knee inflammation.

If you could follow the instructions so far, reach forward to bind the left foot. Flexible students can take the right wrist with the left hand. Inhaling, lift the chest and straighten the arms.

Vinyasa Eight

Exhaling, fold forward over the inside of the left leg. Continue to medially rotate the thigh here. While the right knee keeps contact with the floor, the left sit bone sinks down to meet the floor. Continue to flex the right foot, drawing it deeper into the left groin. The heel should press into the lower abdomen. In females the heel presses into the uterus. This posture is especially therapeutic for the female reproductive system, just as *Janushirshasana* B is therapeutic for the male reproductive system.

The left foot is between a flexed and a pointed position, with the underneath of the leg actively working. The right femur reaches out of the hip joint. Reaching outward along the inside of the right thigh will release the adductors.

As with all postures where the *drishti* is up to the toes, it is essential not to kink the neck. With correct alignment the chin will eventually meet the shin. Never compromise the alignment of the spine to meet illusionary goals; rather, always retain the inner integrity of the posture, and the real goals of yoga will be attained. Stay here for five breaths.

Vinyasa Nine

Inhaling, lift your chest while still holding the foot. Exhaling, take the right leg out of position and place your hands down on the floor.

Vinyasa **Ten**	Inhaling, lift up.
Vinyasa **Eleven**	Exhale, *Chaturanga Dandasana*.
Vinyasa **Twelve**	Inhale into Upward Dog.
Vinyasa **Thirteen**	Exhale into Downward Dog.

Vinyasas Fourteen to Twenty

Repeat the posture on the left.

Marichyasana A

POSTURE OF THE RISHI MARICHI A

Drishti Toes

Vinyasa Seven

Inhaling, jump through to *Dandasana*. Fold the right leg and place the right foot outside the right hip, as far back as possible. Keep about two hands' width, or enough space to fit your torso, between the right foot and the left inner thigh. The right foot is

---

PRACTICAL TIP
The Gift

Marichyasana A is like a forward bend with a handicap. It is very challenging for those with tight hamstrings. The tendency here is to avoid taking weight into the bent leg, but to be propelled instead over onto the straight leg. This defeats the very challenge of the posture: to soften the hip of the bent leg. This posture prepares the hips for the *Kurmasana*s. Such flexibility is needed to perform the action of placing the leg behind the head.

The action of forward bending is performed solely by the hip flexors and is supported by the feet, legs, and trunk. With our hands bound, the temptation to use our arms for assistance to fold forward in the *Marichyasana*s is removed. *Marichyasana* A offers the therapeutic benefit of strengthening these muscles. The handicap becomes the gift.

---

parallel to the left leg and not turned out. With the right arm, reach forward until your shoulder is in front of the knee. Wrap your right arm around the shin, ideally half way between knee and ankle. As your forward bend progresses, you will be able to wrap the arm lower down your shin. Work toward binding the left wrist with the right hand. Inhaling, lift the heart high. The right buttock deliberately leaves the floor.

Vinyasa Eight

Exhaling, tip the pelvis forward and lengthen out your trunk. Keep weight, and thereby action, in the foot of the bent leg. Use both feet, both legs, and both hip flexors to propel yourself forward. Continue to lift your heart and place the chest squarely down on the straight leg. To soften deeper into the posture, once forward ground the right buttock down toward the floor and lift the right knee away from the floor. The heel of the straight leg continues to press down into the floor.

Marichyasana A

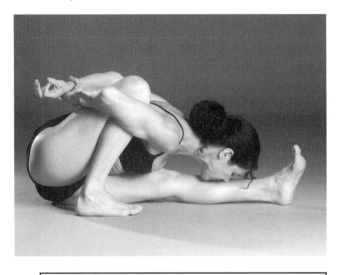

MYTHOLOGICAL BACKGROUND

The Rishi Marichi

Here we start a new group of postures, called the *Marichyasanas*, which first and foremost are hip openers. They are dedicated to the Maharishi Marichi (meaning ray of light). Marichi is one of the six mind-born sons of Lord Brahma and father of the Rishi Kashyappa, who is the ancestor of gods, demons, humans, and animals. Marichi appears several times in the *Mahabharata*, where he celebrates Arjuna's birth and visits Bhishma at his deathbed. In the *Bhagavata Purana* we learn that Marichi performed a ritual to purify Lord Indra from the sin of slaying the Brahmin Vrtra. After the conclusion of his earthly life, Marichi is said to have become one of the stars of the constellation Ursa Major.

Lift your heart away from the knee, but forward toward the left foot. This action not only prevents hunching your back, but also strengthens the back muscles as the trunk extensors are engaged. Hold this posture for five breaths.

Vinyasa **Nine**

Inhaling, come up and release the hands. Exhaling, place the hands down to the floor, keeping the knee behind the shoulder if possible.

Vinyasa **Ten**	Inhaling, lift up.
Vinyasa **Eleven**	Exhale, *Chaturanga Dandasana*.
Vinyasa **Twelve**	Inhale into Upward Dog.
Vinyasa **Thirteen**	Exhale into Downward Dog.

Vinyasas **Fourteen to Twenty**

Repeat the posture on the left.

Marichyasana B
POSTURE OF THE RISHI MARICHI B

Drishti Nose

Marichyasana A and B are almost identical, the only difference being that the leg that is straight in A is in half lotus in B.

Vinyasa **Seven**

Inhaling, jump through and straighten your legs. Bend up the left leg and place it into half lotus in the way described in *Ardha Baddha Padma Pashimottanasana* (page 74). Bend up the right leg, lifting the right sit bone off the floor and drawing the left knee down to the floor. Place the right foot so that the right ankle is in line with the greater trochanter of the femur (the bony outside of the hip joint).

Draw the left knee out to the side until an angle of 45° is reached between both thighs. Be sure to maintain this angle when folding forward. With the knee far out to the side, this posture is a very effective hip opener. Otherwise, it becomes just another forward bend.

With the right arm, reach up to stretch the right waist and then far forward inside the knee, until the right shoulder is in front of the right knee. Stay as low as possible, ideally hooking the shoulder half way between the knee and ankle of the right leg. Now, touching the right outer ribs against the right inner thigh, wrap the arm around the leg and if possible clasp the wrist of the left arm with the right hand. Holding on to the wrist, inhale deeply and lift the chest high.

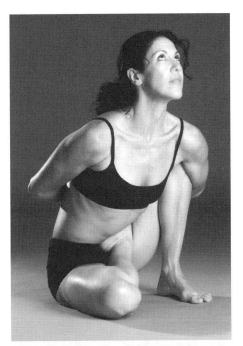

Vinyasa Eight

Exhaling, fold forward, placing your torso in the center between the right foot and the left knee. At the same time prevent the left knee from moving into the center by drawing the right hip joint forward. Rather than bending toward the left knee, fold forward along the inside of the upright right leg, always maintaining contact with the outer ribs.

At the same time rotate the left thigh medially and extend out along the inside of that thigh. Place the forehead and, once that has become easy, the chin down on the floor, without ever compromising the position of the neck. The heart reaches forward to the floor supported by strong abdominals.

A frequent problem encountered in *Marichyasana* B is pain on the outside of the ankle of the leg in half lotus. The pain is caused by excessive inversion

Right, *Marichyasana* B,
vinyasa seven
Below, *Marichyasana* B

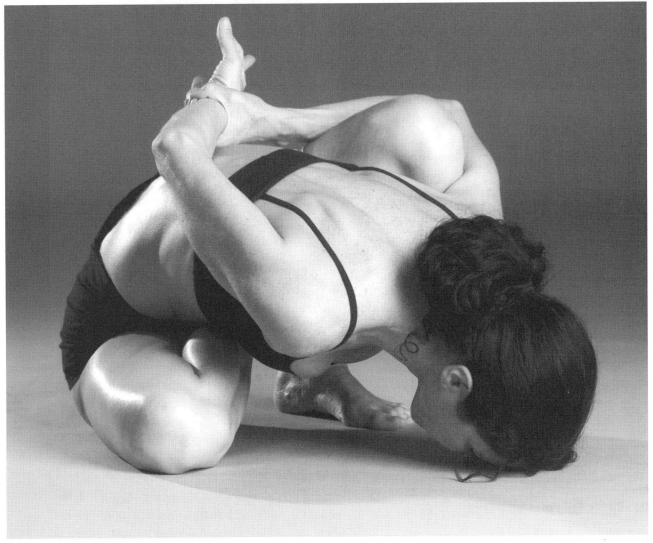

of the ankle, which in turn is brought about by lack of medial rotation of the femur. All lotus and half-lotus postures need to be performed with a medially rotated femur. If this is not done due to a dormant hip joint, then often the knee joint, but in this case the ankle joint, will bear the brunt. The solution is to first avoid the inversion of the ankle by using the peroneus group on the outside of the leg. The everting action of the peronei will return the foot to a pointed, neutral position. The creative tension ensuing has now to be directed into the hip joint, and the femur medially rotated. If this is not possible, study medial rotation more closely in the previous postures. Stay in *Marichyasana* B for five breaths.

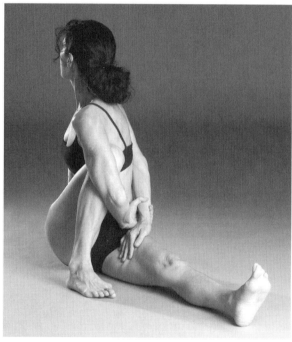

Marichyasana C

Vinyasa Nine

Inhaling, come upright and sit as tall as possible, keeping the hands bound. Exhaling, release the hands, straighten the upright leg first, then take the leg out of half lotus and place the hands down.

Vinyasa **Ten**   Inhaling, lift up.
Vinyasa **Eleven**   Exhale, *Chaturanga Dandasana*.
Vinyasa **Twelve**   Inhale into Upward Dog.
Vinyasa **Thirteen**   Exhale into Downward Dog.

Vinyasas Fourteen to Twenty

Repeat the posture on the left.

Marichyasana C
POSTURE OF THE RISHI MARICHI C
Drishti Side

Marichyasana C is the first sitting twist. The thoracic spine (upper back) from vertebra T1 to T12 is designed to twist. Here, the angle of the facet joints facilitates the greatest amount of rotation possible along the entire spine. Most of the twisting action is performed here. Twisting stretches the intercostal muscles, which lie between the ribs. As tight intercostal muscles are one of the main limitations to backbending, twists are an ideal preparation for it. The lumbar spine, which is very pliable in the forward- and backbending directions, is limited in its ability to twist. This provides necessary stability. Excessive twisting of the lumbar spine can destabilize the low back, so un-square the hips in seated twists and instead direct the twist into the upper back.

Vinyasa Seven

Inhaling, jump through and enter *Marichyasana* C on the same count. Fold the right leg up and place the foot close to the left thigh. Draw the right hip back with the foot until the hips are no longer square. The left leg remains straight. Beginners may place the right hand behind the sit bones (fingers pointing away from them) for support. Soften at the waist. Reach around with the left arm, stretching the waist, and exhaling place the left outer ribs against the right thigh until no gap remains. The left arm wraps around the knee. Clasp the right wrist with the left hand. Turn the head and gaze over your right shoulder.

Sit down and sit up. Ground the sit bones evenly. At the same time the crown of the head rises up to the ceiling. The shoulder blades glide down the back; the heart floats in front. Keep the left foot perpendicular to the floor. Counteract the tendency of the left thigh to roll out by medially rotating the femur.

Let the entire torso twist with the breath. Use the left arm as a lever by pressing it against the right knee. Counteract the tendency of the right knee to cross the midline of the body by engaging the right abductor group, which draws the knee out to the side. Hold *Marichyasana* C for five breaths.

Exhaling, release the posture, spin around, and place the hands onto the floor. You can keep the upright leg in position and hook the right shoulder in front of the knee as in *Marichyasana* A. Lifting in this way builds additional strength. If this is too difficult, lift in the same way as for all other postures.

This posture has a shorter *vinyasa* count:

Vinyasa **Eight**	Inhaling, lift up.
Vinyasa **Nine**	Exhale, *Chaturanga Dandasana*.
Vinyasa **Ten**	Inhale into Upward Dog.
Vinyasa **Eleven**	Exhale into Downward Dog.

Vinyasas Twelve to Sixteen

Repeat the posture on the left.

Marichyasana D

POSTURE OF THE RISHI MARICHI D

Drishti Side

This posture is like *Marichyasana* C with the straight leg in a half lotus.

Prerequisite: The posture should only be performed after one is proficient in *Marichyasana* B.

Vinyasa Seven

Inhaling, jump through to *Dandasana*. Bend up the left leg and place it into half lotus, using the same method, precision, and care described under *Ardha Baddha Padma Pashimottanasana* (page 74). Now bend up the right leg as in *Marichyasana* A, with the right foot in line with the outside of the right hip joint. Take the right hip back with the right foot, un-leveling the hips. If necessary, lift the right buttock off the floor to draw the left knee down to the floor. You are now sitting on a solid tripod, consisting of the left knee, the left buttock and the right foot. This is the same position as the set-up for *Marichyasana* B. Here, instead of bending forward, combine this seat with the twist of *Marichyasana* C.

Place your right hand on the floor behind your sacrum, fingers pointing away from you. Revolve the thorax, aligning shoulders with your bent knee. Place your left elbow on the outside of the right knee. Inhaling, lengthen the entire spine and lift your chest free. Exhaling, use your external and internal

oblique abdominis muscles to glide your arm along your knee, until your left shoulder is on the outside of the right knee. You may need several rounds of breath until the shoulder is in the correct position.

Draw the upright right leg toward the center using your adductor muscles (see figure 17, page 101). If your adductors have a tendency to spasm, place your right hand on the outside of the knee and

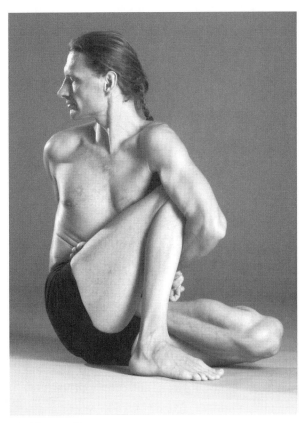

Marichyasana D

draw the knee toward the midline. Rotate the left arm inward, wrap it around the knee, and extend it until it is behind your back. (Extension is defined as returning from flexion, and flexion of the humerus is defined as raising the arm out to the front.) Now reach the right arm behind your back and clasp your fingers or take the left wrist with the right hand.

The left femur spins inward until it has reached its neutral position. Maintaining floor contact with the left knee, let the right sit bone become heavy. Inhaling, lift the front of the chest and sit up tall. Draw both shoulders back and sink the shoulder blades down. With each inhalation lift the heart area to counteract the tendency of compression in this posture. So the length of the spine expands evenly in both directions, the sit bones reach down to the earth and the heart rises up to the heavens. Initiate a spiraling movement in the spine and allow the space created between each pair of vertebrae to inspire an even deeper spiral. Hold this *vinyasa* for five breaths.

Exhaling, release your arms and turn to the front. Straighten the upright leg and then remove the half lotus (never the other way around, as this endangers the knee). Place your hands to the floor.

Vinyasa **Eight**	Inhaling, lift up.
Vinyasa **Nine**	Exhale, *Chaturanga Dandasana*.
Vinyasa **Ten**	Inhale into Upward Dog.
Vinyasa **Eleven**	Exhale into Downward Dog.

*Vinyasa*s Twelve to Sixteen

Repeat the posture on the left.

Note:

• A deposit of adipose tissue (fat) on thighs or abdomen makes this posture very difficult and places strain on the joints.

• Adjustments in *Baddha Konasana* may give the needed openness in the hip joints to do the posture without stressing the knees.

• Proficiency in this posture is essential prior to attempting *Supta Kurmasana*. *Marichyasana* D develops the trunk flexors and extensors and the abdominals, so that *Supta Kurmasana* can be performed safely.

• *Marichyasana* D is one of the three main creators of support strength in the Primary Series.

ANATOMICAL FOCUS
Abdominal Strength

The main action in the following posture is hip flexion. The weight of the legs has the tendency to pull the pelvis anteriorly (forward). This is counteracted by the abdominal muscles, which lift the pubic bone and tilt the pelvis back. For this reason *Navasana* is one of the prime creators of abdominal strength in the Primary Series. It is thereby an important preparation for *Kurmasana*.

Navasana
BOAT POSTURE

Drishti Toes

Vinyasa Seven

Inhaling, jump through to *Dandasana*. Lean back, balancing behind the sit bones and in front of the sacrum. Lift your legs off the floor until there is a right angle (90°) between torso and legs. Attempt to

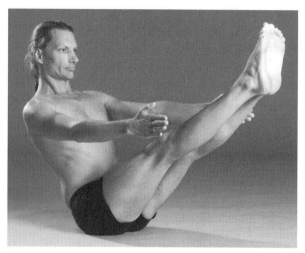

Navasana

have the legs straight. The toes rest at eye level and the feet are pointed. As you decrease the angle between torso and legs, less strength is required.

Extend your arms straight out toward your feet and at shoulder height. Hold them parallel to the floor with the palms facing each other. Draw your arms back into the shoulder joints. Do not collapse the low back. Maintain a straight back and the lift of your heart. Your body is the hull of the boat and your arms become its oars.

If the abdominals are underdeveloped, however, the low back could be put under strain in this posture. For beginners the following approach is suggested:

PHASE 1

From sitting, fold the knees into the chest and hug them. Lift the heart and, keeping the back straight, lift the feet just off the floor. Take the arms into position.

PHASE 2

Continue to increase the angle between the knees and the chest and to lift the feet away from the floor until the lower leg eventually runs parallel to the floor.

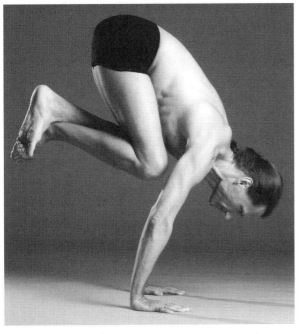

Navasana, vinyasa eight

PHASE 3

Proceed to straighten the legs to a point where the abdominals are fully engaged but the back remains straight.

Vinyasa Eight

Place your palms on the floor beside your hips. Cross your legs and, inhaling, hook the breath into the *bandhas* and push down through the arms to lift your body off the floor. Make a sincere effort here, and don't be satisfied if you cannot yet lift off. For many students, this exercise brings the breakthrough in jumping back. If you can only lift a little bit, keep working until eventually you are able to lift through into *Lollasana*. This movement confers the ability to curl the trunk into a ball. It teaches *bandha* control and is the key to jumping back. (See page 70 for a photograph of *Lollasana*; see also page 90, "Toward *Lollasana*.")

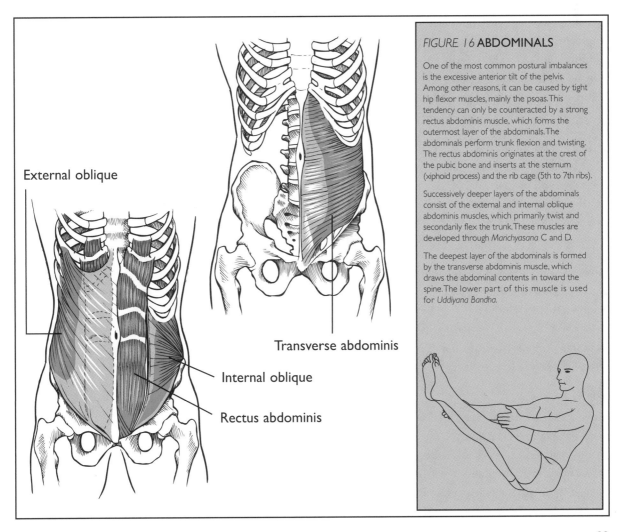

External oblique

Transverse abdominis

Internal oblique

Rectus abdominis

FIGURE 16 ABDOMINALS

One of the most common postural imbalances is the excessive anterior tilt of the pelvis. Among other reasons, it can be caused by tight hip flexor muscles, mainly the psoas. This tendency can only be counteracted by a strong rectus abdominis muscle, which forms the outermost layer of the abdominals. The abdominals perform trunk flexion and twisting. The rectus abdominis originates at the crest of the pubic bone and inserts at the sternum (xiphoid process) and the rib cage (5th to 7th ribs).

Successively deeper layers of the abdominals consist of the external and internal oblique abdominis muscles, which primarily twist and secondarily flex the trunk. These muscles are developed through *Marichyasana* C and D.

The deepest layer of the abdominals is formed by the transverse abdominis muscle, which draws the abdominal contents in toward the spine. The lower part of this muscle is used for *Uddiyana Bandha*.

Exhaling, sit back down.

Repeat the last two *vinyasas* four more times, totaling five sets.

Vinyasa **Nine**	Exhaling, glide into *Chaturanga Dandasana*.
Vinyasa **Ten**	Inhale into Upward Dog.
Vinyasa **Eleven**	Exhale into Downward Dog.

Bhujapidasana

KNEES-ON-THE-SHOULDERS POSTURE

Drishti Nose

Vinyasa **Seven**

On the inhalation, instead of jumping through, jump your feet around your arms. Keep the buttocks lifted in this transition, an action that requires *bandha* control. The key is to keep inhaling as long as you are airborne, which means to inhale until your inner thighs touch your arms. Then wrap your legs around your arms and interlock the ankles, preferably all without touching the feet to the floor.
If this is too difficult, try the following approach:

PHASE 1

Inhaling, hop forward so that your feet land outside your hands. If your hands are as wide as the mat, your feet will be just outside the mat. Without taking the hands off the floor, straighten your legs as much as the hamstrings permit.

PHASE 2

Take the right heel with your right hand and lever the right shoulder behind your right knee. Repeat on the left side. The farther you get your shoulders under your knees the easier it will be to hold the posture. Now replace your hands on the floor as close as possible to your feet.

PHASE 3

Slowly shift the weight back into your hands until your feet come off the floor. If you are comfortable, lift the feet and interlock the ankles. If your knees are close to your shoulders, the posture will be quite easy. If they are down around your elbows, getting the feet off the floor will be strenuous, as your

abdominals must lift higher. Hold the posture for five breaths, then unlock your ankles and straighten your legs while inhaling. Fold back your legs by bending your knees, and jump back from here.

Vinyasa **Eight**

Exhaling, turn the feet so that the toes point backward, ideally without touching the floor. Lower your chest to the floor by bending the elbows back. Eventually place your forehead and, once that has become easy, your chin lightly onto the floor. Done in this way, *Bhujapidasana* is the ideal preparation

---

PRACTICAL TIP
Toward Lollasana

If you have difficulties with *Lollasana*, which is part of the jump back and jump through, use the following approach: Go down on your knees and place one ankle over the other. Now place your hands on either side of the knees and, inhaling, lift your knees off the floor and up to your chest. Count the number of breaths for which you can hold this position. Repeat the exercise daily, attempting to add one breath each day.

When you have reached fifteen breaths, begin lifting your feet off as well. You will find this more difficult and the number of breaths will decrease. Work back up to ten breaths. If you make no progress, practice this exercise more than once a day.

When you have reached ten breaths, start to swing back and forth slowly, keeping your feet clear of the floor. When you can swing for ten breaths, begin to increase the amplitude of the swinging movement. Increase the swing until you can press through from *Lollasana* into Downward Dog without touching the floor.

Now attempt the same movement from sitting. It may take you a few days — or a few years — to execute this movement properly. Be patient.

---

for *Kurmasana*. It awakens the core muscles of the body, particularly the abdominals, the trunk extensors, and the psoas.

Beginners may attempt this full version after

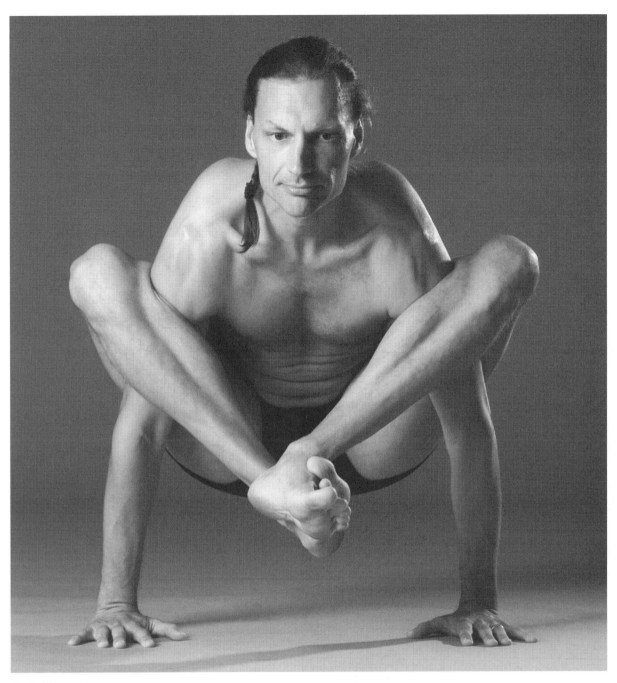

Bhujapidasana, vinyasa seven

they have gained proficiency in the previously described Phase 3. Once you can place your chin down, eliminate the five breaths of the upright version. The last step is to learn jumping straight in and out of the posture.

Vinyasa **Nine**

Inhaling, come up, straighten the arms, and bring the feet forward without touching the floor. Unlock your ankles and work the legs strongly to straighten

them. Point the feet and gaze upward. This transitional posture to exit *Bhujapidasana* is *Tittibhasana* (insect posture).

Exhaling, bend your legs, suck your knees into your armpits, and lift your heels up to your buttocks.

Vinyasa **Ten**

Hold for the duration of the inhalation. This second transitional posture is known as *Bakasana* (crane posture).

91

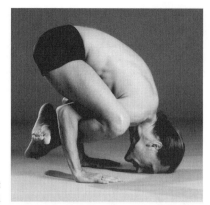

Bhujapidasana
forehead

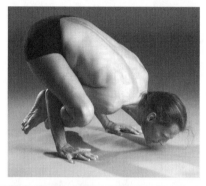

Right,
Bhujapidasana
final version
Below,
Tittibhasana

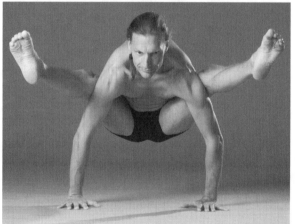

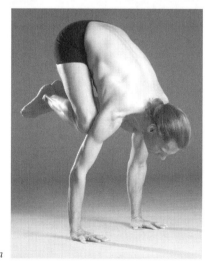

Bakasana

***Vinyasa* Eleven**	Exhaling, glide into *Chaturanga Dandasana*.
***Vinyasa* Twelve**	Inhale into Upward Dog.
***Vinyasa* Thirteen**	Exhale into Downward Dog.

Kurmasana AND *Supta Kurmasana*

TURTLE POSTURE AND RECLINING TURTLE POSTURE

Drishti Third eye

Prerequisites: Proficiency in *Marichyasana* D and *Bhujapidasana*

> **YOGIC CONTEXT**
> ### *Importance of Leg-Behind-Head Postures*
> *Supta Kurmasana* is one of the key postures in the Primary Series. Whereas all other postures in the primary sequence are forward bends or hip rotations or combinations thereof, *Supta Kurmasana* opens an entire universe of leg-behind-head postures. There are three in the Intermediate Series, six in the Advanced A Series, and seven in the Advanced B Series. Leg-behind-head counteracts backbending. These postures invigorate the spine and strengthen the abdominals and trunk extensors; they also develop the chest and increase blood supply to the heart and lungs. As well, they increase humility and decrease pride. This is one of the most important categories of postures. Combined with the sequences of backbends and arm balances, it purifies the nervous system and induces meditation.

Apart from its significance in introducing the leg-behind-head postures, *Supta Kurmasana* creates the support strength that is needed to carry the spine safely in dynamic backbends. For this reason proficiency in *Supta Kurmasana* needs to be recognized as a prerequisite for the drop-back (dynamic backbend from *Samasthiti* and return).

Vinyasa Seven

Proficiency in *Bhujapidasana* is necessary before one attempts this posture. Some progress in *Pashimottanasana* is also required for the hamstring

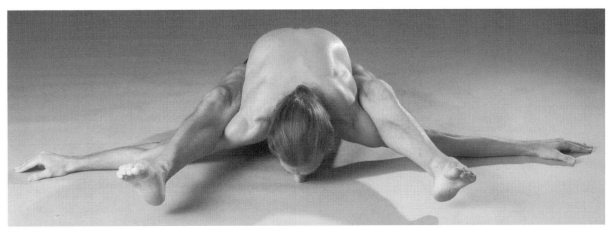

Kurmasana

length needed. Inhaling, jump around your arms as when entering *Bhujapidasana*. With the knees up close to your shoulders, straighten the legs and lift

your shoulders. Palms press down into the floor. Place your head on the floor, first with the forehead and later with the chin, as in *Bhujapidasana*. Point

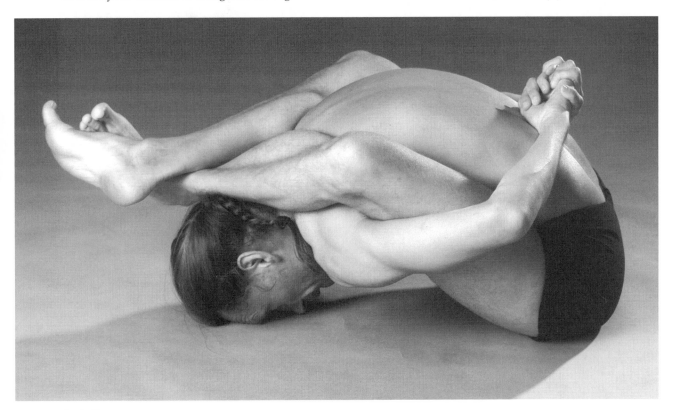

Supta Kurmasana

the buttocks until your legs are parallel to the floor.

Exhaling, slowly lower down like a helicopter, bending your elbows back behind you. On the floor, make another attempt to bring your knees right up on to your shoulders. The legs need to be almost parallel, without a gap between the inner thighs and the sides of the rib cage. Straighten your arms and bring the hands forward until they are in line with

your feet — as with all extreme forward bends this protects the hamstrings and the cruciate ligaments. Straighten the legs and work toward lifting the heels from the floor. Hold *Kurmasana* for five breaths.

If your legs are straight but the heels do not come off the floor, check that your arms extend out in line with your shoulders.

93

If the hands are farther back, there is a tendency for the sit bones to lift off. If you do not have enough space available to extend the arms out to the sides, you can extend them backward with the palms facing up. This version is inferior, however, as there is a tendency for the shoulders to hunch and collapse forward.

It takes a lot of strength to lift the heels off the floor. It is, however, an important aspect of this posture for various reasons:

• The quadriceps and the hamstrings are strengthened, enhancing all other forward bends.

• It improves access to the quadriceps if you have difficulty keeping the kneecaps pulled up in the standing postures.

• The spine is strengthened in preparation for drop-backs.

• Most important, it creates the abdominal strength required for *Supta Kurmasana.*

Do not attempt *Supta Kurmasana* before you have gained proficiency in *Kurmasana.* If the back is greatly rounded in *Kurmasana,* the lumbar discs are in a vulnerable position. The additional weight of the legs behind the head can cause strain if the body is not prepared. The strength required to lift the feet clear of the floor offers the necessary protection.

Vinyasa **Eight:** *Primary Version*

Exhaling, bend up the legs, bring your shoulders farther under the knees, reach your arms around your back, and clasp your hands. If possible take hold of the wrist.

Vinyasa **Eight:** *Intermediate Version*

Students who are practicing the Intermediate Series can come up to sitting and enter *Dvi Pada Shirshasana* to transit into *Supta Kurmasana.* (Do this variation only when you have gained proficiency in *Ekapada Shirshasana.* The weight of two legs behind the head requires considerable core strength.)

To do this, first place the left leg behind the head. Take care to move your knee well behind your shoulder to ensure that you can hook the shin below the C7 vertebra. This prevents the neck from carrying the weight of the legs: it should be borne on the

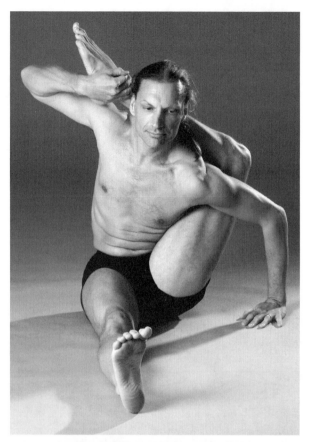

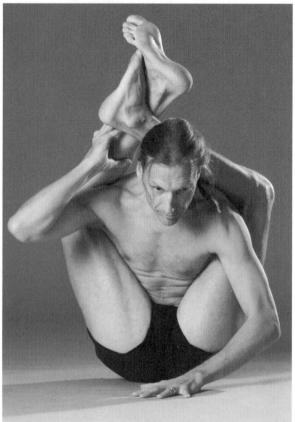

Going into *Supta Kurmasana,* 1 (top) and 2

shoulders and the upper thoracic spine. Exhaling, place the right leg on top of the left leg, ensuring that the left stays behind the head.

Practiced in this way, the posture will not cause more discomfort than carrying a mid-sized backpack. Performed poorly, it can cause considerable irritation of the spinal nerves in the neck, with all the accompanying symptoms.

Vinyasa Nine: *Primary Version*

Inhaling, cross the ankles and place your forehead on the floor. This is the state of *Supta Kurmasana*. Stay in it for five breaths, supporting the spine with a combination of abdominal and back extensor work.

Vinyasa Nine: *Intermediate Version*

Place your hands on the floor and lower your forehead to it, keeping both legs behind the head. Reach around your back and interlock your fingers or take a wrist.

Vinyasa Ten

Release your hands, bring them forward, and place them under your shoulders. Inhaling, lift the entire body off the floor, if possible keeping the legs behind the head. Then, as in *Bhujapidasana*, straighten your legs into *Tittibhasana* (see photograph on page 92).

Exhaling, fold the legs back until the knees rest on the back of the arms. Inhaling, lift up into *Bakasana*, straightening the arms. Point the feet and tuck the heels up under the sit bones. At the end of the inhalation, when you are most buoyant, move into *vinyasa* eleven.

Vinyasa Eleven	Exhaling, glide back into *Chaturanga Dandasana*.
Vinyasa Twelve	Inhale into Upward Dog.
Vinyasa Thirteen	Exhale into Downward Dog.

Garbha Pindasana
EMBRYO-IN-THE-WOMB POSTURE

Drishti Nose

Prerequisites: All postures covered so far, especially *Marichyasana* D.

Vinyasa Seven

Inhaling, jump through and straighten your legs into *Dandasana*.

Vinyasa Eight

Exhaling, fold into *Garbha Pindasana*. Seasoned practitioners may do this on one exhalation; others may prefer to break it down into stages. *Padmasana* and its variations in Western circles have a reputation for causing knee problems. If our hip joints are stiff from a lifetime of sitting in chairs, we cannot expect to learn this posture in a week. It has been mentioned already that Indians traditionally sat on Mother Earth, which opens the hip joints for *Padmasana*. If the hip joints are stiff and we force ourselves into *Padmasana*, the knees may be injured.

The solution is to open the hip joints first (if necessary through years of work), and then attempt this posture. If you are not proficient in *Marichyasana* D, do not attempt *Garbha Pindasana*.

PHASE 1

From *Dandasana* place the right leg into half lotus, precisely following the instructions under *Ardha Baddha Padma Pashimottanasana* (page 73). In short:

- Point and invert the right foot.[16]
- Draw the right knee far out to the right.
- Close the knee joint completely by drawing the right heel into the right groin.
- From here, draw the heel into the navel.

Keeping the heel in the navel, place the right foot into the left groin.

Note: If your right foot rests on the opposite thigh rather than in the groin, and your right heel has lost contact with the navel, do not proceed any further. In this case the flexibility needed to perform the posture is insufficient.

16. For the question as to why we sit only with the right leg first in lotus, refer to *Padmasana* at the end of the sequence.

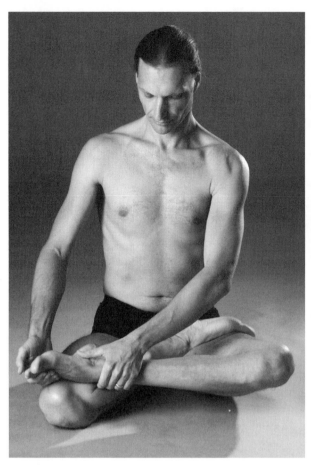 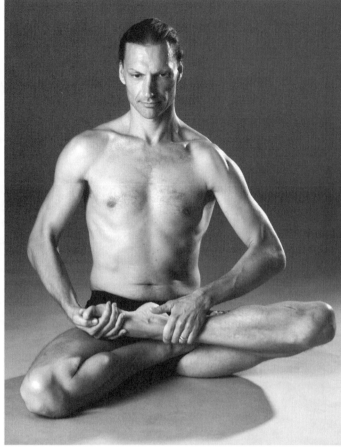

Garbha Pindasana: incorrect (left) and correct method of going into lotus

PHASE 2

Only if the right leg is snugly in the left groin should one proceed further. Most mishaps in lotus posture happen when the second leg, here the left leg, is forced into position. The most precarious way to place the second foot is to bend the leg only to 90° and transit the foot over the right knee to bring it into position. Even flexible students damage their knees with this method.

To protect the knees in lotus and half-lotus pos-tures, first close the knee joint completely, bringing tibia and femur close together. Then move them both as one unit. This method eliminates lateral movement in the knee, which is responsible for meniscus injuries.

To protect the knee of the second leg, visualize *Padmasana* as being two half-lotus postures united. This means that we follow the same steps for the half-lotus posture with the second leg, completely ignoring the fact that the right leg is already in half lotus. Try the following steps:

• Point and invert the left foot.

• Draw the left heel toward the left groin, closing the knee joint completely.

• In therapy situations, first place the left foot under the right ankle. Only proceed further if this position is comfortable. Still keeping the knee joint closed, draw the left knee as far out to the side as possible without moving the sit bones. Gently lift your foot over the right ankle toward the navel.

• From here, draw the foot across into the right groin.

If the movement is performed in this way, the knee joint is completely closed at all times, which means that, on the left side also, the tibia and femur move as a unity. If you experience pain in the knees at any point, reverse the movement to a point were you are pain free and proceed more slowly, paying attention to detail.

Practice the other postures until you have gained the necessary flexibility.

PHASE 3

To prepare for *Garbha Pindasana*, medially rotate the femurs until the front edges of the tibias point down to the floor and the soles and heels face upward and not toward the torso. (Refer to "The Buddha's Lotus" in *Janushirshasana* A, page 79.)

Gently bring the knees close together, to a point where the thighs are almost parallel. This will create the necessary space to insert the arms between thighs and calves. Insert the right hand, with the palm facing toward you, below the calf muscle where the leg is thinnest.

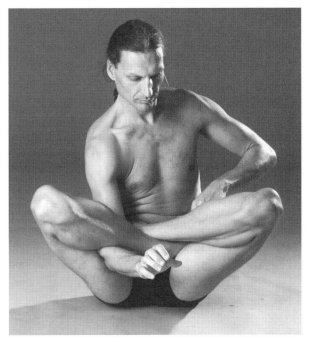

Going into *Garbha Pindasana*

Once you have inserted your right hand between thigh and calf, invert the hand until the palm faces away from you. This will help the elbow to glide through. Do not apply excessive force. Insert the second palm facing toward you and again turn it to allow the elbow to come through. After both elbows are through, bend your arms, place your hands on the chin, and touch your fingertips to your earlobes. Inability to do this often points to weak abdominal muscles, since a significant amount of trunk flexion is needed here. Lift the head and sit as upright as possible, balancing on the sit bones.

You are now in the state of *Garbha Pindasana*, which resembles the curled-up position of an embryo in the womb. Stay for five breaths.

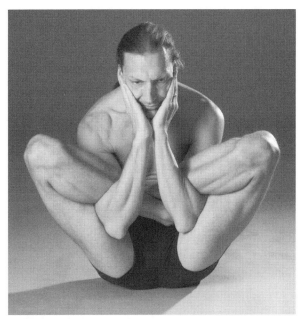

Garbha Pindasana, vinyasa eight, hands on chin

For the second part of the posture, bend the head forward and ideally place the hands on the crown of the head. This rounds the back in anticipation of rolling onto the back.

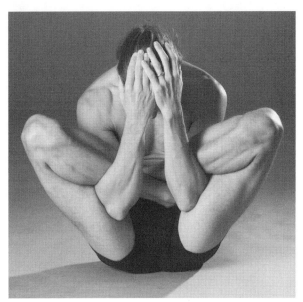

Garbha Pindasana, vinyasa eight, hands on crown of head

Exhaling, roll down on the back and perform a movement similar to that of a rocking chair. When the buttocks are in the air swivel them slightly to the right. This action will turn you, on the spot, in a clockwise direction. Rock nine times, representing the nine months of gestation. Use the inhalation to rock up and the exhalation to roll down. If possible

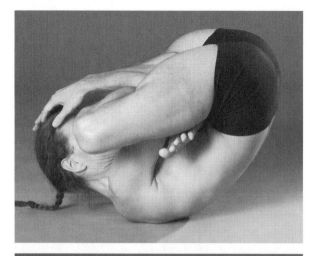

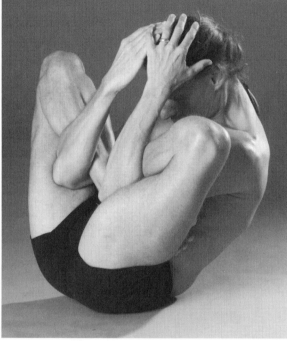

Garbha Pindasana, rolling 1 and 2

keep hold of your head with your hands. Let the movement come out of the connection of breath and *bandha*s.

On the last inhalation, use more momentum and rock up to *Kukkutasana*.

Kukkutasana
ROOSTER POSTURE

Drishti Nose

Inhaling, roll all the way up until you balance on your hands. As soon as the hands are on the floor, lift the head to fade out the movement and begin to balance. You are now in *Kukkutasana*, rooster posture, in which your two hands resemble the feet of the rooster. *Garbha Pindasana* and *Kukkutasana* are very effective in opening the hip joints farther and, if performed correctly, they are therapy for the knees. They strongly improve the quality of one's *Padmasana*. They create support strength, exercise the abdominals, and invigorate the spine; and they are, together with *Kurmasana*, the prime preparation and counterposture for backbending at the end of the series. Stay in the state of *Kukkutasana* for five breaths.

Exhaling, sit down, pull the arms out, and place the hands down.

Vinyasa Nine

Bring the knees as close together as possible, so that they will fit through your arms. Inhaling, swing your legs to the front, and lift your knees high. Suck your thighs into your chest and swing your sit bones through your arms to gain momentum.

Vinyasa Ten

Exhaling, swing back and lift your sit bones high behind you. Keep the legs folded into the chest until the sit bones have reached their highest point. The spine needs to be parallel to the floor or the sit bones even higher than that. Only now let your legs, which are still in lotus, swing through. After your thighs have come parallel to the floor, flick your legs out to land in *Chaturanga Dandasana*.

Note:
• When swinging through, lift your sit bones really high, so that your knees can swing through without knocking the floor.
• If you want to build strength, do the movement slowly, using less and less momentum.

Opposite top, *Kukkutasana*
Opposite lower, jump back from lotus, phases 1, 2, and 3

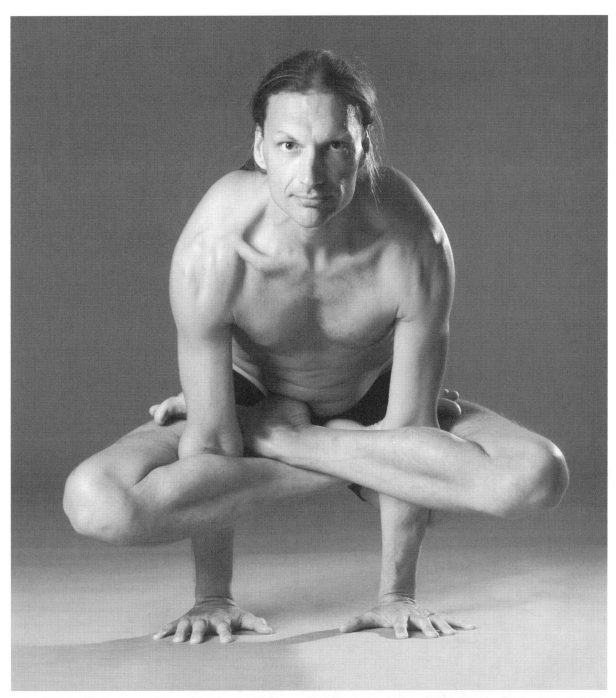

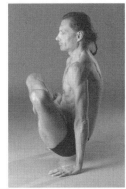
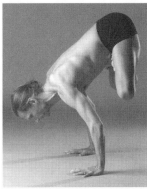
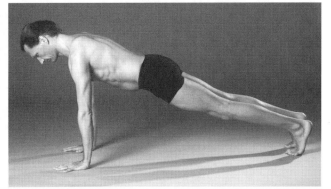

• If you have not yet developed sufficient *bandha* control, or you experience discomfort in your knees, fold out of *Padmasana* one leg at a time. Straighten your legs into *Dandasana* and jump back from there.

Vinyasa Eleven   Inhale into Upward Dog.
Vinyasa Twelve   Exhale into Downward Dog.

Baddha Konasana
BOUND ANGLE POSTURE

Drishti Nose

Vinyasa Seven

Inhaling, glide through to *Dandasana*. Draw the feet toward you until you can draw a straight line through both knees and both ankles, while letting the knees sink out to the side. There is no set distance from pubic bone to heel; it varies from person to person depending on the ratio between length of femur and length of tibia. If your pelvis tilts posteriorly at this point already, elevate the sit bones by sitting on a folded blanket. This will help you to use gravity more.

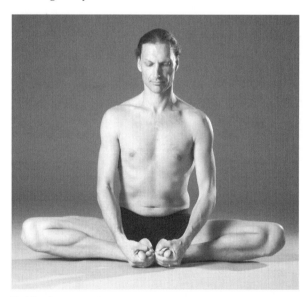

Baddha Konasana, vinyasa seven

Take the feet now by reaching with your thumbs in between the soles and then open the feet like the pages of a book. At the same time, use your abductors (gluteus medius, gluteus minimus, tensor fascia latae) to draw your knees down to the floor. Take a deep inhalation to sit as tall as possible, with sit

bones reaching down into the floor, low back concaved, and heart lifted high.

Vinyasa Eight

Exhaling, fold forward, keeping your back completely straight and the heart lifting forward.

This is a potentially difficult posture, which might not even be mastered through years of adjustments, but it can be mastered through inquiry (*vichara*) and intelligence (*buddhi*). We have to understand that *Baddha Konasana* is two *Janushirshasana* A's put together. If we have understood and practiced *Janushirshasana* A properly, then *Baddha Konasana* will unfold.

Let's recall *Janushirshasana* A. When the right leg is folded back, we:

• point and invert the right foot
• draw the right heel into the right groin
• medially (inwardly) rotate the right thigh bone
• draw the knee down to the floor and backward
• extend out along the inside of the thigh bone.

You need to perform all of those actions in *Baddha Konasana* simultaneously on both sides. In *vinyasa*

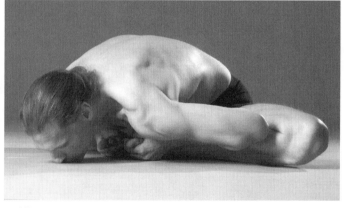

Baddha Konasana

seven you already inverted your feet, which means that the soles face upward. Now point the feet, which leads to the heels moving apart from each other. This lengthens the insides of the thighs. The heels then reach toward the respective groins, which prevents the sit bones from escaping backward as we fold forward. The most important action, however, is the inward rotation of the thighs. The thigh bones should roll forward like the wheels of a cart (with the floor as a reference point). The thigh bone has to inwardly rotate in *Baddha Konasana* to perform the same action as the tibia, which will close and protect the knee joint. The tibia rolls forward until its front edge points straight down. Since we

This is often due to emotions such as fear, pain, and shame held on to in these muscles. These emotions need to be acknowledged and then released with the exhalation. In order to do that, the intensity of

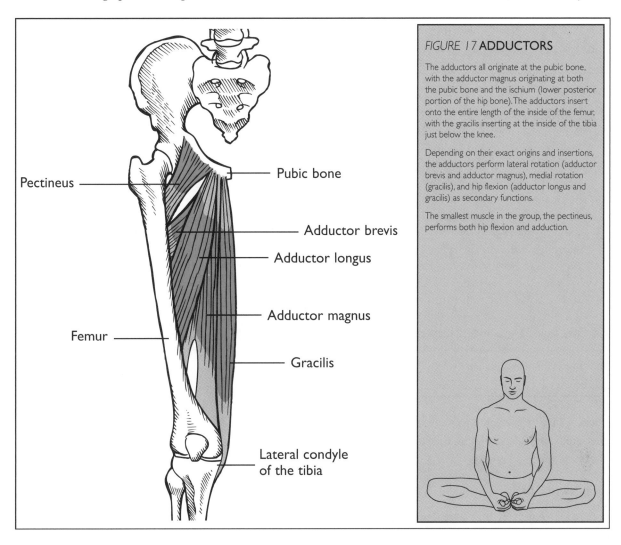

Pectineus

Pubic bone

Adductor brevis

Adductor longus

Adductor magnus

Femur

Gracilis

Lateral condyle
of the tibia

FIGURE 17 ADDUCTORS

The adductors all originate at the pubic bone, with the adductor magnus originating at both the pubic bone and the ischium (lower posterior portion of the hip bone). The adductors insert onto the entire length of the inside of the femur, with the gracilis inserting at the inside of the tibia just below the knee.

Depending on their exact origins and insertions, the adductors perform lateral rotation (adductor brevis and adductor magnus), medial rotation (gracilis), and hip flexion (adductor longus and gracilis) as secondary functions.

The smallest muscle in the group, the pectineus, performs both hip flexion and adduction.

externally rotated the femurs in *vinyasa* seven, we need to reverse this movement now in *vinyasa* eight to work deeply into the posture.

As in *Janushirshasana* A, the knees draw down and backward. Finally, let the thigh bones reach out to the side, a movement that will release the adductors. This isometric movement was initiated already by pointing the feet and separating the heels. Often there is a fear reflex here to suck the thigh bones into the hip joints. This action is, however, performed by the adductors, and will prevent you from opening into the posture.

What prevents most students from going deeply into this posture is chronic tension of the adductors.

the sensation in the posture needs to be still tolerable. If one overstretches one's muscles, a trauma is stored in the tissue. The muscles will prevent one from going again to that point as a mere protective mechanism.

The trunk actions for *Baddha Konasana* are the same as for *Janushirshasana* A and *Pashimottanasana* — drawing in the lower abdomen, lifting the heart forward, drawing the shoulder blades down the back, and letting the crown of the head and the sit bones reach into opposing directions. Press the elbows against the inner thighs to keep the knees grounded. Draw the feet toward you while they maintain their action of pointing and inverting.

If your sit bones lift off and escape backward in the process of folding forward, counteract this by sucking your heels into the abdomen using breath and abdominal muscles. The abdominals can do that by drawing the abdominal contents vigorously in against the spine, which lets the heart leap forward and creates a vacuum into which the heels are

---

PRACTICAL TIP
Tips for Different Skin Types

Practitioners with *vata* skin,[17] which is rather thin, papery, and silken, and easily slips on cloth material, will generally find no problem with wearing long tights. They usually do not sweat a lot, but should they do so they will find it hard to slip through — wet skin on material offers too much friction. Students with *pitta* or *kapha* skin (thick, oily, sticky, and moist skin types) tend to sweat a lot, and they are better off to wear shorts and spray water on the arms and especially the elbows. In cold weather, when heavy sweating is less likely, they can wear long tights and long-sleeved tops. Material on material also slips easily.

---

sucked. Finally place the toes on the chest, wearing them like a necklace. Stay in the state of *Baddha Konasana* for five breaths.

Vinyasa **Nine**

Inhaling, we reverse the movement and sit upright in the same position as the seventh *vinyasa*. The knees draw down, the heart lifts, the low back concaves, the shoulder blades draw down. Exhaling, place your hands down and straighten your legs.

Vinyasa **Ten**

Inhaling, lift up. You will feel the benefit of the abdominals' work, and now fly like a butterfly.

***Vinyasa* Eleven**	Exhaling, *Chaturanga Dandasana*.
***Vinyasa* Twelve**	Inhale into Upward Dog.
***Vinyasa* Thirteen**	Exhale into Downward Dog.

17. *Vata* is one of the three Ayurvedic *doshas*, or constitution types.

Upavishta Konasana

BOUND ANGLE POSTURE

Drishti Nose (*vinyasa* eight), upward (*vinyasa* nine)

Vinyasa **Seven**

Inhaling, jump through to *Dandasana*. Widen your legs to the extent that you can still just hold the outside of the feet, which could be to an angle of anything between 90° and 120°.

If you can't get hold of the outsides whatever the angle, take the big toes instead. Beginners may bend the legs at first to make sure the low back is not rounded and sit on a folded blanket to use gravity when extending forward.

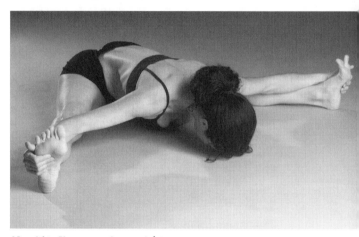

Upavishta Konasana, vinyasa eight

Holding onto the feet, lift through the entire front of the torso. Draw the lower abdomen in and concave the low back. Lift the heart while drawing the shoulder blades down the back.

Vinyasa **Eight**

Exhaling, fold forward. Work the legs strongly by lifting the kneecaps and drawing the heels into the floor to protect the cruciate ligaments and hamstring origins. Keep the thighs in a neutral position, with knees and feet pointing straight up. Fold forward as far as you can while keeping the back straight.

The purpose of the posture is to balance the flow of the principal *vayus* (vital air currents) in the torso.

These different currents of the life force are balanced by exercising *Upavishta Konasana*. It is necessary for this purpose not to jut the chin down to the floor but to lead with the heart forward and down in an even movement. The inner integrity of the spine needs to be maintained as if still standing. Hold this *vinyasa* for five breaths.

Vinyasa Nine

Inhaling, straighten your arms, raise the torso, but still hold on to your feet. Exhaling, fold forward to take momentum. Inhaling, roll up and balance on your sit bones.

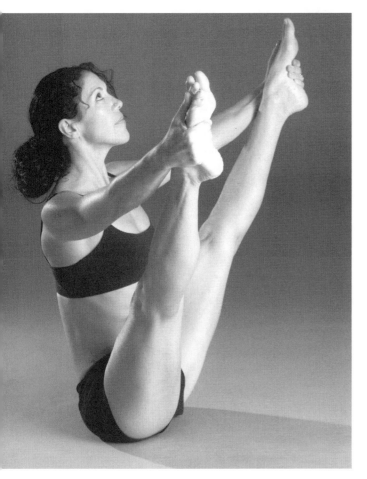

Upavishta Konasana, vinyasa nine

Experienced students can try to hold on to the feet on the way up. You will need flexibility in forward bending and a strong low back. Rapidly move the torso back up through hip extension. When your arms are almost straight, press the legs into the ground using the gluteus maximus and hamstrings. Once the legs lift off, continue the movement by using the hip flexors to actively lift the legs higher. Assist with the arms, which will draw the feet toward the midline. Take your head back to fade out the momentum and balance.

If that method doesn't work, change the grip to the big toes. An even easier version is to let go of the toes, but lift the straight legs up to the hands.

> **YOGIC CONTEXT**
> ### *The Vayus*
>
> The *vayus*, of which there are ten in all, are vital currents within the body. They are *prana, apana, samana, udana, vyana, naga, kurma, krkara, devadatta,* and *dhananjaya.* According to the *Gheranda Samhita*, the first five of these are the principal *vayus.*[18] The *vayus* are pranic currents that can be regarded as subdivisions of *prana,* the life force. The first item within this subdivision is also called *prana,* which is potentially confusing. If the term *prana* is mentioned together with *apana,* then it refers to the *vayu prana.* In the term *pranayama,* however, *prana* refers to the life force itself, which is the sum total of the ten *vayus.*
>
> Besides the ten *vayus,* which we can also call the ten *vatas,* there are ten *kaphas* and ten *pittas* in the body. The reasons why they are not often mentioned is that we can alter the *vayus* through our actions and therefore alter the entire organism. We cannot influence the *pittas* and *kaphas* directly.
>
> In his commentary, Vyasa says about the five principal *vayus,* "Movement of *prana* is limited to the mouth and the nose and its action extends up to the heart. *Samana* distributes [the nourishment from food] to all parts equally and its sphere of action is up to the navel. *Apana* is so called because it carries the wastes away and it acts down to the soles of the feet. *Udana* is the vital force with upward direction and it goes right up to the head. The vital force *vyana* is spread all over the body. Of these forces, the chief is the *prana.*"[19]

Alternatively beginners may sit upright with the spine completely straight, then draw the knees into the chest as for *Navasana* preparation (page 88). Take the toes or the outsides of the feet and proceed to

18. *The Gheranda Samhita* V.61, trans. R. B. S. Chandra Vasu, Sri Satguru Publications, Delhi, 1986, p. 46.

19. H. Aranya, *Yoga Philosophy of Patanjali with Bhasvati,* 4th enlarged ed., University of Calcutta, Kolkata, 2000, p. 315.

straighten the legs as much as you can while keeping the back straight. The focus in the posture needs to be the integrity of the spine and not whether the legs are straight. There is no point in straightening the legs if the low back is rounded and the heart collapses. Hold this *vinyasa* also for five breaths. Then, exhaling, bring the feet together and place your hands on the floor.

Vinyasa **Ten**	Inhaling, lift up.
Vinyasa **Eleven**	Exhaling, *Chaturanga Dandasana*.
Vinyasa **Twelve**	Inhale into Upward Dog.
Vinyasa **Thirteen**	Exhale into Downward Dog.

Supta Konasana

RECLINING ANGLE POSTURE

Drishti Nose

Vinyasa Seven

Inhaling, jump through to *Dandasana*. Exhaling, slowly lie down, keeping the arms at either side of the torso.

Vinyasa Eight

Inhaling, lift the legs, bring the hips over the shoulders, and place your feet onto the floor behind your head. Take the arms over your head, reach for your big toes, and take your legs out wide until your arms are extended straight. Work the spine long, lifting the sit bones up to the ceiling. Work the legs strong and straight. Flex the feet and keep the thighs in a neutral position, neither laterally nor medially rotated. Lift the T1 and C7 vertebrae away from the floor by gently pushing the shoulders and the back of the head into the floor.

Exhaling, create some momentum by rolling the buttocks a little toward the head and push off your toes.

Vinyasa Nine

Inhaling, rock up using the breath. Pause at the pivot point behind your sit bones, as in *Upavishta Konasana*. Lift your heart and your face to the ceiling. Flex the feet completely and contract the quadriceps fully.

Exhaling, resist the pull of gravity, landing on

your calves rather than the heels of your feet, and reach your chest and chin toward the floor.

It is the coordination of movement and breath that gives one control and balance throughout this posture. Complete the inhalation when you reach the point at which you wish to balance. By lifting the heart and face here, the forward momentum is arrested — a moment of silence — before the

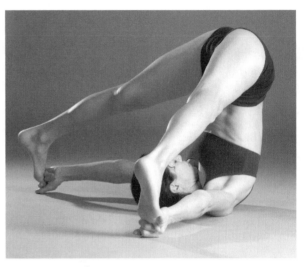

Supta Konasana, phase 1

exhalation completes the forward fold. Keeping the heart and face lifted and the legs strong and straight will make the movement smooth and the landing buoyant.

If there is insufficient flexibility in the hamstrings to keep the legs straight at *Upavishta Konasana*, it is important to release the toes on the descent. Otherwise you will land heavily on your heels and risk a severe stretch of the hamstring muscles.

Done properly, this movement strengthens the back and abdominal muscles and improves the *bandha*s; it can also assist in correcting subluxations of the vertebrae.

Vinyasa Ten

Inhaling, lift your heart while still holding your toes. Exhaling, place your hands to the floor.

Vinyasa **Eleven**	Inhaling, lift up.
Vinyasa **Twelve**	Exhale into *Chaturanga Dandasana*.
Vinyasa **Thirteen**	Inhale into Upward Dog.
Vinyasa **Fourteen**	Exhale into Downward Dog.

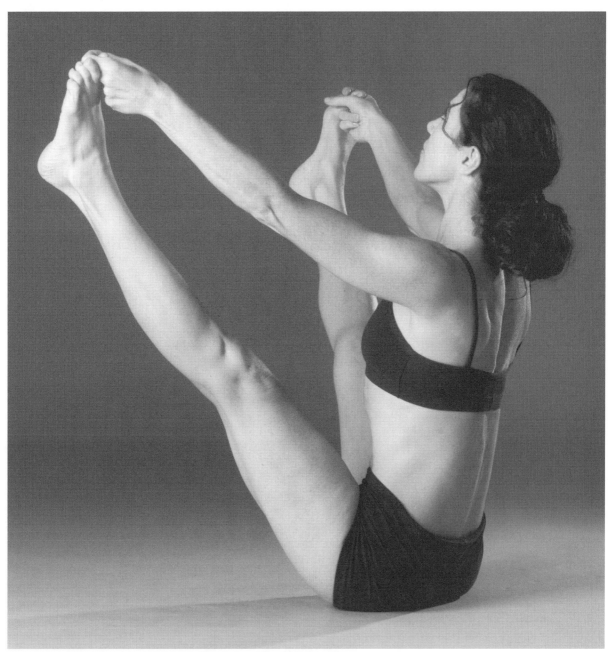

Supta Konasana, phases 2 (above) and 3

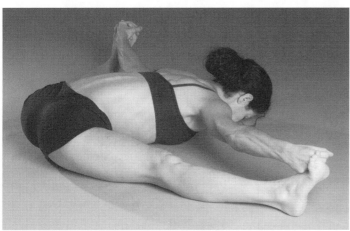

Supta Padangushtasana
RECLINING HOLD-THE-BIG-TOE POSTURE

Drishti Toes and to the side

Vinyasa Seven

Inhaling, jump through. Exhaling, lie down in a slow, controlled movement. This uses the hip flexor muscles eccentrically, which have to lengthen slowly against the pull of gravity; you would otherwise land on your back with a thud. Now place both hands on your thighs.

Vinyasa Eight

Inhaling, lift the right leg without bending it and take your big toe.

Vinyasa Nine

Exhaling, lift your torso up to meet your leg rather than drawing the leg down toward your trunk. Ideally, lift the entire spine off the floor. This makes *Supta Padangushtasana* more of a strength-building exercise than one for enhancing flexibility. Keep the left leg straight and in contact with the floor. The heart lifts up to the knee, the chin eventually meets the shin, and the gaze is lifted to the toes. Hold the state of *Supta Padangushtasana* for five breaths.

Vinyasa Ten

Inhaling, lengthen the hip flexors and abdominals eccentrically and thereby lower the torso and head down to the floor.

Vinyasa Eleven

Exhaling, and still holding the big toe, draw the right leg out to the right side. The entire length of the spine and the underneath side of the left leg maintain contact with the floor. Continue the side-ward movement of the right leg only to the extent that you can keep the left buttock grounded. The left hand on your hip may aid you with this. It is the heel of the right foot that leads the movement down toward the floor. This causes the right femur to rotate medially. This action is necessary to counteract the opposite tendency (lateral rotation of the thigh), which avoids stretching and lengthening the adductor muscles of the inner thigh. The adductors need to lengthen eccentrically on the way down,

a movement that can teach us a lot about *Baddha Konasana*.

On completion of the movement, lift the head a little off the floor and replace it to gaze out to the left side. Work the left leg strongly to stay anchored, while extending out through the bases of all toes of the left foot. In the final version, shoulders, buttocks, and feet are all touching the floor. Traditionally this posture is ascribed the power to correct the length of the extremities in relation to the torso. Hold this *vinyasa* for five breaths.

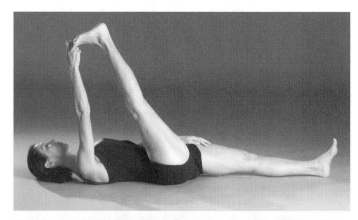

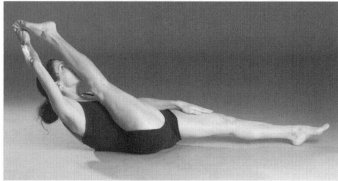

Supta Padangushtasana, vinyasa eight (top) and *vinyasa* nine

Vinyasa Twelve

Inhaling, lift the leg back to the center, a movement that combines adduction and lateral rotation of the femur. Bring the gaze back to the toes.

Vinyasa Thirteen

Exhaling, lift the torso, repeating the movement of the ninth *vinyasa*.

Vinyasa Fourteen

Inhaling, lower the torso to the floor, repeating the movement of the tenth *vinyasa*.

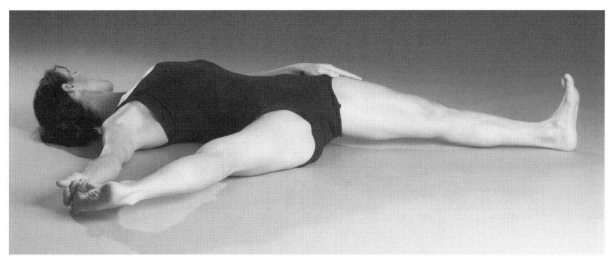

Supta Parshvasahita (*vinyasa* eleven of *Supta Padangushtasana*)

Vinyasa **Fifteen**

Exhaling, release the big toe and draw the right leg down to the floor. Until we reach 90° of hip flexion (leg pointing up to the ceiling), this movement is hip extension, which is performed here by the gluteus maximus against gravity. From then on, the work is carried on by the hip flexors lengthening eccentrically, which prevents the leg from falling uncontrolled to the floor. On conclusion of the movement, both hands lie on top of the thighs.

*Vinyasa*s Sixteen to Twenty-Three

Repeat the same movements on the left side. At count twenty-three we arrive at lying on the floor.

Vinyasa **Twenty-Four:**
Version for Experienced Students

Inhaling, lift your legs off the floor by flexing the hip joints and place your hands about your ears, tucking the fingers under the shoulders. Continue this movement by flexing the trunk, using your abdominal muscles. Momentum combines these movements with those of the upper body; when only the shoulders remain on the floor, push your hands into the floor as if straightening out the arms. Keeping the legs strong and the hips supported away from the floor, roll over into *Chaturanga Dandasana*. Keep the gaze at the tip of the nose throughout.

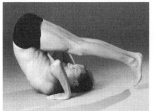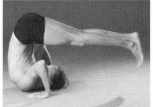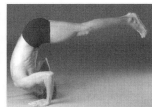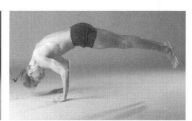

Above from left, *Chakrasana*, phases 1 to 4; right, phase 5

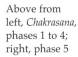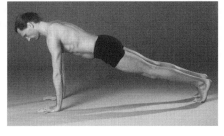

All postures that end with lying on the floor are exited through a movement called *Chakrasana* (wheel posture). Do not attempt *Chakrasana* when a whiplash or reversed neck curvature is present.

Vinyasa **Twenty-Four:**
Version for Students with Moderate Experience

Place a blanket under your shoulders to elevate T1, C7 and C6. On the last of the exhalation, lift your legs off the floor. After you have transited through 30°, inhale and take your legs over while you flex your trunk. Exhaling, place the feet down behind the head in *Halasana* (plough posture) and place the hands under the shoulders. At the end of the exhalation, when your chest is completely deflated,

107

roll over and, inhaling, push your hands into the floor to transit into *Chaturanga Dandasana*.

Considerable upper-body strength is required to avoid excessive pressure on the musculature of the neck. Your teacher should assess whether you are prepared for this transitional move. Beginners may abstain from this transition entirely. Alternatively, draw your knees into the chest, rock up to sitting, and transit through your normal *vinyasa*.

Vinyasa Twenty-five   Inhale into Upward Dog.

Vinyasa Twenty-six   Exhale into Downward Dog.

Ubhaya Padangushtasana
TAKE-BOTH-BIG-TOES POSTURE

Drishti Upward

Vinyasa Seven

Inhaling, glide through to *Dandasana* and, exhaling, lie down.

Vinyasa Eight

Keep the feet together and, taking your arms over your head, grasp both big toes. Lengthen the spine and reach the sit bones up to the ceiling. Straighten the arms and legs, flexing the feet. Exhaling, draw the buttocks over your head by flexing the trunk to create some momentum.

Ubhaya Padangushtasana, vinyasa eight

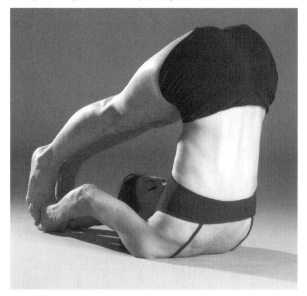

Vinyasa Nine

Inhaling, roll up, pointing the feet. To roll smoothly over the back, curve the low back sufficiently by drawing in the lower abdomen. Continue the upward movement by using the connection of inhalation and *bandha*s. Arrest the forward movement by lifting

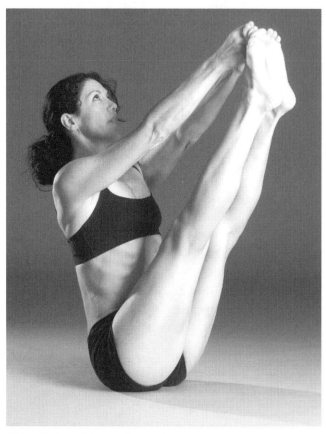

Ubhaya Padangushtasana, vinyasa nine

your heart and your face to the ceiling, coming to balance behind the sit bones. Concurrently the inhalation is completed at the balance point, flowing into an exhalation, while keeping the final position of balance. Lengthen the back of the neck and draw the shoulder blades down. Gaze upward and hold *Ubhaya Padangushtasana* for five breaths.

Exhaling, place your hands down. The feet stay, hovering in their final position.

Vinyasa Ten   Inhaling, lift up, curling into a ball.

Vinyasa Eleven   Exhaling, glide back into *Chaturanga Dandasana*.

Vinyasa Twelve   Inhale into Upward Dog.

Vinyasa Thirteen   Exhale into Downward Dog.

Urdhva Mukha Pashimottanasana

UPWARD-FACING FORWARD BEND

Drishti Upward

Vinyasa **Seven**

Inhaling, glide through to *Dandasana*; exhaling, lie down.

Vinyasa **Eight**

Inhaling, take your legs over and place your feet on the floor behind your head.

In this posture, take hold of the outside of the feet and point them. Lengthen and straighten the spine by lifting the sit bones toward the ceiling. Draw in the lower abdomen and breathe deeply into the chest.

Exhaling, flex the spine and roll over your toes until your feet are flexed.

Lower left, *Urdhva Mukha Pashimottanasana, vinyasa*s eight (top) and nine; below, final position

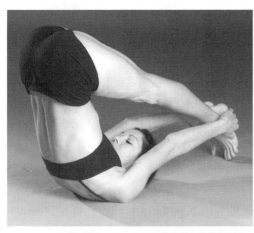

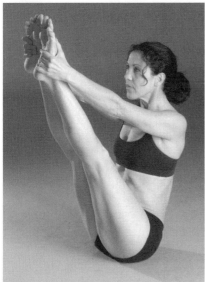

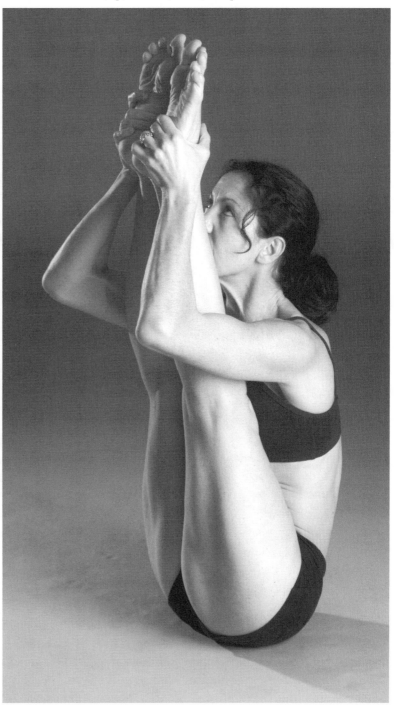

Vinyasa Nine

Inhaling, push off your feet and roll up until you balance behind your sit bones. This movement takes more hamstring flexibility, or alternatively more momentum, than the previous posture. Again, lift your heart, take your head back, and arrest the inhalation to capture the point of balance.

Exhaling, draw your legs in toward the torso, closing the gap between them. Deepen the groins, point the feet, and gaze up to your toes. Hold this *vinyasa* for five breaths.

Exhaling, release the feet, leave your legs in position and place your hands on the floor.

***Vinyasa* Ten**	Inhaling, lift off and swing through, clearing the floor.
***Vinyasa* Eleven**	Exhaling, lower into *Chaturanga Dandasana*.
***Vinyasa* Twelve**	Inhale into Upward Dog.
***Vinyasa* Thirteen**	Exhale into Downward Dog.

Setu Bandhasana

BRIDGE POSTURE

Drishti Nose

Vinyasa Seven

Inhaling, glide through to *Dandasana*. Exhaling, lie down.

Vinyasa Eight

With the buttocks grounded, arch your chest up to the ceiling and place the crown of your head on the floor. Keep the heels together and laterally rotate the femurs until the outer arches of the feet touch the floor. Now bend the knees so that the heels are approximately twenty inches from the buttocks, still keeping the heels together. This distance will vary greatly, depending on flexibility and leg length. Finally, cross your arms upon the chest and place each hand in the opposite armpit.

Vinyasa Nine

Inhaling, extend your legs and lift the buttocks off the floor. Roll onto your forehead and gaze toward the nose. Do not contract the muscles in the back of the neck (the neck extensors — trapezius,

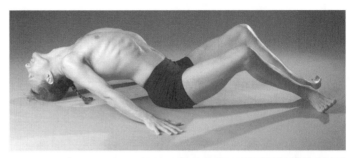

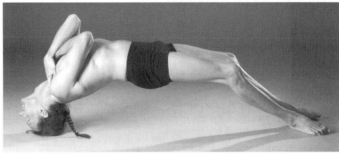

Top, *Setu Bandhasana, vinyasa* eight, variation for beginners; above, *vinyasa* nine, final version

levator scapulae, splenius capitis) but keep the neck flexors (scaleni, sternocleidomastoideus) active to control the amount of extension and thereby protect the neck (see "The Paradox of Active Release," page 73). Open the front of the throat. Lift your chest up into your arms with the elbows rising toward the ceiling, rather than taking the weight of the arms onto the chest. Keep the hip joint extended by using your buttocks (gluteus maximus) rather than your hamstrings, which easily spasm in this posture. The body becomes a bridge, arching from the feet to the head.

VARIATIONS FOR BEGINNERS

If you have suffered a whiplash injury, have other neck problems, or your neck is not sufficiently strong, it is suggested that you stay in *vinyasa* eight until the condition improves.

If you wish to go a step further, from *vinyasa* eight take your arms out to the side, palms down. With the arms in this position, straighten your legs. This arm position assists in carrying the weight of the torso and provides greater stability. Do this version for some time to allow your neck to strengthen.

To progress even deeper into the posture, from *vinyasa* eight place the hands on the floor on either side of your head, fingers pointing toward the feet. You can now carry part of the weight with your arms while you explore rolling farther toward your

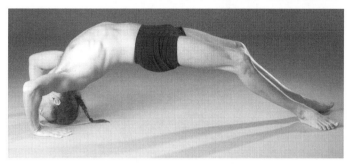

Setu Bandhasana, vinyasa nine, variations for beginners:
top, arms out to side; above, hands beside head

forehead. Again, allow yourself the time to feel
competent in this version before attempting the
final arm position.

If performed correctly *Setu Bandhasana* realigns
the neck.

Vinyasa **Ten**

Exhaling, exactly reverse the movements that took
you into the posture. Do not roll back down off your
head, which would place too much pressure on the
cervical vertebrae. Instead, retain the back arch and
place the buttocks down close to your head. Now
lift the chest and head and lie down, straightening
the legs and returning them to a neutral position by
medially rotating the thighs.

Vinyasa **Eleven**

This is the second posture that, when completed,
has us lying on our backs. As in *Supta
Padangushtasana*, exit this posture through
Chakrasana. If this is too difficult, rock up to sitting
and hop back to *Chaturanga Dandasana*.

Vinyasa Twelve   Inhale into Upward Dog.
Vinyasa Thirteen Exhale into Downward Dog.

Urdhva Dhanurasana
UPWARD BOW POSTURE

Drishti Nose

Prerequisite: K. Pattabhi Jois contends that students
need to be able to perform all postures up to this
point proficiently before embarking on intense backbending. He explains that a subtle nerve (*nadi*) at the
base of the skull can be damaged if backbending is
undertaken without this preparation.

Forward bending and opening the hip joints
create a platform from where we venture into more
complex actions. *Marichyasana* D, *Supta Kurmasana*,
and *Garbha Pindasana* create the core strength that is
necessary before attempting more intense backbending exercises, like dropping back from standing.

Please note that *Urdhva Dhanurasana* is absent not
only from *Yoga Mala* but also from other old lists of
the Primary Series. The inclusion of *Urdhva
Dhanurasana* in the Primary Series appears to be a
later interpolation.

Vinyasa **Seven**

Inhaling, glide through to *Dandasana* and lie down.

Vinyasa **Eight**

Exhaling, bend the legs and draw the heels toward
the buttocks. Place the feet down parallel and hip-
width apart. Now place the hands on the floor on
either side of your head, middle fingers parallel and

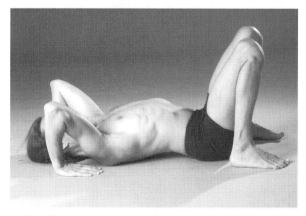

Urdhva Dhanurasana, vinyasa eight

pointing toward the feet. Spread your fingers. With
the last of the exhalation, lift the torso off the floor
just half an inch or so.

Vinyasa **Nine**

With the inhalation, in a flowing movement straighten your arms and legs and raise the torso into the air. Do not suck the air in, but breathe in smoothly. Do not thrust the body up, which can lead to strain of the shoulder joints, the sacrum, and the spinal fascia.

There is a tendency for many students to turn out the feet and to splay the knees open to the sides with the thighs rolled out. This is a compensation for the sacrum. If the piriformis spasms from overuse, the sacrum can no longer float in the sacroiliac joints and becomes fixed.

The subtle movements of the sacrum act as a pump, which stimulates the flow of cerebrospinal fluid between the protective layers of the spinal cord. Our brain floats in cerebrospinal fluid, which is responsible for nourishing it and the spinal cord, as well as protecting it by acting as a shock absorber.

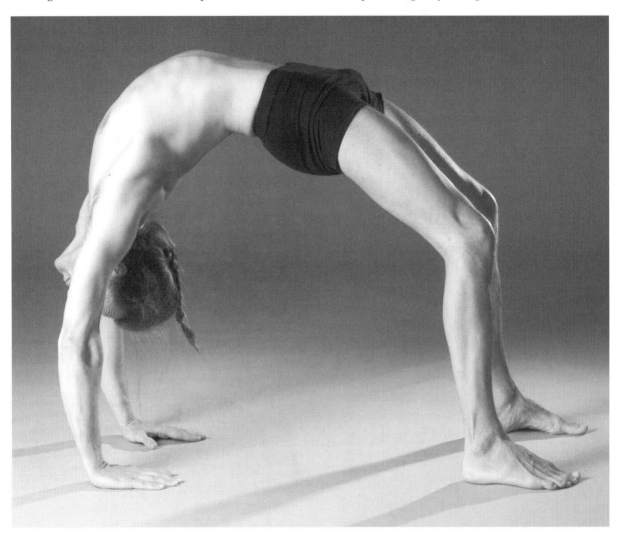

Urdhva Dhanurasana, vinyasa nine

stiffness in the quadriceps and/or psoas muscles. By opening into the inseams of the legs, more space is gained without having to stretch the hip flexors. Although this may achieve a short-term goal, in the long run it can lead to jamming the sacrum, which leads to low-back pain. Rolling out the thighs engages the lateral hip rotator muscles, one of which, the piriformis, originates via ligaments at

Jamming the sacrum not only impairs vertebral motion (domino effect) but also inhibits the flow of vital cerebrospinal fluid. This creates difficulties for everything from doing the daily chores to engaging in the subtle work of meditation.

This tendency to turn out the feet and thighs is counteracted by medially rotating the femurs until a neutral position of the legs is found. Medial rotation

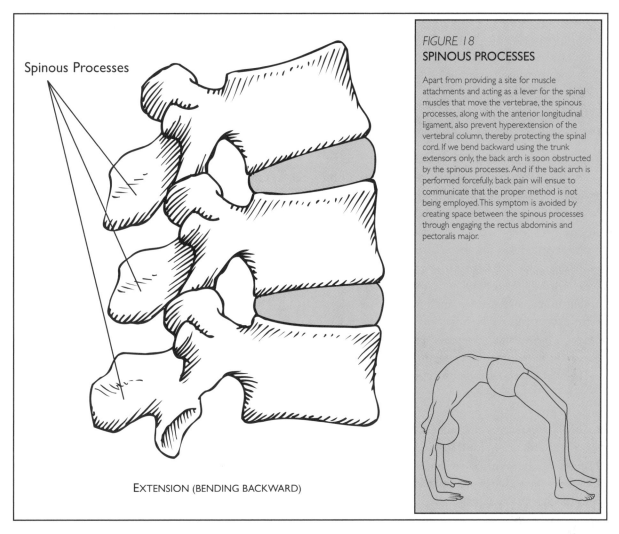

Spinous Processes

EXTENSION (BENDING BACKWARD)

FIGURE 18
SPINOUS PROCESSES

Apart from providing a site for muscle attachments and acting as a lever for the spinal muscles that move the vertebrae, the spinous processes, along with the anterior longitudinal ligament, also prevent hyperextension of the vertebral column, thereby protecting the spinal cord. If we bend backward using the trunk extensors only, the back arch is soon obstructed by the spinous processes. And if the back arch is performed forcefully, back pain will ensue to communicate that the proper method is not being employed. This symptom is avoided by creating space between the spinous processes through engaging the rectus abdominis and pectoralis major.

of the femur is achieved by the tensor fascia latae, gracilis, semitendinosus and semimembranosus (two of the hamstrings), and the gluteus minimus muscles. With this leg position, the hip flexor muscles (rectus femoris and psoas) will be stretched, which is necessary for real progress in backbends. All four corners of the feet will then be equally anchored.

To open the chest we again need to prevent the compensation of the armpits turning out to the side. This is achieved through lateral rotation of the humerus, which is performed by the infraspinatus muscle.

Before animals walked upright, the spine was horizontal like a table, evenly supported on all four corners by four limbs. With an upright stance, the pelvic girdle, the thorax, and the shoulder girdle protect most of the spine not only from attackers but also from overzealous yoga students. One area that conspicuously lacks any protection, however, is the lumbar spine. Since the low back is the softest

region, the novice will freely "push" into it, trying to "conquer" the backbend.

Instead, breathe into those areas that are tight, usually the chest and the front of the thighs, and soften and release them. Simultaneously, support those areas that are weak and soft. This is usually the low back, which needs to be protected by the firm corset of abdominal muscles (external and internal obliques, rectus and transverse abdominis). Additionally, the low back and neck already assume a natural lordotic curve (see figure 1, page 23), and overcontraction of these areas in backbends can lead to muscle spasm.

Similarly to the case of Upward Facing Dog, cultivate the support strength of the four pillars: your arms and legs. Once the torso is lifted into the backward arch, the work of the arms and legs conspires to lift the spine higher into the air, lengthening the trunk and alleviating any compression of the vertebrae.

Imagine your trunk as a canopy billowing up, mounted on four strong and anchored supports. Protect the neck by lengthening rather than contracting it and releasing the crown of the head in the direction of the floor.

To Progress Deeper into Backbending:

Once you have lifted into *Urdhva Dhanurasana* and feel you have reached your limit, release some of the tension on those muscles that transported you into the posture and instead engage their antagonists. Around the shoulder girdle, this means releasing the trapezius and deltoideus muscles by engaging the pectoralis major and latissimus dorsi. Along the trunk, release the erector spinae and quadratus lumborum by engaging the abdominals, especially rectus abdominis. At the hips, release the gluteus maximus by engaging the psoas and, in the legs, release the hamstrings by engaging the quadriceps.

This method of releasing the opposites is important for the following reasons:

- The back extensors contract and shorten the back. This is a useful action for transiting into *Urdhva Dhanurasana*, but it has its limitations. Continued beyond the objective of arching the back, the movement pinches the spinous processes of the vertebrae together, which prevents any further backward movement.

- To create a deeper backbend, we therefore need to lengthen the spine and back. This action is performed by the rectus abdominis, psoas, and pectoralis major, all on the front of the torso.

- When pushing up into a backbend, the main muscles that are overcontracted are those in the low back, this being the softest area of the spine. The quadratus lumborum is released and lengthened by engaging the psoas and rectus abdominis.

- At the commencement of yoga practice, the rib cage of the practitioner often has a wooden and dormant quality. Yogic breathing and backbends help to make it soft and pulsating, ensuring healthy functioning of the vital organs in the thoracic cavity and increasing tidal volume — the amount of air exchanged during normal respiration. With engagement of the pectoralis major muscles, the chest awakens and will open.

How to Achieve These Movements:

Maintain the support of those muscles that carried you into the posture (back extensors, shoulder flexors, hip extensors, and leg flexors) and then engage their antagonists to move deeper into the posture. To engage the pectoralis major in order to open the chest and armpits, make a swiping movement with your hands toward the end of the mat. This action brings the sternum toward the wrists or beyond, as the armpits and chest open.

Now, without compensating, walk your hands in toward your feet. Here engage the quadriceps as if you wanted to flex the hip joint. In this position, however, the hip joint cannot flex, as flexion is prevented by the hip extensor muscles. The quadriceps therefore deeply release and their work straightens the legs. Take up the space gained by bringing hands and feet closer together. Now come up onto the tips of your toes and lift your chest high above your shoulders. Keeping this newly gained height, lengthen your heels down to the floor again.

Engage your abdominal muscles now and use this contraction to lift the entire torso up to the ceiling. Engaging your abdominals will draw the spinous processes of the vertebrae apart. Deepen your backbend now by creating space underneath you.

Ensure throughout that the armpits, thighs, knees, and feet do not roll out. Take the stretch into the quadriceps and the rest of the front of the body.

Feel how the inhalations taken into the front of the chest and underneath the collarbones soften and open the rib cage. During the entire backbend the gaze is toward the nose. This *drishti* helps to prevent overcontracting the neck. Rather than taking the head back to look down to your hands, drop the crown of the head and lengthen the back of the neck.

Engage the latissimus dorsi, which works together with the pectoralis major to extend the arms. The latissimus dorsi also has the capacity to depress the entire shoulder girdle (drawing the shoulder blades down the back). With this function it is the antagonist to the trapezius and levator scapulae muscles. By depressing the scapulae, the trapezius is released and the neck and upper back lengthen. The action of the latissimus dorsi together with the pectoralis major draws the spinous processes of the thoracic spine apart. This arches the chest and enables you to open behind the heart.

Yoga students are sometimes seen standing in *Samasthiti* with a proudly swelled chest as if attending an army parade. The military attention posture

are right in the middle of everything: that everything just is and nothing needs to be conquered. This stance relates to suspended mind, which occurs when the breath enters the central channel, which is also called the heart, the devourer of mind.

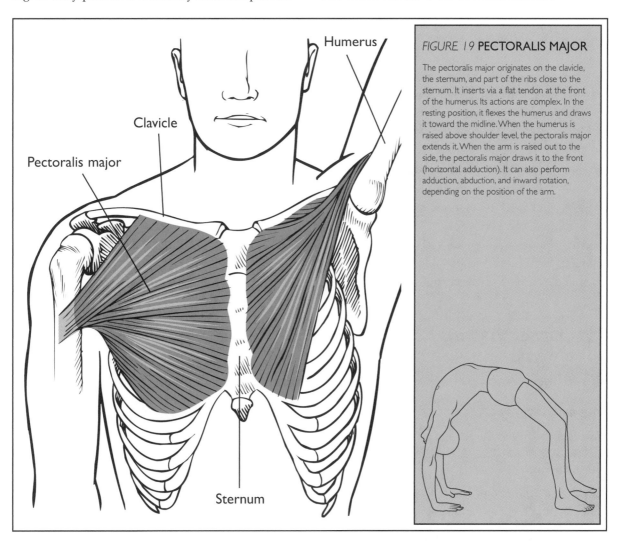

FIGURE 19 **PECTORALIS MAJOR**

The pectoralis major originates on the clavicle, the sternum, and part of the ribs close to the sternum. It inserts via a flat tendon at the front of the humerus. Its actions are complex. In the resting position, it flexes the humerus and draws it toward the midline. When the humerus is raised above shoulder level, the pectoralis major extends it. When the arm is raised out to the side, the pectoralis major draws it to the front (horizontal adduction). It can also perform adduction, abduction, and inward rotation, depending on the position of the arm.

consists of lifting and stretching the rib cage forward as character armor and fortification. This is achieved by hardening behind the heart, which gets us ready for combat. Anatomically this is done through contracting the trapezius and rhomboideus. The rhomboideus adducts the scapulae (pulls the shoulder blades in toward the spine).

In yoga the area behind the heart needs to stay as open as the sky. Closing off behind the heart makes us focus on what needs to be conquered in front of us. This is a function of the solar mind (related to Surya Nadi, the solar energy channel). In contrast, opening behind the heart allows us to see that we

To stay open behind the heart in this particular posture we need to release the rhomboids by contracting their antagonist muscle, serratus anterior. Serratus anterior has widely fallen into disgrace and misuse. It is this muscle that sets the shoulder blades wide whenever weight is borne in the hands; it is therefore also a key muscle in Downward Dog and the arm balances. In all of these postures, the position of the shoulder blades needs to be depressed (latissimus dorsi) and abducted (serratus anterior).

The vigorous action of latissimus dorsi has a side effect, which is inward rotation of the humerus (arm bone). The "lats" share this effect with subscapularis and teres major. This medial rotation of the humerus lets the armpits flare out to the sides, an action that allows the shoulders to move up to the ears and ultimately decreases the backbend. This action needs to be counteracted by infraspinatus.

Caution: The proper alignment of the armpits must be assessed by a qualified teacher. The action of outward rotation, if overdone, can lead to chronic inflammation of the shoulder joint, especially in the case of someone who already has permanently outwardly rotated humeri.

Vinyasa **Ten**

Exhaling slowly, come down. Look up to the ceiling and place the back of the head down. Repeat *vinyasa*s eight to ten twice more, each time working deeper into the backbend.

After completion, we counteract the heating, stimulatory effects of backbending with the cooling, pacifying effects of forward bending.

Pashimottanasana

INTENSE WESTERN STRETCH

Drishti Toes

Vinyasa **Seven**

Inhaling, rock up to *Dandasana*.

Vinyasa **Eight**

Exhaling, reach forward and hold your feet. Inhaling, lift your chest and look up.

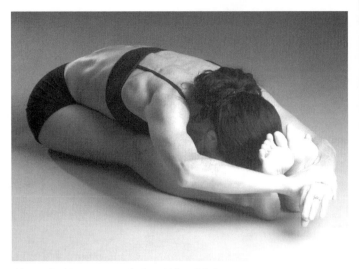

Above, *Pashimottanasana*; below, *Tadaga Mudra*

Vinyasa **Nine**

Exhale into *Pashimottanasana*. The posture can be held much longer here than at the beginning of the sequence. Especially after a long or strenuous practice it can be held for twenty or thirty breaths as a restorative *asana*.

Vinyasa **Ten**

Inhaling, lift your head and straighten your arms. Exhaling, lie down in *Tadaga Mudra*. *Tadaga* means tank or pond, and it is the stillness of a pond after the activity of backbends that is emulated here. The *mudra* resembles *Samasthiti* lying on one's back. Keep all the main muscle groups engaged and your eyes open. Hold *Tadaga Mudra* for ten breaths or until your breath has returned to its normal, resting ratio. The breath during the finishing *asana*s needs to be calm.

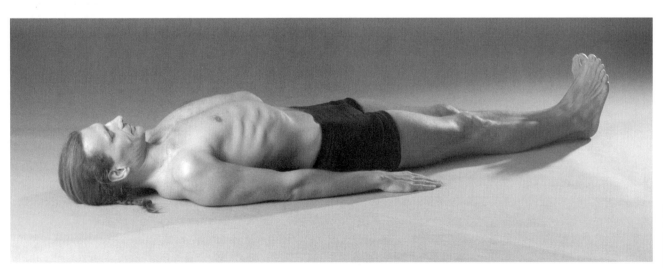

For *Sarvangasana, Halasana, Karnapidasana, Urdvha Padmasana, Pindasana, Matsyasana,* and *Uttana Padasana, vinyasa* seven is uncounted, since we are already lying on our backs.

Sarvangasana
All Limbs Posture

Drishti Nose

Vinyasa **Eight**

From *Tadaga Mudra*, lift your legs off the floor (hip flexion). The abdominals need to be well developed for this to be possible with legs straight. The weight of the legs will have the tendency to draw the pubic bone down in front, to tilt the pelvis anteriorly (forward), and thereby to concave the low back. This needs to be counteracted by contracting the rectus abdominis. If your abdominal muscles are not strong enough to hold the pubic bone down, lift the legs with bent knees.

Continue the lift until the hips come off the floor, extend the legs straight up to the ceiling, and point the feet. Keep the legs active and all postural muscles engaged to prevent the blood pooling down toward the head. Inversions are not relaxation postures.

Place the hands onto the low back with the forearms parallel. As you progress, slowly move your hands up toward the shoulder blades to open the chest. Proceed with care, as this increases neck flexion.

None of the cervical vertebrae should be in contact with the floor. Excess pressure on the neck can lead to headaches, wrist pain, a loss of natural lordotic neck curvature (see figure 1, page 23) and/or the condition called forward head (see under *Samasthiti*, page 23). If you already have forward head, abstain from *Sarvangasana* until you have corrected the condition through backbending. To take

Right, *Sarvangasana*

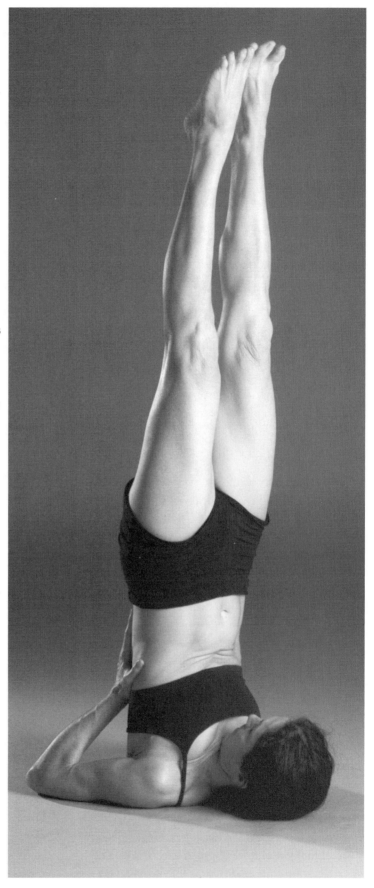

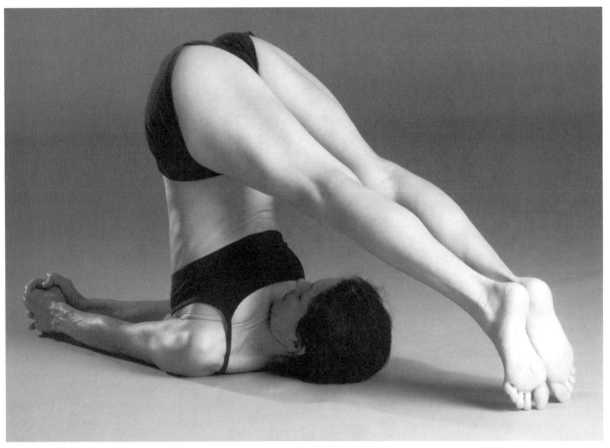

Halasana

weight off the neck, gently press the elbows, shoulders, forearms, and back of the head into the floor. If you cannot keep the back of the neck off the floor, use one or two folded blankets under the shoulders and elbows.

Create a feeling of lightness and reach the entire torso and legs up to the ceiling. If your feet are over your head, shift them to come in line with your torso. This will take weight away from the head and toward the elbows.

Sarvangasana provides a great vantage point for viewing the freely fluctuating stomach area versus the non-oscillating area of the lower abdomen from the application of *Uddiyana Bandha* with *Ujjayi Pranayama*.

Sarvangasana improves blood circulation and keeps the blood vessels, the heart, and the lungs youthful. It has a general toning affect and is rejuvenating. After strenuous practice this posture can be held for longer periods. Inversions are not practiced during menstruation because they can interrupt normal menstrual flow. High blood pressure and wrist pain are contraindications for *Sarvangasana*.

Halasana

PLOUGH POSTURE

Drishti Nose

Vinyasa Eight

Exhaling, from *Sarvangasana* lower your straight legs slowly down toward the floor. Do this only by flexing the hip joints and without bending the back. If your feet do not reach the floor due to stiff hamstring muscles, keep them hovering above the ground. In stiff students, especially those with underdeveloped abdominal muscles, arching the back here with the great weight of the legs places excessive stress on the intervertebral discs of the spine. This could lead to a disc bulge if one forces the feet down.

Let the sit bones reach up to the ceiling. Touch the legs down lightly by carrying most of their weight with the back. Keep drawing up on the kneecaps. Initially you can flex your feet to reach the floor; once established in the posture, point the feet. Interlock the fingers, straighten the arms, and draw the hands down toward the floor. Lift all cervical vertebrae off the floor. Use *Uddiyana Bandha* to distribute breath into the chest.

Karnapidasana
KNEES-TO-THE-EARS POSTURE

Drishti Nose

Vinyasa Eight

Exhaling, from *Halasana* bend the legs around the back and place the knees next to the ears. Release the knees down toward the floor. Keeping the hands interlocked as in *Halasana*, point your feet and bring them together. This is the strongest trunk flexion in the sequence. Breathe freely although the chest is compressed.

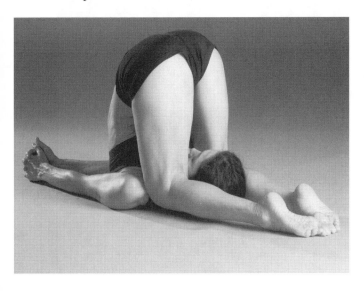

Urdhva Padmasana
UPWARD LOTUS POSTURE

Drishti Nose

As with some other postures, there is some confusion concerning the *vinyasa* count in *Urdhva Padmasana*. *Yoga Mala* states that we arrive at count eight in the state of this *asana*, whereas Ashtanga Yoga lists the posture as *vinyasa* nine. I have followed *Yoga Mala*, since it represents the older source.

Vinyasa Eight

Inhaling, from *Karnapidasana* straighten your legs back up into *Sarvangasana*, extending the spine first and then the hip joints.

Vinyasa Nine

Exhaling, place first the right leg and then the left into *Padmasana*. This posture should only be attempted after proficiency in *Padmasana* is gained. At first use the assistance of one hand while the other stabilizes the posture.

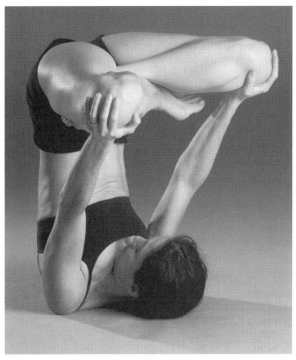

Left, *Karnapidasana*; above, *Urdhva Padmasana*

Once in *Padmasana*, bring your thighs parallel to the floor and place the hands under your knees. Now balance on the solid tripod of your shoulders and the back of the head. Keep the cervical vertebrae off the floor by grounding down through the three corners of your tripod base while reaching the sit bones up to the ceiling.

Pindasana
EMBRYO POSTURE

Drishti Nose

Vinyasa Nine

Exhaling, fold the lotus down into the chest. Draw your knees closer together so that the thighs become parallel. This will draw the feet farther up into the groins. Reach around your thighs and clasp your hands or, if possible, your wrists. It is more difficult here to lift the lower cervical vertebrae off the ground. Rolling down a little onto the upper back can alleviate the problem.

Matsyasana
FISH POSTURE

Drishti Nose

Vinyasa Nine

Inhaling, release the arms and lower the back down to the floor. Extend the hip joints and place the knees onto the floor. Holding the feet, lift the chest up to the ceiling, arch the back, and place the crown of your head on the floor. Keeping hold of the feet, straighten your arms and continue to lift the heart to the ceiling. *Matsyasana* opens the throat and enhances the lordotic curvature of the neck, these having been reversed during the shoulder-stand sequence. Seen from the top, the posture has the shape of a fish, with the head and the shoulders forming the head of the fish, the bent legs representing the tail and the arms the dorsal and caudal fins.

Uttana Padasana
INTENSE LEG POSTURE

Drishti Nose

Vinyasa Eight

Inhaling with your torso and head held in the same position as for *Matsyasana*, unfold your legs from lotus and straighten them out 30° over the floor. Extend your arms out at the same angle with the palms together. The abdominals work strongly here as they carry the weight of the legs, which will want to tilt the pelvis anteriorly. Breathe into the chest, as breathing into the abdomen would destabilize the low back. This is not a posture for beginners. The abdominal muscles need to be prepared by slowly adding on the preceding postures of the Primary Series.

Vinyasa Nine

Inhaling, lift the head and straighten the neck. Exhaling, lower the legs over the head into *Halasana*. Place the hands down on either side of the head

and, exiting the posture via *Chakrasana*, lift over into *Chaturanga Dandasana*.

Vinyasa **Ten**   Inhale into Upward Dog.
Vinyasa **Eleven**   Exhale into Downward Dog.

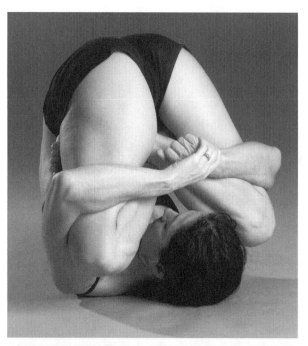

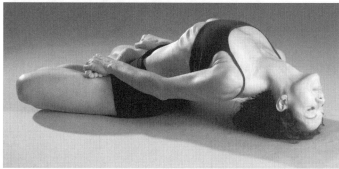

Top, *Pindasana*; above, *Matsyasana*

Shirshasana
HEADSTAND

Drishti Nose

Vinyasa Seven

Inhaling, bend the knees and, exhaling, place the elbows down onto the floor. Check for the correct width of your elbows by wrapping your hands around them: at the correct distance your knuckles will be on the outsides of the elbows. Without changing the position of your elbows, release the grip of your hands and interlace your fingers. Place both

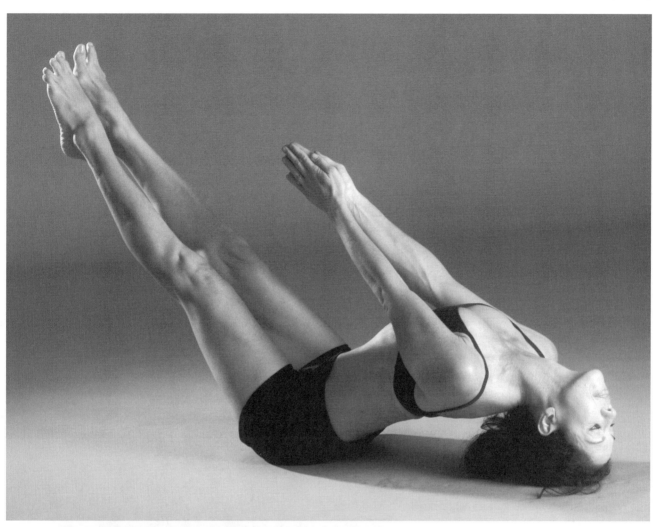

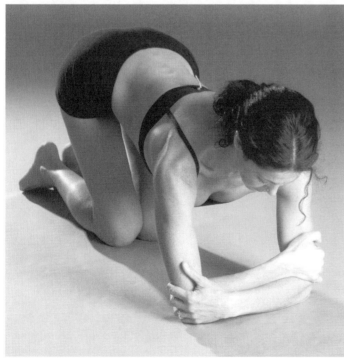

little fingers on the floor — not on top of each other — and separate your wrists. Be sure to keep your hands and wrists upright (perpendicular to the floor) by not rolling over onto the backs of your hands. This forms a strong tripod for support and balance. Keep the shoulders broad and the neck long and press the floor away with your forearms. This is the grounding action necessary in *Shirshasana*. The underneath side of the wrists is the point of balance.

Stability in a headstand depends on the distance between your fingers and the center point between your elbows. The more the elbows flare out to the sides, the shorter this distance becomes, and the headstand becomes accordingly less stable.

Top, *Uttana Padasana*
Left, *Shirshasana, vinyasa* seven

121

If your humeri (arm bones) are not longer than the distance between the base of your neck and the crown of your head, the described arm position will compress the neck. If this is the case, press the heels of your hands together and allow the elbows to come apart. This will position your head more centrally in the triangle and the humeri will be perpendicular to the floor. This better accommodates the length of the upper arms, but the shortened stance makes this arm position less stable and thereby more challenging.

Place the highest point of your head down onto the mat with the back of the head resting against your palms. If instead you were to balance on your forehead, you would induce excessive cervical curvature and compress the vertebrae of the neck. The point of the head, which is the highest point in *Samasthiti*, needs to touch the floor. In fact most instructions for *Samasthiti* and *Shirshasana* are identical.

To come to the upside-down position, straighten your legs and walk the feet in toward the head. Keep the grounding of your tripod as you walk your feet in as close as possible while extending your sit bones high toward the ceiling. The sit bones will travel backward beyond the head, so that the back is slightly in extension. Now take all of your body weight onto your arms: the head should only lightly touch the floor. K. Pattabhi Jois instructs students not to place weight on the head, and in *Yoga Mala* he declares that, if we hold *Shirshasana* by carrying the body weight on the head, this will impinge on our intellectual development. Furthermore there is the possibility of damaging the subtle *nadi*s in the brain.[20]

Vinyasa Eight

Inhaling, slowly raise the straight legs up toward the ceiling, extending the hip joints by engaging the gluteus maximus. Breathe slowly and keep the lower abdomen firm. Rapid breathing, especially into the abdomen, destabilizes all inversions. Keep your hands relaxed to the point that you can still wriggle your fingers. If the fingers are squeezed together in an attempt to hold the posture what often follows is that too much weight is placed on

20. K. Pattabhi Jois, *Yoga Mala*, 1st English ed., Eddie Stern/Patanjala Yoga Shala, New York, 1999, p. 126.

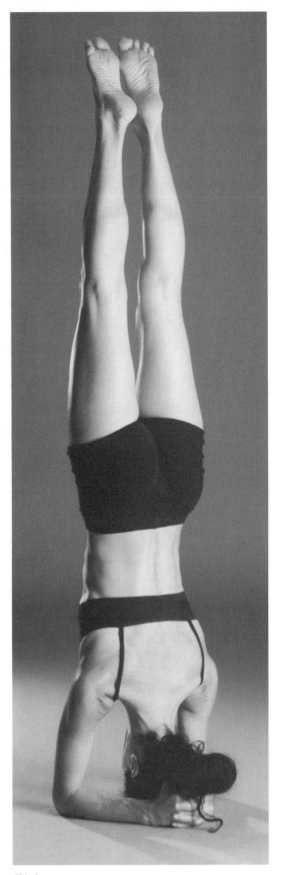

Shirshasana

the elbows and the elbows are positioned too widely. To balance, press the wrists down into the ground and evenly distribute your body weight between the elbows and the hands.

Set the shoulder blades wide (abduction of the scapulae by serratus anterior — see *Urdhva Dhanurasana*, page 111). Then draw the scapulae toward the hips by contracting the latissimus dorsi. Initially this movement can be difficult without placing more weight on the head, as it requires a developed latissimus dorsi muscle.

To open the chest, reach the armpits toward the wall in front of you. This will eliminate the hump that might exist in the upper back around T6. The entire trunk and the legs are kept active and reach to the ceiling. The feet are pointed (plantar flexion).

Performed in this way, *Shirshasana* is a great posture for meditation. Open yourself to the fact that it is easier to maintain than standing on your feet! We have forgotten how much effort we put into learning to walk. The center of gravity is much lower in *Shirshasana* than when standing on one's feet, and therefore balancing is easier. The arms, elbows, head, and hands cover a much larger area than the feet, which potentially makes the posture steadier than standing upright.

Much was said in medieval Hatha scriptures about the capacity of the headstand and shoulder stand to "conquer" death and gain immortality. This is thought to happen in the following way: The subtle moon is situated in the body inside the head, precisely at the upper back of the soft palate. This is also the end of the *sushumna*, called *brahmarandhra*, the gate of Brahman. Anatomically this location is close to where the cranium joins the spine. From this "moon" the cooling nectar of immortality, called *amrita* (*mrta* = death, *a-mrta* = deathlessness), is thought to trickle down. This nectar is also utilized in other techniques such as *Nabho* and *Kechari Mudra*.

The subtle "sun" in the body is located in the stomach, where the gastric fire (*agni*) is seated. The nectar of immortality exuded by the moon trickles down onto the sun, where it is consumed by its gastric fire. When the nectar is eventually exhausted, death is imminent. With the body inverted in space, the sun is placed above the moon. Gravity now

inhibits the flow of *amrita*, so that it can be reabsorbed. Immortality or extension of the life span was thought to be the result. The preoccupation with physical immortality is, however, a fairly recent development in yogic history. As Mircea Eliade has shown,[21] it only gained momentum after 1000 CE. In the original yoga tradition, immortality was gained by realizing that which itself is deathless: the *purusha* (consciousness).

The identification with the body is called egoism. The body is a manifestation of our past experiences,

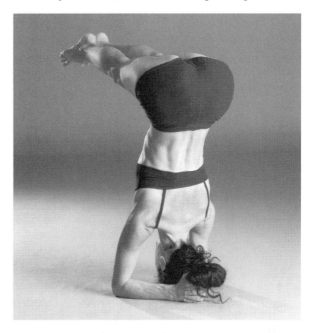

Urdhva Dandasana (see next page)

including our hurts, ambitions, and limitations. Why would we endeavor to hold on to the bars of our prison cell forever, when we could be free? Why should we carry a huge anvil on our shoulder when we could spread our wings and fly? The body is a statement that "I am separate from deep reality (Brahman)," as Shankara has sufficiently demonstrated. According to the *Samkhya Karika*, "As a potter's wheel continues its movement even after the potter has ceased his effort, so the body will complete its natural course. Then after true knowledge is gained, no more physical manifestation will happen." The body is surrendered when the ocean of infinite consciousness is entered. This is yogic immortality. The ancient yoga has been taught in

21. Mircea Eliade, *Yoga — Immortality and Freedom*, 2nd ed., Princeton University Press, Princeton, New Jersey, 1969.

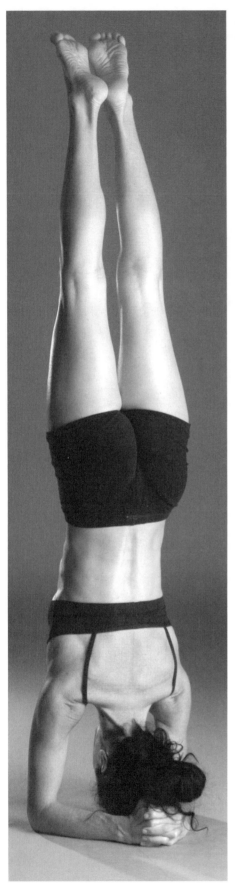

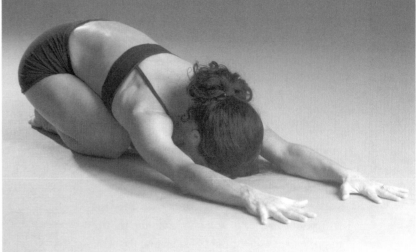

Left, *Shirshasana* lift off; above, *Balasana*

this way in the *Upanishads*, and by the great masters such as Kapila, Patanjali, Vyasa, and Shankara. Medieval attempts to seek freedom by the very thing that binds us are manifestations of the Kali Yuga.

Shirshasana is a very useful posture for purifying the blood, the heart, and the lungs. It also helps to develop an awareness of the center of the body, which is useful in all other postures. Slowly extend the time spent in *Shirshasana*, twenty-five breaths being sufficient at first. After a longer, more strenuous practice more time in *Shirshasana* is recommended.

Vinyasa **Nine**

Exhaling, lower your legs, keeping them straight, until they are parallel to the floor. This posture — *Urdhva Dandasana* (inverted rod) — develops the hip extensors (mainly gluteus maximus) and the back extensors (erector spinae and quadratus lumborum). The sit bones have to travel backward beyond the back of the head to keep the balance. The spine is held slightly in extension and the chest is open. Point the feet (plantar flexion) in this posture. Gaze to the nose and hold the posture for ten breaths.

Vinyasa **Ten**

Inhaling, lift the straight legs back up into *Shirshasana*. From here lift the head off the floor completely. This is initiated by pressing the elbows into the floor (flexion of the shoulder joint). You are now in a forearm balance with the crown of the head pointing straight down and the fingers interlocked. First look to the nose and later lift the chin to the sternum and look up to the navel. Open your chest and draw the shoulder blades out to the sides and up toward the ceiling. Hold *Uddiyana Bandha* strongly and hold the posture for ten breaths.

This posture is the ideal preparation for *Pincha Mayurasana* in the Intermediate Series. For those who want to perform the handstand later, the ability to hold the head clear off the floor in *Shirshasana* is a necessary preparation.

Vinyasa Eleven

Exhaling, gently replace your head to the floor and lower your straight legs to land silently on the floor. Bend the knees, take your hips back to rest on your heels, and place your forehead down on the floor. With your arms outstretched above your head, gently draw the shoulder blades down to release the neck muscles. We prostrate and surrender ourselves in this posture (*Balasana*, the child pose). *Balasana* facilitates pressure exchange in the head after *Shirshasana*. Depending on the length of the headstand, we may hold *Balasana* for between ten breaths and two minutes. K. Pattabhi Jois stresses that, if one does not keep the head on the floor for some time to allow for pressure exchange, damage to the brain and nervous system can occur.

Vinyasa Twelve

Inhaling, straighten the arms and legs. Exhaling, lower into *Chaturanga Dandasana*.

Vinyasa Thirteen   Inhale into Upward Dog.
Vinyasa Fourteen   Exhale into Downward Dog.

Padmasana
LOTUS POSTURE

Drishti Nose

Padmasana is the principal yoga posture. Such benefits as the destruction of all diseases, to conquering death, to crossing the ocean of conditioned existence are all enthusiastically ascribed to it.

Vinyasa Seven

Inhaling, jump through to *Dandasana*.

Vinyasa Eight

Exhaling from a straight-legged position, fold first the right leg into *Padmasana*. To do this safely, flex the right knee joint completely by drawing the right heel to the right buttock. If this is not possible, do not attempt *Padmasana*, but instead sit cross-legged. If you

can touch your heel to your buttock, let the right knee fall out to the side, pointing and inverting the right foot. Now draw the right heel into the right groin to ensure that the knee joint remains completely flexed in this abducted position. From here lift the right heel in toward the navel, bringing the knee closer to the

> **YOGIC CONTEXT**
> Padmasana: *Right Leg First*
>
> Why is *Padmasana* traditionally done only by first placing the right leg and then bringing the left leg on top? When asked this question, K. Pattabhi Jois quoted the *Yoga Shastra* as saying, "Right side first and left leg on top purifies liver and spleen. Left leg first and right leg on top is of no use at all." He also explained that the lotus done in this way stimulates insulin production.
>
> Contemporary teachers have suggested performing *Padmasana* on both sides to balance the body. Improving the symmetry of the body is achieved through the standing postures. However, the postures that strongly influence the abdominal and thoracic cavities, such as *Padmasana, Kurmasana, Dvi Pada Shirshasana*, and *Pashasana*, do not have the function of making the body symmetrical, but of accommodating the asymmetry of the abdominal and thoracic organs. To accommodate the fact that the liver is in the right side of the abdominal cavity and the spleen in the left, the right leg is first placed into position with the left leg on top. As leg-behind-the-head postures develop the chest, to place the left leg first in *Kurmasana* accommodates the fact that the heart is predominantly in the left side of the thoracic cavity.

midline. Keeping the heel in line with the navel, place the ball of the foot into the opposite groin.

Repeat these steps on the left, as if the right leg were still straight. First flex the knee joint completely until the underneath of the thigh touches the back of the leg over its entire length. Drawing the knee far out to the left, lift the left foot over the right ankle in toward the navel. Do not lift the left foot over the right knee, as this would mean opening the left knee joint, which would induce lateral movement into the knee during the transition.

Sitting in *Padmasana*, inwardly rotate your femurs until the front edges of the tibias point downward and the soles and heels of the feet face upward. In this way the knee joints are completely closed and thereby protected. Do not sit in *Padmasana* and retain the initial lateral rotation of the femurs used to enter the posture.

YOGIC CONTEXT

The Importance of Baddha Padmasana

Baddha Padmasana is a very potent meditation posture. In the scriptures it is suggested that the yogi prepare a seat from *kusha* grass, place a deerskin or, better, a tiger skin over it, and a clean white cotton cloth on top. This set-up was suggested to me on several occasions during my studies in India. Such an elaborate meditation seat is used for the purpose of insulation. Energy always flows from the highest to the lowest potential. As the earth is receptive, the energy will flow from the body of the yogi into the ground. For this reason, insulation is suggested to preserve energy for the rising of *kundalini*. *Mula Bandha* is done for similar reasons. It prevents energy leaking out from the base of the spine.

The habit of yogis to meditate in the Himalayas must be seen in a similar light. The higher up into the mountains we go, the more the receptive pull of the earth decreases and the easier it is for *kundalini* to rise. We most readily lose energy from the palms of our hands and the soles of our feet. For this reason the soles are turned up away from the ground in *Padmasana*. In *Baddha Padmasana* the hands are connected to the feet, and in this way an energy circuit is created. All energy is now recycled within the body, apart from the energy that leaves through the nine sensory gates (two eyes, two ears, two nostrils, the mouth, the generative organ, and the anus).

With your left arm, reach around your back and take the big toe of the left foot with the palm facing downward. The foot that is on top is bound first. Now bind the right big toe with your right hand, placing the right arm on top of the left arm on your back. This is *Baddha Padmasana*. If you experience difficulty binding, cross the arms above the elbows

rather than the forearms. This induces opening of the shoulders and the chest. A tight pectoralis minor muscle is the greatest obstacle here.

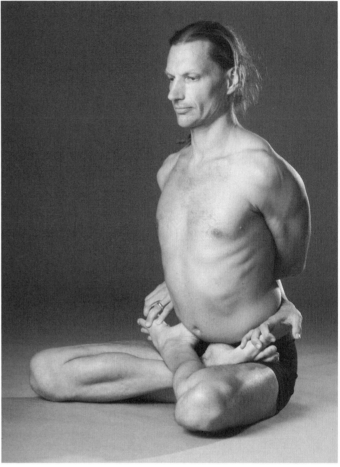

Baddha Padmasana

If you still encounter difficulties binding, look at the following areas:

• Hip rotation — the more we can inwardly rotate the femurs and bring the knees closer together, the more the feet will slide up into the groins. This brings the feet closer to the hands and thereby makes binding easier.

• Shoulder flexibility — if the shoulders are freed up, we can more easily roll them back to reach for the toes.

• We need to wrap the arms around the waist. The thinner the waist, the easier the task. Shedding excess weight can work miracles here, as is the case in *Kurmasana*.

Inhaling, lift the chest high, draw the shoulders back, and gaze upward.

Vinyasa **Nine**

Exhaling, fold forward, placing the forehead on the floor, and gaze toward the nose. With increasing proficiency you can place the chin onto the floor. Do not achieve this by jutting the chin forward and creasing the back of the neck. This blocks off energy and prevents *kundalini* from rising. Keep the back of the neck long and gaze up between the eyebrows.

- Ring finger represents *manas* (mind).
- Little finger represents *kaya* (body).

Placing your thumb and pointing finger together seals the intention of realizing that your true nature (*atman*) is nothing but infinite consciousness (Brahman).

You are now in the classic position for meditation. It is preferred over the simple cross-legged position. In *Padmasana* we sit on a solid base of sit bones,

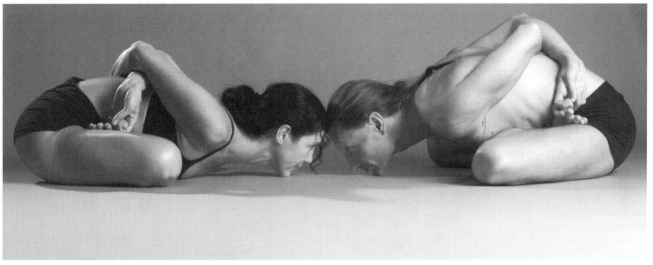

Yoga Mudra

Keep inwardly rotating the thigh bones here and let the crown of the head and the sit bones reach in opposite directions. The shoulder blades follow the sit bones. This posture is *Yoga Mudra* (seal of yoga), and it is one of the most effective ways of sealing within the body the energy cultivated during the practice. Hold the posture for ten to twenty-five breaths, depending on the length of your practice, while focusing on the *bandha*s.

Vinyasa **Ten**

Inhaling, come up, let go of the feet, and place the hands on the knees, palms facing upward in a receptive attitude. Keep the arms straight to align the shoulders and to make the spine steady. Place the hands into *Jnana Mudra* (seal of knowledge) by joining the thumb and pointing finger and extending the other fingers. The significance of the fingers is as follows:

- Thumb represents Brahman (infinite consciousness).
- Pointing finger represents *atman* (true nature).
- Middle finger represents *buddhi* (intellect).

thighs, and knees. This enables us to retain the natural double-S curve of the spine as if we were standing upright in *Samasthiti*.

Not only is this correct positioning of the spine required for *kundalini* to rise, it also promotes alertness. If we simply sit cross-legged, there is the tendency for the pelvis to tilt posteriorly, the heart to collapse, and the head to sink down toward the chest. Effort is required to avoid this slouching, which quickly leads to fatigue. If fatigue is present, meditation becomes difficult. Meditation is brightness and luminosity of the mind. If the mind is torpid during meditation, detrimental effects will result. (A more detailed discussion of meditation is given in part 4.)

To keep the mind alert, we need a posture in which the head can effortlessly be kept in line with the neck and the spine for an extended period of time. *Padmasana* is the ideal posture for this purpose.

Drop the chin slightly. Direct the gaze gently down toward the tip of the nose. Stay for at least twenty-five slow breaths.

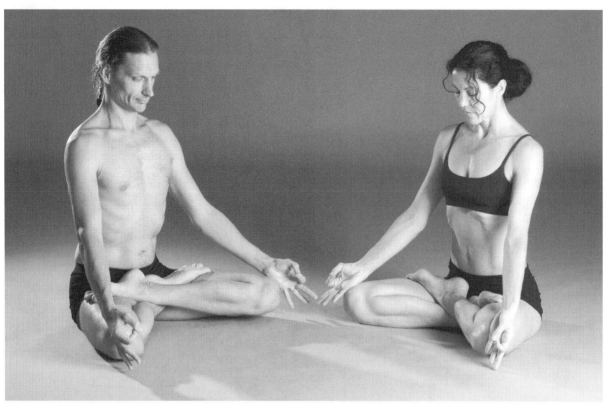

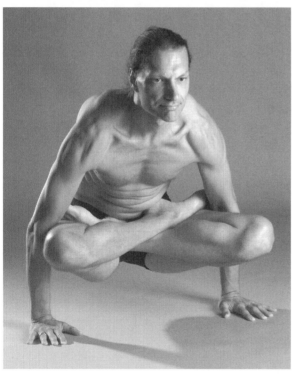

Top, *Padmasana* with *Jnana Mudra*
Above, *Utpluthi*

Vinyasa Eleven

Place the hands down on either side of the thighs with the fingers spread. Inhaling, lift the entire body off the floor into *Utpluthi* (uprooting).

The spine needs to curl to lift up, which involves flexing the trunk. This action is performed by the abdominal muscles, mainly the rectus abdominis. The shoulders are supporting by depressing the shoulder girdle (latissimus dorsi). Keep the breath ratio normal. This posture increases *bandha* control and helps in understanding the *vinyasa* movement. This is one of the best postures for restoring energy. It eliminates fatigue at the end of the practice.

Hold *Utpluthi* for twenty-five breaths, gazing toward the nose.

Vinyasa Twelve

Exhaling, swing through, fold out of lotus, and lower into *Chaturanga Dandasana*. The movement and its possible variations have been described under *Kukkutasana*, *vinyasa*s nine and ten (page 98).

Vinyasa Thirteen Inhale into Upward Dog.
Vinyasa Fourteen Exhale into Downward Dog.
Vinyasa Fifteen Inhaling, jump through.
Exhaling, lie down.

Shavasana
TAKE REST

No *drishti*, as eyes are closed.

K. Pattabhi Jois refers to this posture as "Taking Rest." Yogic literature, however, refers to it as *Shavasana* (corpse posture) or *Mritasana* (death posture). According to the *Hatha Yoga Pradipika*, "Lying down on the ground, like a corpse, is called *Shavasana*. It removes fatigue and gives rest to the mind."[22] The *Gheranda Samhita* agrees: "Lying flat on the ground like a corpse is called *Mritasana*. This posture destroys fatigue, and quiets the agitations of the mind."[23] Both treatises attribute to this posture not only recuperation but also the important function of calming the mind.

The Physical Importance of Relaxation

Shavasana is defined as the complete relaxation of body and mind. The relaxation of the body is important for the assimilation of *prana*. *Prana* occurs in the atmosphere. Attempts have been made to compare *prana* to solar wind and alpha rays.[24] The practice is most beneficial at sunrise and sunset, because pranic levels are then highest.[25] Only through accumulated *prana* is it possible to sustain the body for a long period of time. There are testimonies of yogis having been buried underground for up to a year and still being alive when disinterred. Although such feats are not the purpose of yoga, they are interesting in this context. Life is primarily sustained by *prana*,

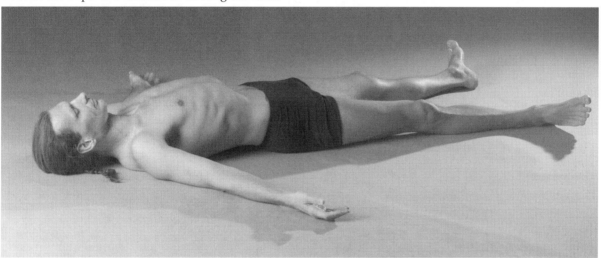

Shavasana

Shavasana is an intrinsic part of yoga practice. Through the practice we heat and purify the gross (physical) body and the subtle (energetic) body. After practice, the body needs time to cool and settle. To jump up immediately and commence our daily pursuits can make one agitated and nervous. The calming, centering, soothing effect of yoga practice can only arise when proper rest is taken afterward.

During the practice we are absorbed with doing; in *Shavasana* it is time to be established in non-doing, time to simply be. The mystical state that is the goal of yoga cannot be reached through activity; instead it arises through the cessation of all activity. This cessation is allowed during *Shavasana*.

22. *The Hatha Yoga Pradipika* I.34, trans. P. Sinh, Sri Satguru Publications, Delhi, 1915, p. 37.

23. *The Gheranda Samhita* II.11, trans. R.B.S. Chandra Vasu, Sri Satguru Publications, Delhi, 1986, p. 15.

and the Ashtanga Vinyasa practice is designed to store it in the body. The *Ujjayi* method turns the epiglottis into a valve, which increases the pranic pressure inside the body. The *bandha*s work like filters that skim the *prana* from the air we breathe. If we continue activity immediately after practice, the accumulated *prana* slowly leaks out of the body and is lost.

Shavasana gives us the chance to assimilate this *prana*. Through relaxation, the body, after it has been prepared through practice, becomes a receptive

24. Andre van Lysbeth, *Die grosse Kraft des Atems*, O.W. Barth Verlag, Munich, 1991.

25. From this we can infer that the pranic level is related to the position of the sun. This makes it likely that *prana* originates from the sun. Many religions and cultures worship the sun as a deity and the giver of life.

sponge that soaks it up. *Shavasana* is literally a bath in atmospheric *prana*. For this to happen we must let go completely.

The Mental Importance of Relaxation

The posture is called *Shavasana* because it prepares us for death. It teaches us to completely surrender and let go. When the time comes to die, this ability to completely cease doing — to surrender totally — will enable us to abandon all identification with this body, this personality, and this ego. Then we can separate from this life as easily as a cucumber separates from the vine.[26] Only the concepts we have of ourselves that cause us to desire some things and reject others, the I-am-ness, make us believe that this is our body. It is not ours at all. Have we created it? Even after centuries of scientific research we still cannot understand all aspects of the body, nor can we create a body. We have no certificate of ownership. When it is time to leave this world behind, we surrender this body back to nature (*prakrti*). Our body is created by nature and not by us, as *Yoga Sutra*s IV.2 and IV.3 affirm.

There is a Zen *koan* that says:

> Butterfly takes off
> To cross the lake
> I come back to myself

There has been much deliberation concerning the meaning of this *koan*. One reading is to equate the butterfly with the thought. If we let go of it, if it leaves us to cross the lake, then we can return into the self. If we hold on to it, then we are one with the fluctuations of the mind (sutra I.4). If we let the butterfly take off then we can abide in our true nature (sutra I.3).

But the butterfly can also be equated to the body and the lake to the division between life and death. The body crosses this division; I do not. If I manage to let go of the body, then I will abide again in my true nature — the eternal, immutable consciousness. If I hold on, this return is not possible, and I will seek a new embodiment.

In *Shavasana* all effort, all determination, all will fall away from us. This falling away, this complete surrender, simulates the process that needs to occur at death. We can say that each *Shavasana* is a preparation for the moment when not us but our corpse is doing the posture. Death may be frightening if we think we are the body. If we surrender, if we hand ourselves over, then it is an invitation to return to the true and natural state, which is consciousness. Following Lord Krishna's suggestion in *Bhagavad Gita*, we "surrender the sense of agency, since only a fool believes himself to be the doer."

The ancient masters taught that we are not the body, which is subject to death, but rather that we are the unborn, uncreated and unchanging. The death of the body invites us to come back to our true nature, which is consciousness. This letting go of artificial identification with what is impermanent is *Shavasana*. *Shavasana*, when done properly — as the letting go of everything — shows us what we truly are. Both the *Yoga Sutra* and the *Bhagavad Gita* state that the pure existence, pure awareness, pure being that is left at the end of the body is without beginning and end.

> It cannot be cut by knives,
> It cannot be pierced by thorns,
> It cannot be burned by fire,
> It cannot be drowned in water.
> It is eternal, the true self.

---

26. This metaphor is used in a traditional Indian prayer. The separation between the cucumber and the vine is peaceful and without external force, whereas fruit growing on a tree or bush is violently torn off by gravity.

Part 3

THE HISTORY AND LINEAGE OF YOGA

The history of yoga may be understood in terms of four phases. These could be further subdivided in the interests of greater precision, but for our present purposes that would involve us in too much detail. I am approaching this discussion from a historical perspective because it is one that Western readers can relate to. The four phases of yogic history I am calling "naturalism," "mysticism," "philosophy," and "technology."

Phase One — Naturalism

At the dawn of time, people lived in harmony with themselves and nature. The average person had contact with the truth inherent in us, our divine nature. Religion or philosophy was not needed very much because people saw truth, beauty, and value within themselves and their surroundings.

The scriptures compiled in this age were called the *Veda*s, of which the most important is the *Rig Veda*. It comprises hymns in appreciation of life, the body we have been given, and the earth we live on. It is because people lived simple and natural lives that I call this age "naturalism."

During the age of naturalism most people used the mind like a muscle: you flexed it only when there was work to do. When there is no work for the mind, it is suspended (*nirodha*). At this time people naturally abided in their true nature.[1] It is this suspension of mind that is characteristic of the phase of naturalism.

Over time, however, the harmonious period of naturalism began to decline: people lost contact with their true nature and simultaneously the power of the priestly caste increased.

By the end of this vedic phase, religion had become no more than a stale establishment, and people had to pay the priests to sustain even some type of contentment.

1. *Yoga Sutra* I.3.

Phase Two — Mysticism

The second phase started when a great number of people turned their backs on society and went into the forest to search within themselves for the lost happiness. Most had lost the suspended mind (*nirodha*) and now had a single-pointed mind (*ekagra chitta*). The disadvantage of the single-pointed mind compared to the suspended mind is that it thinks constantly. However, in contrast to the predominant mind of today, it has the huge advantage of still being able to think about one subject until a clear solution is arrived at.

During this phase there were many masters called *rishi*s (seers) who had attained freedom through meditation, and many students gathered around them. In fact, if we believe various passages of the *Ramayana* and *Mahabharata*, some of the forests were then as densely populated as the cities.

In this phase many could still quiet their minds by meditation. Often just listening to a teacher prompted people to awaken. The teachers living during this period were *nirodha*s, meaning they taught from a suspended mind. They offered a spontaneous insight into the nature of reality. It takes a student whose mind is at least single-pointed (*ekagra*) to spontaneously understand such a teacher. In other words the student needs to have a "mature soul." I put this in quotation marks because the true self is eternally free and unchangeable. It does not increase or decrease in maturity.

The scriptures compiled in those days were the *Upanishad*s, which are mystical dialogues between master and student. "Upanishad" means sitting near the master, while "mysticism" means that the hidden or the inexpressible is being expressed. The mere use of the word "hidden" indicates that we had largely lost the knowledge of our true nature by then, whereas in the vedic age, the age of naturalism, nothing was hidden. Gradually, the age of mysticism declined.

Phase Three — Philosophy

When the age of philosophy dawned, the majority of people had lost their ability to focus and now had a distracted mind (*vikshipta chitta*). A person with a distracted mind cannot understand a teacher with a suspended mind (*nirodha chitta*). The distracted mind, which is also called a confused or oscillating mind, needs a teacher with a single-pointed mind to explain systematically what has to be done. An individual with a distracted mind can no longer grasp truth spontaneously.

One teacher who rose to the challenge was the Rishi Kapila, who created the first systematic philosophy of mankind, the *Samkhya*. Since the truth could not be found spontaneously anymore, it had to be reached in systematic steps. Kapila's great achievement was that he created a meditation system that guided students to freedom using a completely rational scientific method totally free of any religious influence. His appearance marked the beginning of the age or phase of philosophy.

During this phase there appeared many great teachers who offered very different solutions. Although superficially at odds, all of the solutions or systems they offered were crystallizations of the one truth uttered by the *rishi*s of the *Upanishad*s. Most of the new schools of philosophy that emerged subsequently, such as Buddhism, Yoga, Vedanta, and Tantra, used the *Samkhya* of Kapila as a foundation and built on it.

Almost a thousand years after Kapila there came another great teacher, Patanjali. Very little is known about his life, but mythology offers us a story about him. Lord Shiva once gave a discourse on yoga to his consort, Uma. Because it was highly secret, a remote jungle location was chosen for the occasion. Shiva had just finished his discourse when he heard a noise in the shrubs. On investigation he found the thousand-headed serpent of infinity, Ananta, trying to get away. Shiva apprehended Ananta and told him that, as a punishment for secretly listening, he was sentenced to go to the humans and impart to them his new knowledge.

Setting out immediately on his new task, Ananta approached a village. As soon as they saw the thousand-headed serpent, some villagers ran away while others started hurling stones at him. When Ananta went back to Lord Shiva and told him what had happened, Shiva explained that humans would be frightened by the appearance of a thousand-headed serpent, and suggested he take on human form. Following this advice, and having taken the name Patanjali, Ananta was readily accepted by humans. Because he is seen as a manifestation of the serpent of infinity, Patanjali is traditionally depicted as being half-human, half-snake.

Ananta himself is seen as the perfect yogi. One of his jobs is to provide a bed for Lord Vishnu. Vishnu can be incredibly heavy at times, so the bed needs to be very strong. At the same time, a very soft bed needs to be provided for the Lord. For this dual task, Ananta was very well suited, his coils being soft and strong simultaneously. In this way Ananta exemplifies the meaning of *Yoga Sutra* II.46, "sthira sukham asanam" — the posture needs the dual quality of firmness and softness.

Patanjali was not only the author of the *Yoga Sutra*, however. The Rishi Vyasa says, in a hymn praising Patanjali:

> Let us bow before the highest of all sages, Patanjali
>
> who instructed on yoga to give clarity of mind
> who instructed on grammar to give clarity of speech
> and who instructed on medicine to give health to the body.

Patanjali was also the author of the *Mahabhasya*, the great commentary on Panini's grammar. The *Charaka Samhita*, one of the principal treatises on *Ayurveda*, is also attributed to Patanjali.

Western scholars believe, however, that these three scriptures were written by three individuals, there being reason to believe they appeared in different centuries. The traditional view is that many of the great masters, such as Patanjali, were in fact *siddha*s or perfected beings who were either immortal or could manifest whenever they chose to. If we accept that Patanjali managed to transform himself from the thousand-headed serpent of infinity into a human being, it is not difficult to believe that he was able to manifest where and when he chose to.

Some time after Patanjali there came the next

master in the lineage, Vyasa. He appears to have been immortal, since it cannot otherwise be explained how he could have produced such a vast body of writing. His birth name was Krishna Dvaipayana, but he is known as Veda Vyasa or just Vyasa. Veda Vyasa means "the divider of the *Veda*." When at the beginning of the fourth age, the Kali Yuga, the memory of mankind had degenerated so much that nobody could memorize the vast entirety of the *Veda*, Vyasa divided it into four (*Rig*, *Yajus*, *Sama*, *Atharva*) and allocated the parts to different *gotra*s or family lineages that were charged with protecting them. He is thus credited with preserving the *Veda*.

Vyasa is said to have created the 100,000 verses of the *Mahabharata*, the largest single piece of literature produced by humanity,[2] as well as the *Bhagavad Gita* and the *Brahma Sutra*, the most influential philosophical treatises in India today. He is believed also to have compiled the thirty-six *Purana*s, which consist mainly of mythological material.

The reason why Vyasa remains so important for us today is that he authored the authoritative commentary on the *Yoga Sutra*, the *Yoga Bhasya*. It has become so important that his commentary and the *Yoga Sutra* together are regarded as one book. If it was not for Vyasa's commentary, the rather cryptic sutras of Patanjali could no longer be understood. In other words it is due to Vyasa that we know what Patanjali meant.

All historical commentators who came after Vyasa, with the exception of King Bhoja, accepted his commentary and commented on it rather than on the *Yoga Sutra* directly. Vyasa was possibly the most important master in Indian history, and tradition ascribes to him divinity. It is said that he comes during every world age to restore ancient knowledge. Vyasa was an all-round genius, and we could call him the Leonardo Da Vinci of Indian philosophy.

Today, surprisingly enough, we find twentieth-century authors who write, in their interpretations of the *Yoga Sutra*, that they disagree with Vyasa or other ancient authorities. As modern-day practitioners we should allow ourselves to "disagree" with such

towering intellectual and mystical giants only when we have risen to their state. Otherwise it will be difficult to reap the precious fruit of yoga.

Another important side of Vyasa that we have to understand is that he wrote authoritative texts on seemingly opposing schools of thought. He founded for example the philosophical school of Vedanta by compiling the *Brahma Sutra*, but he contributed to a rival school, that of Samkhya/Yoga by compiling the "Commentary on the *Yoga Sutra*." Western scholars are very confused by the notion that one and the same person could write commentaries on opposing schools of thought, and they usually propose that there were two or more Vyasas. The truth is most Vedanta masters, such as Gaudapada, Shankara and Vachaspati Mishra, wrote commentaries on yoga — which, viewed superficially, is an opposing school of thought — while yoga masters provided commentaries on Vedanta. The reason for this is that all philosophical systems are only representations of the one truth taught in the *Upanishad*s — they are versions of the truth but never the truth itself. A true mystic knows this. Although one might have a favorite system, he or she is still capable of realizing the truth in other systems and can make a contribution to them.

Scholars who have not had a mystical experience cannot understand this: they are still caught up in the game of right or wrong. According to the logic of consciousness, thesis (a certain position), antithesis (the opposing position), synthesis (the incorporation of both), and the negation of all these positions can be held simultaneously, since none of them can be true. Truth is only consciousness, which has no position and no right or wrong, but only awareness. If this is truly realized, the goal of yoga is reached.

The next teacher concludes the age of philosophy. His name is Adi Shankara, but he is often called Shankara Bhagavatpada (after his master), Govinda Bhagavatpada, or Shankaracharya, the last of these meaning the teacher Shankara. He founded four monasteries whose abbots still carry the title Shankaracharya today. Some scriptures that are attributed to Shankara were actually written by abbots; nevertheless, he did leave behind a vast body of writings.

Shankara was a true genius. When he was twelve, his master assigned him the task of writing

2. Earlier in this essay the *Ramayana* was mentioned in conjunction with the *Mahabharata*. It was written down after the *Mahabharata*, but is set in a much earlier time.

commentaries on the principal *Upanishads*, and they remain authoritative. His main work is the *Brahma Sutra Bhasya*, a commentary on the *Brahma Sutra*. Today he is mainly known as a teacher of Advaita Vedanta, which was his chief subject.

Shankara's great contribution to yoga is his commentary on Vyasa's commentary on Patanjali's *Yoga Sutra*, called *Vivarana*.[3] One of the best descriptions of Yoga philosophy, it is a worthy expression of Shankara's genius. With him the age of philosophy drew to a close, and the world experienced an even further decline.

Phase Four — Technology

While most people in the age of naturalism had a suspended mind (*nirodha chitta*), in the age of mysticism a single-pointed mind (*ekagra chitta*), and in the age of philosophy a distracted mind (*vikshipta chitta*), the average person in the last age has an infatuated mind (*mudha chitta*).

"Infatuated" here means obsessed with one's own body, wealth, appearance, and family relations. Connected to these are materialism and vanity. Important here is that the infatuated mind identifies with the body. Materialism is the philosophy that reduces human beings to their bodies. Obsession with wealth results from preoccupation with the whims of the body, while vanity is preoccupation with one's external appearance. Obsession with family relations means relating more to people who share one's gene pool.

This last phase is called the age of technology. The Sanskrit word *tantra* means "technique." Since philosophy and, to a greater extent, mysticism and naturalism now went right over people's heads, the new types of teaching were concerned only with techniques: how one does things.

The scriptures of this age, which describe mainly technique and do not emphasize philosophy, are called *tantra*s, and there are between seven and eight hundred of them. Westerners know the *tantra*s mostly for their excursions into explicit sexual technique, but to reduce the *tantra*s to those rare passages does not do them justice. It does show us, however, how the infatuated Western mind works. Most yogic treatises

written after Shankara, such as the *Shiva Sutra*, the *Hatha Yoga Pradipika*, the *Shiva Samhita*, and the *Gheranda Samhita*, to name but a few, are in fact *tantra*s.

The philosophical school of yoga was maintained during the age of technique by a number of masters. Vachaspati Mishra, who commented on Vyasa's commentary and all other traditional systems of philosophy, made outstanding contributions in the tenth century. Vijnanabhikshu, who also commented on Samkhya and Vedanta, wrote one of the most important commentaries, the *Yoga Vartikka*, in the fifteenth century. The most recent of the important contributions is the excellent commentary on Vyasa's commentary written by Hariharananda Aranya in the twentieth century. All of these writings have been consulted in preparing the present text.

The Importance of the Four Ages for Today's Practitioner

According to the *Puranas*, humanity started out in the golden age (the vedic age) and, through progressive ages of degeneration, we are now in the dark age (Kali Yuga). If we look at the development of yogic scriptures we can recognize these stages.

In the golden age people had a suspended mind (*nirodha chitta*), which means they thought only when necessary and at other times abided in the heart, the divine source. In the second age, people had single-pointed minds (*ekagra chitta*) and, through a few instructions given by a master who had a suspended mind himself, they could return to the source. In the third age people's minds shifted down into a confused state (*vikshipta chitta*). The masters who taught in this period worked on getting individuals back into the single-pointed state. In the fourth age, the period we live in now, people's minds have degenerated into the infatuated, materialistic state (*mudha chitta*). Teachers today first have to teach that there is an eternal, immortal sacred core to us, which the confused mind is still able to remember but the infatuated mind has forgotten.

For the study of philosophy this means that we must first understand what was taught by teachers who also lived like us, in the age of the infatuated mind. They include Vachaspati Mishra, Vijnanabhikshu, and Hariharananda Aranya. With this

3. As a commentary on a commentary, it is referred to as a subcommentary.

understanding, we unlock the teachings of the masters of the age of philosophy (= confused mind) like Patanjali, Vyasa, and Shankara. After internalizing these, we can understand even earlier teachers like Yajnavalkya, Vasishta, and Kapila (single-pointed mind). If we understand their simple message of the heart we have arrived home at the suspended mind, where our true nature is recognized.

Involution Versus Evolution

We can say that, on an individual level, the yogi has to reverse the historical development that the human race has undergone. Similarly we can say the yogi has to reverse the movement of evolution of the universe on an individual level. The philosophy of Samkhya describes the process of evolution of the world as a down-and-out movement. Evolution here starts with the highest and most subtle, the state before the Big Bang (*prakrti*).

This source of nature evolves into intelligence. From intelligence comes ego. From ego comes space. From space comes air. From air comes fire, from fire comes water, and from water comes earth. Each evolute becomes coarser and grosser than the previous, subtler one.

In the human body these steps are represented through the *chakra*s, with pure intelligence referring to the *Sahasrara chakra*, pure I-am-ness or ego to the *Ajna chakra*, space to the *Vishuddha chakra*, air to the *Anahatta chakra*, fire to the *Manipura chakra,* and water to the *Svadhisthana chakra*. Finally the element earth is represented through the lowest *chakra*, the *Muladhara*. This whole process is called evolution, but it comes with a degeneration of awareness. When the *Muladhara* is reached, the world is manifest and self-knowledge is lost. This movement of evolution is directed downward and outward.

The yogic process of involution reverses this to an in-and-up movement. We go in and up through the *chakra*s of earth, water, fire, air, and space, and then reabsorb ego into intelligence and intelligence into its origin, *prakrti* (nature). Then we abide in the pristine state of consciousness and awareness, which is the state of freedom and ecstasy.

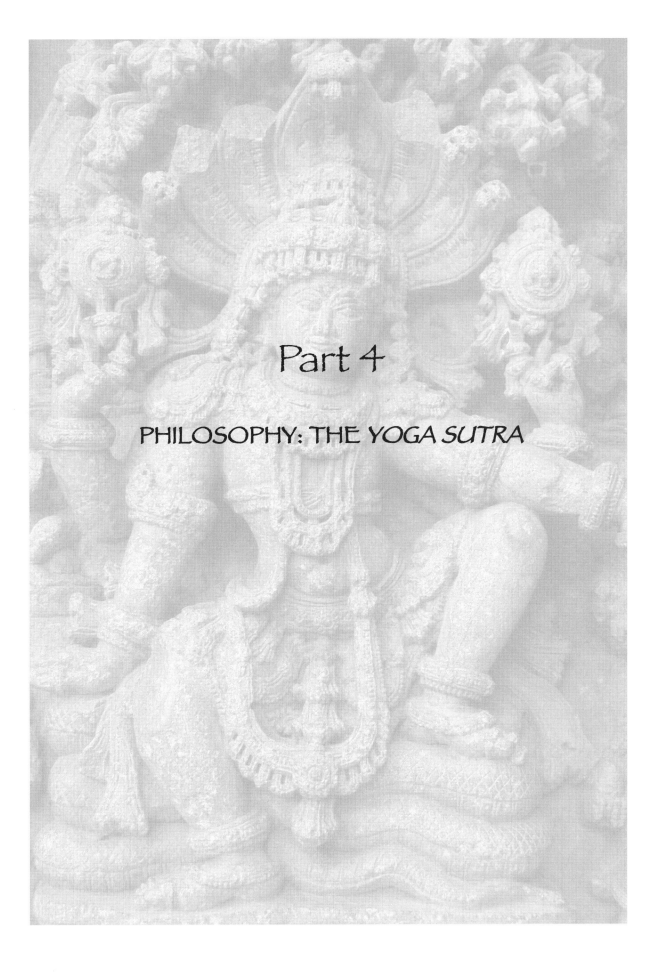

Part 4

PHILOSOPHY: THE *YOGA SUTRA*

Chapter I: On *Samadhi*

अथ योगानुशासनम् ॥ १ ॥
1.1 Now then authoritative instruction in yoga.

The word *atha*, translated here as "now then," signals the start of an authoritative treatise. The *Brahma Sutra*, for example, starts with the stanza "athato brahmajninasya" which means "Then therefore inquiry into consciousness." Patanjali's treatise on grammar, the *Mahabhasya*, starts with "atha sabdanusasanam," which means "Now then inquiry into sound." What is implied with the use of *atha* is that the author is not relaying someone else's understanding but has mastered the subject as set out in the text. In other words, the author is in a position to make such a statement. This is reflected in the fact that all later generations of yogis have accepted Patanjali as an authority.

The term *yoga* is then defined. According to Panini,[1] the term *yoga* can be derived from either of two roots, *yujir yoge* and *yujir samadhau*. If we derive it out of *yujir yoge* it means "union" or "bringing together." The *Bhagavad Gita* accepts this meaning.

1. Panini is the leading authority on classical Sanskrit grammar. In his *Ashtadyayi* he listed two thousand word roots and, out of these, with the help of rules called *guna* and *vriddhi*, we can form verbs, nouns, various endings, and the like. According to Western scholars he lived around 500 BCE; according to Indian tradition, however, he lived more than six thousand years ago. Patanjali wrote a commentary on Panini's *Ashtadyayi* called the *Great Commentary* (*Mahabhasya*). In India it is generally understood that Patanjali the yoga master and Patanjali the grammarian are one and the same person, though some Western scholars doubt this. In this text we follow respectfully the traditional Indian view. It is in the context of its tradition that yoga must be understood.

The *Gita* teaches that there is one deep reality underlying all phenomena, which is the Supreme Being. Yoga here means to unite oneself with or merge into this underlying or deep reality. All scriptures and meditation systems that propose one truth contained in all appearances, and therefore take yoga to mean union, are called nondualistic (meaning not-two) or monistic (from *mono* — one).

The second root out of which we can derive the term *yoga* is *yujir samadhau*, which gives it the meaning of "contemplation" or "absorption." It is this meaning that the *Yoga Sutra* follows. The basic concept of the *Yoga Sutra* is that there are two separate realities, nature (*prakrti*) and consciousness (*purusha*). Yoga here means the contemplation that enables us to discriminate between the two. Scriptures and meditation systems that distinguish between two essential categories, and therefore take yoga to mean contemplation, are called dualistic. This will be covered in detail later.

We know that the *Yoga Sutra* employs the second meaning of the word *yoga* (i.e., the meaning of absorption/contemplation) because of a clear statement by the Rishi Vyasa. In his commentary on the *Yoga Sutra* — *Yoga Bhasya* — he explained every sutra with such clarity that no misunderstanding was possible. It is mainly through the work of Vyasa that we know the meaning of the sutras. Many of them are so concise and cryptic that they cannot be understood without his explanations. It has been mentioned that Vyasa's commentary is so important that it and Patanjali's sutras together are regarded as virtually one book.

For today's yoga student it is vital to realize that the historical school of yoga does not consist only of Patanjali's sutras but also of Vyasa's commentary and various other subcommentaries as well. The authoritative subcommentaries are those of Vachaspati Mishra (ninth century CE), Shankara (eighth century CE), and Vijnanabhikshu (fifteenth century CE). The authoritative twentieth-century commentary, by Hariharananda Aranya, is outstanding in its depth. All yoga masters after Vyasa accepted his commentary and wrote subcommentaries on it.[2]

The Rishi Vyasa states in his commentary on sutra I.1 that yoga means absorption/contemplation (*yogah samadhih*). He also explains that contemplation is a potential of the mind (*chitta*). This potential is dormant in most and needs to be trained and developed. Yoga, then, is the science of training the mind, and it is for those who are *in need* of this training. There are those who do not need the training but can see the one true reality in all appearances. They can bypass yoga and go instead to the Vedanta, which is the science of consciousness, explained by the Rishi Vyasa in the *Brahma Sutra*.

Those who do not realize their true nature are advised to take up the study of yoga. Yoga is the process that prepares a clouded mind for self-knowledge. In other words, the study of yoga starts by us admitting our ignorance and knowing that we first have to change ourselves before we can see the truth.

Neither of the two paths described in the *Brahma Sutra* and the *Yoga Sutra* is right or wrong. Rather, they apply to different students. For the advanced soul, the path of the *Brahma Sutra* (Vedanta) is recommended. For a more confused student, the clarifying of the mind through yoga is recommended first.

Vyasa goes on to say that mind (*chitta*) occurs in five different states. Every person will have a dominant tendency toward one of these states, but gradual change is possible. It is very important that we understand these five states well. Out of this understanding comes a great comprehension of the path and teachings of yoga and how yoga knowledge was conceived in the first place.

The five states of the mind are the restless (*kshipta*), infatuated (*mudha*), distracted (*vikshipta*), one-pointed (*ekagra*), and suspended (*nirodha*) mind. To explain these five states we have to look briefly at the three qualities of the mind.

As mentioned before, yoga states that there are two separate entities that are both real and eternal — nature (*prakrti*) and consciousness (*purusha*). The closest idea in Western science to describe *prakrti* is

the state before the Big Bang or the state before the universe manifested. *Prakrti* has also been translated as "creation" (although *prakrti* itself is eternal and uncreated) or "procreatress" — the matrix that procreates, brings forth everything.

Prakrti is said to be stirred into action by the proximity or closeness of consciousness (*purusha*), and it manifests the world with the help of its three qualities (*guna*s). They are:

> *Tamas* — heaviness, inertia, mass
> *Rajas* — movement, energy, dynamics
> *Sattva* — light, intelligence, wisdom.

Together, the three *guna*s form all phenomena and objects. We can compare them in some ways to the elementary particles proton, neutron, and electron in Western science, which miraculously form all 105 elements and thus all matter. We cannot stretch this comparison too far, though, since the *guna*s form also ego and mind.

With the restless (*kshipta*) state of mind, *rajas* is predominant. This mind is associated with hyperactivity, excess movement, and one thought chasing the next. It is said that this type of mind can only reach concentration through intense hatred, such as in destroying one's imagined enemies. The restless mind is very unsuitable for yoga, and one dominated by a restless mind rarely takes it up. If they nevertheless do so, it is often only in the hope of gaining magical powers to vanquish their enemies.

With the second, infatuated (*mudha*) state of mind, *tamas* is predominant. This mind is often dull, stupefied or deluded, and infatuated with the body, wealth, family, tribe, or nationality. Because the *tamas guna* makes the mind heavy, one cannot look further than any obvious objects of identification such as those just mentioned.

The infatuated mind is not suitable for yoga, and the only way it can concentrate is through intense greed. If somebody with such a mind-set takes up yoga, it is usually for physical gain (so that the body looks better) or monetary gain (to be able to work harder or achieve more).

With the third state of mind, the distracted (*vikshipta*) mind, no *guna* is predominant. Rather, any one of the three (*rajas*, *tamas*, or *sattva*) takes over, depending on impulse. This state of mind can

---

2. With the exception of King Bhoja (tenth century), who wrote his explanation (called *Raja Martanda*) directly on Patanjali's sutras.

also be called confused or oscillating, and it is typical of people who identify with being "New Age." They see everything as being true and meaningful and believe that "all have to live according to their truth." If something happens it is "meant to be," although possibly we were just too unfocused to achieve a certain result.

Those dominated by the distracted mind are opportunist agnostics — believing there are many truths and that the one truth cannot be known. Rather, one's mind-set is merely adjusted according to circumstances in order to stay comfortable. The distracted mind has glimpses of the truth, but with the next obstacle it is thrown off track and holds onto another idea.

When in the grip of the distracted mind we often hold on to beliefs, since we cannot permanently recognize deep reality or truth. This type of mind is unsuitable for higher yoga, such as *samadhi*, as it can achieve concentration only randomly and it loses it quickly.

The fact that yoga is a science that enables us to directly perceive and realize the deepest layer of reality means that the holding of beliefs is contradictory to yogic examination. If we hold on to beliefs, we will always superimpose them onto reality and so never arrive at the correct conclusion. Realistically speaking, most yoga students start with distracted minds and most of one's yogic life is spent attempting to transform the distracted mind into the one-pointed state.

In the fourth — one-pointed (*ekagra*) — state of mind, *sattva* is predominant. Through yoga, the mind is made more and more sattvic. If the state of pure *sattva* is achieved, that is pure intelligence. This intelligence is necessary to see reality as it is. According to sutra III.55,

> When the intelligence is as untainted as consciousness, this will lead to liberation.

Somebody who is born in a state of one-pointedness can become free after a comparatively short phase of practice and study. This state of mind is suitable for *samadhi*-based-on-an-object (*samprajnata samadhi*), which is the lower type of *samadhi*. It is through this type of *samadhi* that many of the great masters conceived and compiled their teachings. However, the feat should not daunt us. As the master Vijnana-bhikshu said, "Transformation of the mind can be gained only gradually, and not all at once."

The last state of mind is *nirodha*, "suspended." In this state there is no predominance of any quality. Instead, one's mind is reabsorbed into its source, which is nature (*prakrti*). Somebody in this state of mind permanently rests in his or her true nature, which is consciousness. The type of *samadhi* achieved here is objectless *samadhi* (*asamprajnata samadhi*), which is the higher form. The suspended mind (*nirodha chitta*) is the goal of yoga. Masters who had this type of mind conceived the *Upanishad*s, which are the highest scriptures. It is because the mind does not interfere with intelligence that *nirodha*s can see to the bottom of their hearts and hear the divine truth. For this reason the *Upanishad*s are considered as revelation and of divine authority.

In this first sutra, the theme of yoga is introduced. There are many important terms and concepts, and they can be confusing in the beginning. If this is the case it is better to go back and read the description of this sutra again before going on to the next. Don't be daunted if reading seems laborious at first. The outcome is worth the effort.

योगश्चित्तवृत्तिनिरोधः ॥ २ ॥
1.2 Yoga is the suspension of the fluctuations of the mind.

In this second sutra, Patanjali defines yoga. It requires little reflection to realize that, in the light of this definition, the reading of yoga as union doesn't make sense. Rather than union, yoga is defined here as the effort or discipline that transforms the mind into a clear surface capable of reflecting whatever it is directed at.

Consider the following. If the surface of a lake is still, you can use it as a mirror to reflect objects. If you throw a stone into the lake, ripples appear that distort the reflected images. The lake represents the mind and the ripples are the fluctuations of the mind or mind waves. While these mind waves can be appropriate for the purpose of survival, they present an obstacle if we want to recognize our innermost nature. The mind waves have to cease and the mind has to become still in order for us to reflect on our deepest core. What exactly the fluctuations or mind waves are will be discussed in sutras I.5–11.

We turn next to Patanjali's concept of mind. The Sanskrit word *chit* refers to that which is conscious. The term *achit*, with the negating prefix "a," refers to what is unconscious. By using the term *chitta* (and not *antahkarana*, which followers of Samkhya usually use) Patanjali expresses the notion that the mind is unconscious, or in other words consciousness is not contained in the mind.

In many ways Patanjali does not present a philosophy of his own, but a psychology or what Georg Feuerstein calls a psycho technology.[3] Where philosophical questions are concerned, Patanjali completely accepts the findings of the Samkhya, with one exception (Ishvara), which we will discuss later. The similarities between Yoga and Samkhya are so striking that S. Dasgupta says, "The Samkhya of Kapila and the Yoga of Patanjali are so similar that they can be regarded as two modifications of the same system."[4]

The founder of Samkhya was the Rishi Kapila, who lived according to Western scholars around 1300 BCE.[5] Tradition places him much earlier than that. Samkhya means order, number, or enumeration, and it is humankind's first attempt to explain the entire creation as one coherent system. I therefore like to call it the ancient mother of all systematic philosophies.

During Patanjali's time and the time of the *Bhagavad Gita*, Samkhya was still the dominant philosophy. Today it has gone out of fashion somewhat, but it is important to remember that most Indian philosophies of today, such as Vedanta, Yoga, Buddhism, and Tantra, have used Samkhya as a foundation and built upon it. If we understand Samkhya, we will easily understand all of these later approaches.

Unfortunately the scripture compiled by Kapila, the *Shastitantra*, is lost. To fill in the gaps that Patanjali leaves, we have to resort to the *Samkhya Karika* of Ishvara Krishna, which was written much later than Kapila's text. The *Samkhya Karika* is an absolute must for every yoga student.[6] At only seventy-three stanzas it is relatively short, and this makes it relatively accessible. Mind in the *Samkhya Karika* is called *antahkarana*, which means inner instrument. Opposed to that is the outer instrument, the body.

The inner instrument is made up of three constituents:

1. *MANAS*

This is the mind or thinking principle. The word "man" is derived from *manas*. It collects sensory input, compares it with previous data, and makes a decision as to what the object cognized probably is. But a rope in the darkness can be mistaken for a snake, or a post in the distance for a man. The mind speedily processes sensory data for the purpose of survival, and in this process accuracy is lost. For example, if we are crossing a street and hear a loud mechanical noise approaching, we move quickly. The mind tells us it is likely the noise comes from a truck, and we should therefore not wait and inquire more deeply into what the noise actually is. In such a situation we are likely to react before we recognize that the sound is really an airplane flying overhead or a construction machine nearby. The mind is constantly telling us to react, and as a result we hardly ever take the time to stop and understand what is really happening.

2. *AHAMKARA*

This is ego or egoity. *Aham* means I and *kara* means caster or maker. Together they mean I-maker. The ego is the agent that owns the perceptions of the thinking principle. Ego says, "It is 'I' who is perceiving the approaching truck, and it is 'I' who has to proceed to the safety of the footpath, otherwise 'I' will be dead."

3. *BUDDHI*

This is intellect or intelligence, the term being derived from the verb root *budh*, which means to awake. In yoga, intellect means seat of intelligence.

3. G. Feuerstein, *The Yoga Tradition,* Hohm Press, Prescott, Arizona, 2001.

4. S. Dasgupta, *Yoga as Philosophy and Religion,* Motilal Banarsidass, Delhi, 1973, p. 6.

5. G. Feuerstein, *The Yoga Tradition.*

6. See G. J. Larson, *Classical Samkhya,* 2nd rev. ed., Motilal Banarsidass, Delhi, 1979; or *Samkhya Karika of Isvara Krsna,* trans. Sw. Virupakshananda, Sri Ramakrishna Math, Madras.

In our example, intelligence is the agent that, for example, manages to comprehend iron ore and fire to the extent that it can conceive an internal combustion engine and build a truck. It is the intellect (*buddhi*) that is the locomotive of yoga. Yoga is the process of refining, sharpening, and enhancing the intellect until we can realize consciousness (*purusha*) itself. This will be looked at in more detail in the third and fourth chapters of the *Yoga Sutra*.

The last term in this sutra is *nirodha*. This is often translated as "control" or "restraint," which does not make sense in the context of yoga. It can also send students on the wrong path. If we restrain or control the mind, there must be an entity that controls it. This entity must be active, so it can't be consciousness, which does not interfere in the world but is a pure witness. Furthermore, this entity must have willpower at its disposal in order to suppress the mind. The only entity available to perform such an act is the ego. The process of suppressing, controlling, and restraining the mind will strengthen the ego. However it is the ego that stands in the way of realizing consciousness.

The way to realize consciousness is through a passive suspending, calming, and ceasing of mind waves, which is possible only through insight, wisdom, intelligence, and knowledge. Sutra I.16 declares that the state of *nirodha* is produced by complete surrender, which is nothing but supreme detachment (*paravairagya*). We will therefore translate *nirodha* as suspension or cessation, since it does not imply an external aggressor like the term "control."

The state of suspended mind (*nirodha chitta*) produces objectless or superconscious *samadhi* (*asamprajnata samadhi*). Sutra II.45 states that *samadhi* also results from surrender to the Supreme Being. Shri T. Krishnamacharya, the teacher of Shri K. Pattabhi Jois, believed that this was the prime way of reaching *samadhi*.

All of these notions show that *samadhi* is an act of surrender, detachment, realization, and knowing through appeasing, stilling, suspending, and silencing the mind waves. Using terms like control, suppression, and restraint to explain *nirodha* implies the agitation of the mind by the use of ego and willpower. Done in this way, meditation will lead not to liberation but to egomania.

In this second sutra, Patanjali also states that only the highest form of *samadhi* constitutes yoga proper. The two forms of *samadhi*, the lower objective (*samprajnata*) *samadhi* and the higher objectless (*asamprajnata*) *samadhi*, are so different that Patanjali could have divided them into two separate limbs. Instead of separating them, however, he defines yoga in this sutra as objectless *samadhi* and in sutra III.3 he defines objective *samadhi*. Objectless *samadhi* can be understood in the following way: This highest form of *samadhi* is our true and natural state — consciousness abiding in consciousness. It is not an experience; rather it is eternal, uncreated, without beginning, and without end. It cannot be practiced and cannot be produced. It is our core, our origin and our destiny. It is our abode right now, but due to ignorance we do not know it. This highest *samadhi* is the goal, and it is the true yoga.

The eight limbs, which include objective *samadhi*, are steps that will lead us back to our source. For this reason, yoga is defined here as the natural state of suspension of mind (*nirodha*), and *samadhi* is defined in sutra III.3 as recognizing an object exactly as it is. In summary we can say that objectless (*asamprajnata*) *samadhi* is the goal and the true state of yoga. The practicing of objective (*samprajnata*) *samadhi* is the path to that goal.

तदा द्रष्टुः स्वरूपेऽवस्थानम् ॥ ३ ॥
I.3 Then the seer abides in his own nature.

Meditation is the act of involution or going inside. The first step in meditation is to observe one's body. From this observation, we realize that the observer or seer and the seen are different. We now know that we are not the body but, rather, we have a body.

The next step is to observe the mind. Once this observation is established, we reject identity with the mind because we, the seer or observer, must be located outside the seen. From here we start to observe the next deeper layer, the ego. This is challenging at first, but with meditation experience and practice we soon observe, isolate, and study that faculty within us that says "I." Using the metaphor of a computer, the ego (*ahamkara*) is the operating system on which the applications body and mind (*manas*) are run. The body and mind function only against the backdrop of ego. In fact, according to Samkhya, body and mind evolve out of ego.

When we become capable of observing ego, we come to know that we are not the ego, but again a deeper lying agent. This next layer is intelligence (*buddhi*). In our metaphor, intelligence is like the computer hardware. This hardware can exist for itself, but the operating system (ego) and the applications (body and mind) cannot function without hardware. According to Samkhya, ego evolves out of intellect (*buddhi*). Intellect comes before and is a deeper layer than ego. It does not know the notion of "I." Intellect is pure intelligence.

Now we go one step further with our meditation. Intelligence, once sharpened, can be observed. Then the intellect can realize that an external agent is observing it. This external agent is called consciousness (*purusha*) or the self (*atman*) and consists only of awareness. Since awareness is without form or quality, we cannot observe or see it. This consciousness is the seer, the deepest and ultimate layer. This was confirmed as fact by the ancient *rishi*s and liberated masters. It can be tried and tested by any meditator.

The sutra now says that, when one is in the state of true yoga and the fluctuations of the mind are stilled, this seer, which is awareness, abides in its own nature. It would be easier to understand if Patanjali had said then the seer experiences itself, but that would be an incorrect use of words for the following reason.

A human being is an interface between consciousness (*purusha*) on the one hand and manifestation (*prakrti*) on the other. Because consciousness, which is our core, perceives but cannot be perceived, we project ourselves out into the world of phenomena. We then believe we are the phenomena, such as the egoic body/mind.

To abide in one's nature simply means to stop projecting oneself outward. Projecting outward means to identify with the perceived. Giving up this projection is to abide in the core, which implies watching the world and one's body/mind go by. The nature of the seer is awareness. To abide in one's nature as awareness means simply to know that we are awareness and not to lose sight of that.

If you have not understood the preceding paragraph, reread it until you do. It holds the secret of yoga. Sometimes the ideas discussed and the use of terse terminology can cause difficulty for the reader, but if I do not set out the facts precisely, the essence of the teachings will be lost. In the words of the late Professor S. Dasgupta, "I have tried to resist the temptation of making the English happy at the risk of sacrificing the exactness of the philosophical sense: and many ideas of Indian philosophy are such that an exact English rendering of them often becomes hopelessly difficult."[7]

What follows is a brief summary of the concept of this sutra.

At our core is a state of permanent, infinite bliss and awareness, which is called our true nature, truth, the natural state, consciousness, or the self. We do not perceive this state because we erroneously identify ourselves with mental activity. Once mental activity (*vrtti*) ceases, we return to our natural state.

Vyasa makes an important statement in his commentary when he says that consciousness always abides in itself, although it appears not to do so. Vijnanabhikshu illustrates this in his subcommentary *Yoga Varttika* through the following example. If we look at a crystal and no object is close by, we will see the crystal as it is. If we place a red rose next to the crystal, the crystal will take on the color of the rose to an extent that, when we look into the crystal, we will only see the rose. However, the truth is that the crystal has not changed its nature at all in this process.

Similarly, consciousness abides in itself during objectless *samadhi* (*asamprajnata*). The truth is that it always abides in itself, but does not appear to. Like the crystal, it appears to be colored by objects. And, like the crystal, when we remove the object, we realize it is unchanged.

7. S. Dasgupta, *Yoga as Philosophy and Religion.*

वृत्तिसारूप्यम् इतरत्र ॥ ४ ॥

1.4 At other times it appears to take on the form of the modifications of the mind.

The "other times" referred to are when the seer does not abide in its true nature as consciousness. Rather, at those times the seer appears to take the shape of whatever the content of the mind is.

As explained in the previous sutra, we have to remember that this only *appears* to be so. In reality the crystal is unchanged while it reflects the red rose. But, since the crystal itself is colorless, what we perceive when we look at it is the color and structure of the rose and not the crystal itself. In other words, the quality of red-rose-ness seems to be superimposed onto the crystal to the extent that we believe the crystal to be a red rose.

Similarly, when thought waves cause ripples on the surface of the lake of the mind, the color and form of those objects are superimposed onto our true nature, which is pure awareness or consciousness. The mind attracts objects like metal to a magnet, and causes erroneous impressions. Since these objects and thoughts possess color, form, structure, and quality, the awareness that illuminates these objects is wrongly perceived as having those attributes. This is the cause of human misery and suffering.

The other day I saw a bumper sticker on a car that read, "I listen to the little voices in my head." We think millions of thoughts every day, and modern psychology now accepts that we have not one but thousands of egos and personalities. In fact, every moment changes us, and a slightly different personality, *vasana*, manifests.

Our many different thoughts and personalities are like the little voices in our heads. They can become a problem if we erroneously connect these thoughts with I-am-ness (*asmita*), which is also called ego. For example, the thousands of thoughts we have every day do not trouble us as long as we do not attach ourselves to them or own them. Even a saint might think about murder or using heroin, but he won't own them because he has no attachment to them. The problem starts when a person identifies with the thought of murder or heroin

addiction. Only when this happens can the action follow. This identification or attachment is the wrong knowledge (*viparyaya*) of us as being the phenomena. This wrong knowledge can persist only when the right knowledge (*pramana*) — that we are awareness only — is not cognized (recognized).

The fastest way to keep our communities safe, our prisons empty, and our judges and police out of work is to teach people meditation and yogic philosophy. If we permanently know ourselves to be eternal and infinite, and to have unchangeable awareness — all of which are total freedom — then the identification with the activities of the mind is interrupted.

If this identification persists, there is nothing that stops us from listening to the voices in our heads. The voices told Adolf Hitler to kill six million Jews; similar voices told Josef Stalin to kill twenty million of his own people. White man listened to these voices and killed millions of people of color worldwide. The voices told Christians to kill millions of "infidels" via the Inquisition and Crusades. All these acts are summarized in J. Krishnamurti's statement "The history of mind is the history of atrocities."

All of these acts were, and continue to be, committed today because we identify ourselves with the voices in our heads. Because the mind is a survival tool, it always tries to dominate others in order to preempt an attack. The mind leads us to competition and warfare. To project oneself out and become one with the fluctuations of the mind leads to mental slavery. In the yogic sense, mental slavery does not mean being manipulated by somebody else but, rather, being duped by one's own mind. We are slaves to our own minds. These are strong words, but their use is justified by a brief look back into the gallery of victims that the terror regime of mind has claimed.

Consciousness, on the other hand, is qualityless. The consciousness in me is the same consciousness as the consciousness in anybody else. Realization of consciousness leads to peace and the wish to do good for all.

वृत्तयः पञ्चतय्यः क्लिष्टा अक्लिष्टाः ॥ ५ ॥

1.5 There are five types of mind waves, which can be troublesome or untroublesome.

Prior to this sutra Patanjali has defined the concepts of freedom and slavery to the mind. Now we move on to analyze the term "fluctuations" (vrtti). It is important here to explain the main ideas that Vyasa laid out in his commentary and the terms that he expected the reader to know.

In the second chapter of the *Yoga Sutra*, Patanjali describes the five different modes of suffering (kleshas). They are ignorance, egoism, desire, aversion, and fear. Vyasa begins his commentary with two important observations. The first is that troublesome mind waves arise out of these five modes of suffering (kleshas). It is important to understand that they do not arise out of peace, happiness, and contentment. His second observation is that the troublesome types of mind waves are those that give rise to a subconscious imprint (samskara). Let us look at the concept of the subconscious imprint in yoga.

If we get angry, this emotion leaves an imprint on our subconscious. The next time we get into a similar situation, the mind compares it with data accumulated in the past, and in this case the subconscious tells us to "get angry again." If we hurt somebody as a result of being angry last time, the tendency will be to do so once more. The difference between an imprint (such as the one described above) and a memory is that we cannot consciously access the imprint. Every experience or emotion has the tendency to repeat or remanifest itself again and again, due to its leaving an imprint and a tendency in the subconscious. This is a great problem for repeat offenders.

For the yogi, these subconscious imprints are very important because the imprints (samskaras) that we create today determine our actions tomorrow. These imprints originate from *vrtti*, but they can produce new mind waves. The fluctuations continue to produce new subconscious imprints, and in this way, as Vyasa says, the wheel of mind waves and subconscious imprints goes on revolving.

For this reason, the yogi concentrates on making the mind one-pointed (ekagra) or suspended (nirodha).

One-pointed means only those thought waves that are conducive to yoga are present; suspended means no thought waves are present at all.

Troublesome mind waves are the ones that lead us to perceiving reality wrongly (viparyaya). This in turn produces ignorance (avidya), egoism (asmita), and suffering (duhkha). The untroublesome mind waves are the ones that lead to perceiving reality correctly (pramana). This leads to discriminative knowledge (viveka khyateh) and freedom (kaivalya).

प्रमाणविपर्ययविकल्पनिद्रास्मृतयः ॥ ६ ॥

1.6 The five fluctuations of mind or mind waves are correct perception, wrong perception, conceptualization, deep sleep, and memory.

The difference between fluctuations of the mind (vrtti) and subconscious imprints (samskaras) is that the fluctuations are conscious and can be consciously accessed and remembered. Why dreamless sleep is included will be explained later.

The *Mandukya Upanishad* speaks of four states of mind — waking, dreaming, dreamless sleep, and the transcendental state that in yoga is called *asamprajnata samadhi*. If the dreamless or deep-sleep state is mentioned in this sutra, why not the waking and dreaming states also? The answer is simple. The *Mandukya Upanishad* is a vedantic scripture that deals mainly with consciousness or the transcendental state. The other three states of mind — waking, dreaming, dreamless sleep — are described as illusionary and unreal.

The *Yoga Sutra* on the other hand is a treatise that studies mind and then gives instruction on how to change it in order to make it fit to realize consciousness. For this purpose, Patanjali has broken down the waking and the dreaming states into their main constituents.

In the waking state we should perceive correctly, but usually there is a mix of right and wrong perception with conceptualization. The dream state is mainly one of conceptualization interspersed with right and wrong perception.

Why this breakdown is important will be clearer after the description of the individual thought waves.

प्रत्यक्षानुमानागमाः प्रमाणानि ॥ ७ ॥

1.7 Correct perception (*pramana*) is made up of direct perception, inference, and valid testimony.

Correct perception refers to the process whereby a certain object is presented and the mind identifies it correctly. Cognition is perception and the subsequent process of identification. The mind identifies by comparing objects cognized in the past with the present one. We can arrive at correct cognition in three ways:

The first and most important is direct perception (*pratyaksha*). Direct perception is of two kinds: perception through the senses and supersensory perception. Sensory perception means we directly perceive an object with our senses and identify it correctly.

This rarely happens, as the mind modifies all sensory input. For example, when rays of light enter our eye through the lens, they cross over and the object is depicted on the retina upside down. For this reason babies have difficulty in grabbing objects; but, through data entering the mind via the tactile sense, the mind eventually decides to turn around the images received by the eye. In other words, the two senses provide a nonidentical image of reality and the mind simulates what it believes to be most likely.

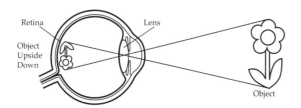

The image projected onto the eye's retina is inverted.

Another example: where the optical nerve enters the eye there is a blind spot on the retina. Moving a white paper with a black spot through one's field of vision can make this apparent: at some point the black spot disappears. This happens because the mind does not receive sensory data from this area so it fills in the blind spot with whatever it believes to be there. In this case it fills it in with the color of the surroundings, which is white.

This illustrates the way the mind works. It simulates reality according to what it believes to be most likely. According to mind, what is likely is what it collected in its surroundings or in the past. In yoga we call this the coloring of the objects through the past and the environment.

This is exactly how racism, sexism, nationalism, and other types of prejudice come about. If we have heard of people of a certain ethnic background behaving in a certain way, upon meeting any of them the mind will project that behavior onto them and will be less open to the realization that they are individuals who might behave completely differently.

A second type of direct perception is more important for the yogi. Sensory perception does not help us when we want to perceive deep reality (Brahman) or consciousness (*purusha*) or even simply objects-as-such. (The term "object-as-such" means an object perceived as it truly is, without the mind projecting onto it.) Since mind modifies sensory input, the truth within us cannot be perceived by the senses.

Mind produces a map of the world in our heads. Necessarily, the world cannot be contained in that map. If you compare for a moment the city in which you live to the street directory, you realize that the street directory is only a poor simulation of reality. It is helpful for getting around, but it is not the city as such.

If we want to experience our true nature, we have to shortcut the mind in what is called the mystical experience or *samadhi*. In *samadhi*, reality is experienced directly, without being manipulated by the mind. More about that later. For now, let us go back to the three types of correct perception.

The second type of direct perception is inference or deduction (*anumana*). From the presence of smoke, fire can be deduced. From a coconut falling off a palm tree we can deduce gravity. From the existence of life, we deduce the presence of consciousness, and from fear of death the previous experience of death. Deduction uses reasoning and correct logic. The effectiveness of deduction depends on the quality of the intellect.

Like all manifestations of nature (*prakrti*), the intellect is made up of dullness (*tamas*), frenzy (*rajas*), and wisdom (*sattva*). Inference can be used successfully only if the intellect is dominated by *sattva*. It can be made wise (sattvic) through the practice of yoga and study of the scriptures.

The third type of correct perception is valid testimony (*agama*). It is of two kinds: testimony of an expert and testimony of the sacred texts. If we cannot experience a fact directly and can't deduce it through reasoning, the way out is to ask someone who has firsthand experience. Criminal investigation, for example, relies heavily on witnesses. The witness is only helpful if he or she has observed at first hand.

If we want to know about yoga, we have to seek the testimony of a yoga expert. Such a person is called a *yoga-acharya* (*yogacharya*). *Acharya* means:

> One who has studied the necessary scriptures
> One who has practiced the suggested methods
> One who has succeeded in the methods
> One who can communicate what has been experienced.

Among other things, this means a Vedanta master who has experienced *samadhi* but has not studied and practiced yoga is no authority on yoga. It is important that this be noted, because students often believe that having the mystical experience suddenly makes one an authority on everything. Strangely enough, mystics sometimes believe it themselves.

On the other hand, if a Vedanta master has had the mystical experience and has studied and practiced yoga, he is an authority on Vedanta and Yoga. This is the case with the masters Vyasa and Shankara. If we look at our definition of the *yogacharya*, we realize it will be difficult to find such a person. They are very rare indeed.

If we want to perceive reality as it is and we can't experience *samadhi*, our intellect is not developed for inference, and we can't find a *yogacharya*, then only the second type of valid testimony can help us.

This is the testimony of sacred scriptures (*shastra*). But not all scriptures will do. Sacred scriptures dealing with liberation are called *moksha shastra*. There are many *moksha shastra*s, the most important probably being the *Upanishads*, the *Bhagavad Gita*, the *Brahma Sutra*, and the *Yoga Sutra*, but there are many others. Out of these, the *Yoga Sutra* is the authoritative yoga *shastra* (scripture dealing with yoga).

If we want to learn about yoga, there is no way around the *Yoga Sutra*. Apart from being our only reliable testimony if we do not know a liberated yoga master, the study of the *Yoga Sutra* has several interesting consequences.

Through this study and subsequent application, we will soon be able to recognize who is an authentic *yogacharya*. This study will also make the intellect sattvic, so that we can use it for deduction. Most important, however, the study leads in due time to *samadhi*, which is the direct view of reality (*pratyaksha*). This means that the study of sacred texts leads to all three forms of correct cognition.

विपर्ययो मिथ्याज्ञानम् अतद्रूपप्रतिष्ठम् ॥ ८ ॥
1.8 Wrong perception is the erroneous superimposition of an image onto an object.

In the case of wrong perception, we perceive an object and the mind then compares the sensory input with data collected in the past and identifies the object wrongly.

For example, we see a post in the distance, but believe it to be a man. We see a rope lying on the floor in the darkness and believe it to be a snake. We perceive our body and believe it to be our true nature. The problem with wrong perception is that, as soon as the error is made, the right perception is not available anymore. The mind arrives at its conclusions very quickly to ensure survival.

As soon as we have made up our mind that the rope is a snake we will retreat into safety and not probe more deeply. In many cases we are happy with our first judgment about a situation, which often is a prejudice based on past experience in a similar circumstance.

Many cases of wrong perception are insignificant, but many others end up causing the five forms of suffering — ignorance, egoism, desire, aversion, and fear.

As examples, skin color, nationality, gender, social status, and religion are, according to yoga, attributes belonging to nature (*prakrti*) and therefore not our true essence, which is consciousness. If I wrongly perceive them to be essential aspects of my self, if I identify with them, I am susceptible to conflict with individuals or groups that have different attributes. There is nothing wrong with belonging to a certain group as long as I do not forget my true nature as consciousness. If I take belonging to a social group as my true, innermost identity, automatically I will be pitched into conflict with individuals who do not belong to it. If we recognized that social or national identity has nothing to do with who we really are, conflict would be at an end. Because it creates this and many other forms of suffering, wrong perception must be overcome.

The good thing about wrong perception is that it is destroyed if right perception is achieved. In our example of the snake, if we meet somebody who tells us that what we thought was a snake is a rope, and we go back to have a second look and see that it really is a rope, at that moment the wrongly superimposed image of the snake disappears. The object, in this case the rope, does not change; it is only our simulation of the object that changes from snake to rope and from wrong to correct. Wrong and right cannot coexist.

शब्दज्ञानानुपाती वस्तुशून्यो विकल्पः ॥ ९ ॥
1.9 Conceptualization is knowledge of words, which are empty of objects.

Wrong and right perceptions are both based on the perception of an actual object. In conceptualizing we are using words, but there is no object to which they refer. If we talk about the goodness or badness of a certain person, we are referring to a set of actions performed by that person, and from that we believe we are perceiving goodness or badness. In reality, there is no such thing as goodness or badness: there is only a collection of individual good or poor choices.

If an enterprise decides to give itself a new corporate identity or image, the strategy might consist of getting a new logo, running a new advertising campaign, giving the car fleet a new color, and putting a new tune on the answering machine. All this together might form the concept of corporate image, but in fact there is no object of corporate image as such. There are only individual occurrences, which we sum up into a concept.

Our language relies heavily on conceptualizations.

To some extent they are useful, but often they are confusing. One often hears the exclamation that something was or was not "meant to be." This implies the vague notion of destiny, which is a mere concept. There is nothing in nature that refers to the concept of destiny.

Another frequently heard phrase is, "It's all for the good." One could, with the same accuracy, say "It's all for the bad." To allocate goodness or badness to a random occurrence is a mere conceptualization in an attempt to cope with change. Although concepts are helpful in getting us going, eventually they have to be abandoned in yoga in order to experience truth. As an example of a helpful concept, Vyasa mentions consciousness. Consciousness is a mere word: there is no such object as consciousness. Consciousness is the experiencer, the seer that is pure awareness. Awareness is that by which objects are perceived. It cannot be perceived, since it is not an object. If it was an object, it could not be awareness, which is pure and attributeless. This will be explained in detail later.

For now it will suffice to understand that the word "consciousness" is a concept, since there is no object that it refers to. Consciousness is the subject, and for this reason it cannot be an object of perception. Without the concept of consciousness, however, liberation itself would be inaccessible for most. Without this concept the teacher could not even explain to the student what to look for.

The concept of consciousness, together with the concept of liberation, will dissolve as soon as we abide in consciousness. To abide in consciousness is not contained in the words "abiding in consciousness." If we do not use the words, though, we cannot communicate.

अभावप्रत्ययालम्बना वृत्तिर्निद्रा ॥ १० ॥
1.10 Deep sleep is that fluctuation of mind in which the waking and dreaming experience are both negated.

That dreamless sleep is treated as a separate fluctuation might seem strange at first, but there are several reasons for it. Vyasa explains that when we wake up, we say things like "I slept soundly," "I slept poorly," or "My sleep was heavy." This indicates that there is a memory whether lightness (*sattva*), activity (*rajas*), or dullness (*tamas*) was predominant in our mind. In other words there is cognition of our mental state during sleep and recognition of it afterward. If there was no such cognition in the first place, we could not remember the quality of our sleep afterward.

How then can the state of mind during sleep be described? Patanjali answers this by saying that, in this mind state, both the waking and the dreaming world are negated. I have mentioned already the *Mandukya Upanishad*. Here the sacred syllable OM is described as having four quarters. The first quarter of the OM, the A, represents the waking state; the second quarter, the U, represents the dream state; the third, the M, represents the dreamless sleep; and the fourth quarter, the silence after the OM, represents the transcendental or fourth state (*turiya*). The master Gaudapada has explained the *Upanishad* in his *Mandukya Karika* and created the foundation of the system of Advaita (nondualist) Vedanta.

Gaudapada says the waking state is unreal because it is negated in the dream state, whereas the dream state is unreal because it is negated in the waking state. When we are awake, we believe the dream experience to be unreal; when we are dreaming, we believe the waking world to be unreal. Therefore, Gaudapada concludes, both are unreal. In the deep-sleep state, both the waking and the dream state do not exist, whereas during waking and dreaming the deep-sleep state is nonexistent. Therefore, says Gaudapada, all three are illusionary.

A similar idea is expressed in a riddle the ancient Taoist master Chuang Tzu once gave his students. After he woke up from an afternoon nap, he told his students that he had just dreamed of being a butterfly. His question was whether he really was Chuang Tzu who had dreamed he was a butterfly or whether he was rather a butterfly who was now dreaming he was Chuang Tzu.

The question cannot be convincingly answered, since all the supporting evidence for the proposition that Chuang Tzu is really Chuang Tzu can be derived only from the waking state. The experience of the waking state was, however, negated by the dream experience of being a butterfly. Chuang Tzu asked his students to bring evidence of his true identity from a third, impartial, unaffected reality.

Since they could not, Chuang Tzu could not be convinced that he really was Chuang Tzu.

It is the impartial, unaffected reality that Gaudapada is interested in. This true reality is, according to him, the transcendental state (*turiya*), which is always there. In it there is awareness of the other three states, but in the three there is no awareness of the fourth, the transcendental state. In yoga we would call the transcendental state objectless *samadhi*, but apart from that Patanjali does not agree with Gaudapada regarding the unreality of the three states. They both agree, however, that waking and dreaming are both negated in deep dreamless sleep.

Patanjali says that the dreamless sleep fluctuation is an obstacle that has to be overcome eventually, since it is opposed to permanent objectless (*asamprajnata*) *samadhi*. For liberation to occur, objectless *samadhi* has to become permanent. If the deep-sleep fluctuation were still present, it would make objectless *samadhi* impermanent.

अनुभूतविषयासंप्रमोषः स्मृतिः ॥ ११ ॥
1.11 Memory is the keeping in one's mind of objects experienced previously.

The yogic definition of memory (*smrti*) pertains only to those mental conditions that we can access consciously. The unconscious ones are treated under subconscious imprint (*samskara*).

Memory is any recollection of the previous four fluctuations, which are correct perception, wrong perception, conceptualization, and sleep.

Sleep is a fluctuation that is deduced by accessing memory. Since we are usually unconscious when we sleep, we can't experience it directly. We know its state of mind from memory.

Correct perception, wrong perception, and conceptualization are called so only when the condition occurs initially; after that they are called memory. Since with both correct and wrong perception an object is present, we can easily distinguish them from memory.

Conceptualization that does not refer to an object in fact often overlaps with memory. Unless we conceive a concept right on the spot, it often contains memorized beliefs.

अभ्यासवैराग्याभ्यां तन्निरोधः ॥ १२ ॥

1.12 The suspension of these fluctuations is through practice and detachment.

After the initial definition of yoga (sutra I.2), all terms involved (yoga, mind, fluctuations) have been defined, apart from suspension, which is treated now.

Patanjali says here that the mind waves will cease through the application of the combined means of practice and detachment. The important word here is "and," since the application of only one of the two leads to extremes of the mind. If we only practice, then we tend to develop beliefs like "Our practice is the only correct practice," "Only Ashtanga Yoga is the correct yoga," "Only Mysore style is the correct form for a yoga class," "Only the God that I worship is the true God," "Capitalism is the only proper economic system," and "Democracy is the only proper political system."

All these statements have in common the belief that there is one truth that excludes all others. In yoga we call this a solar attitude. It is dominant when the *prana* flows through the solar energy channel (*pingala*), which begins at the right nostril. We may also call it a tendency to fundamentalism. It prevents us from recognizing that a position different from our own valid view could also be right. It is a trap of the mind, which believes to have figured out reality by imposing a particular extreme reality tunnel on it.

We fall into the opposite trap, however, if we do not practice but only apply detachment. We develop beliefs like "All paths lead to the same goal," "It's all yoga," "Everything is holy and sacred," "Everybody has to live their own truth," "Everybody has to do their own thing," and "All statements, philosophies, and religions are valid." These statements have in common the belief that there are many truths, which cancel out the one truth. In yoga we call this a lunar attitude, dominant when *prana* flows in the lunar (*ida*) channel, which starts at the left nostril. A lunar attitude makes us surrender our tools before we use them, and we therefore won't be able to change ourselves. According to the lunar attitude, I don't have to change because I am okay as I am; in fact everybody is okay. The lunar extreme makes it impossible for us to recognize wrong views, and especially it disables us for rejecting views and values — which might be okay in general, but they aren't the right ones for us.

If everybody is okay, why does 50 percent of humankind live in poverty? Why did we live for thousands of years in permanent warfare? Why are our prisons and mental wards full, and why does planet Earth shake itself as if in an attempt to shake off humankind gone mad? We can call the lunar attitude relativism. Since everything is true only from a certain angle, we won't have to worry about anything really. Relativism is a trap of the mind, which believes to have figured out reality by imposing on it an extreme reality tunnel. Reality according to yoga is not to be found in either extreme of the mind. It is to be found resting in the center, unchallenged by the extremes of the mind.

The center has many names in yoga, such as Brahman, *purusha*, and *hrdaya*, the heart. One of the names is *sushumna*, the central energy channel. When the *prana* flows in the central energy channel, the mind is free of solar and lunar extremes, which means that the thought waves are suspended. To reach this state, Patanjali suggests the combined application of practice and detachment. This is paradoxical, since the two are in some ways opposed. They need to be, otherwise the mind could figure out what is going on, and then that would be just another simulation of reality and not the truth.

For the paradox to stay intact we have to avoid two attitudes. One is to practice detachment. Detachment is the opposite of practice: it is to loosen one's hold on things. One cannot practice letting go; one just lets go and surrenders. The other is to practice detachment from one's practice. If you detach yourself from your practice, only detachment is left and you fall back into relativism. It's just another trick of the mind.

तत्र स्थितौ यत्नोऽभ्यासः ॥ १३ ॥

1.13 Practice is the effort to attain steadiness in the suspended state.

After Patanjali has pointed out the dual strategy to suspend the mind waves, he now defines its two aspects, beginning with practice. We might have had the suspended state (*nirodha*) in glimpses, but that's not enough. We have to attain steadiness in it. Steadiness means that *nirodha* flows peacefully, according to Vyasa. The effort to remain in that peaceful flow is called practice (*abhyasa*). This effort needs to have the qualities of vigor and enthusiasm. We might be surprised to hear a Vedanta master, Vyasa, who is the author of the *Brahma Sutra*, recommend effort, vigor, and enthusiasm to stay in the peaceful flow. But Shankara, another Vedanta master, confirms Vyasa's statement by declaring that effort, vigor, and enthusiasm are synonyms here.[8]

Patanjali's sutras and Vyasa's commentary remind us also of the following verse of Shankara: "The aspirant should carefully practise this [meditation], which reveals his natural bliss until, being under his full control, it arises spontaneously…"[9]

All three masters show a subtle and deep understanding of how the "natural bliss," the "peaceful flow," the "suspended state," arises spontaneously when it is preceded by effort, practice, and vigor. This teaches us two facts. One is that in days of yore the gap between Vedanta and Yoga was much smaller than modern-day Vedanta masters want us to believe. The second is that "just spontaneously being in the moment and making no artificial effort whatsoever," which some contemporary masters teach and which accommodated the beliefs of the hippie generation so comfortably, is not based on the teachings of Vyasa and Shankara, the founders of the school of Vedanta. Just being natural spontaneously is a very advanced state that follows after years of practice and study. It is not following one's whims, which is only slavery of the mind. As will be explained in more detail later, inner freedom (*samadhi*) is attained through outer structure and discipline,

which is called practice. The lack of outer structure and discipline advocated by some modern teachers, who clearly draw masses of listeners, leads to inner dogmatism and limitation.

स तु दीर्घकालनैरन्तर्यसत्कारासेवितो दृढभूमिः ॥ १४ ॥

1.14 One becomes firmly established in practice only after attending to it for a long time, without interruption and with an attitude of devotion.

We might practice for a while and then all at once find our past conditioning overwhelms our practice efforts. We may suddenly develop anger, greed, pride, lust, and envy, and wonder how that can be after all this yoga. How can we avoid succumbing to such impulses?

Patanjali suggests it is by being firmly established in practice. This cannot happen all of a sudden: we are bound to have a yoyo practice at first. We may make good progress one moment and the next moment find ourselves back in our old conditioning. To really become established one needs to practice for a long time, without interruption and in a devoted way.

What does a long time mean? A year is not a long time. A decade is more to the point. Several decades would be realistic. The ancient *rishi*s are usually depicted with long beards, and they are said to have reached freedom from bondage after a lifetime of study and practice. True, some teachers have reached incredible wisdom at a young age: for example Shankara composed the *Brahma Sutra Bhasya* when he was twelve. That this is not the normal course of events is reflected in the fact that he is considered in India to be of divine origin.

The average yogi cannot expect to be established in truth through a few years of practice. A "long time" means we make a commitment to practice, however long it takes, and are not perturbed by any setbacks. The *Bhagavad Gita* explains that all actions are performed by the Supreme Being only, and so the fruits or results of those actions belong only to the Supreme Being. If I can admit that the one practicing is not I, then I will not expect results.

---

8. *Shankara on the Yoga Sutras*, trans. T. Leggett, 1st Indian ed., Motilal Banarsidass, Delhi, 1992, p. 97.

9. *Aparokshanubhuti of Sri Sankaracharya*, v. 125, trans. Sw. Vimuktananda, Advaita Ashrama, Kolkata, 1938, p. 68.

According to Patanjali, it is *prakrti* (nature) that practices, and we are only looking on. The *Bhagavad Gita* has it that the Supreme Being operates *prakrti*, and so performs all actions. In both approaches, if we give up the idea of ever getting anywhere with our yoga, then we have arrived at the destination, the present moment, now. However long the practice may take does not matter anymore, since we have arrived already.

To practice without interruption means to do one's formal practice daily. Some really clever people have said, "Yes, but if you are tired, exhausted and don't have the time or energy to do your practice, doing it will have a detrimental effect anyway." This is a reasonable thought, but we should ask ourselves why we are exhausted and have no energy and time. Possibly we spend too much time running after money, or our social life takes up too much energy. Alternatively, we might have eaten too late or too much the day before or have not rested enough. H. Aranya says that uninterrupted practice means constant practice. He is not referring to one's formal practice but to mindfulness and watchfulness.

The last of Patanjali's three parameters for establishment in practice is to practice with an attitude of devotion. An example of practicing with a bad attitude is to practice because one thinks one has to, for whatever reason, but actually hates what one does. This could be because:

> We think we have to get our frame into shape, so that others desire us.

> We think that, when we exercise postures more proficiently than others, we are superior to them. (The same can be said about practicing meditation and *samadhi*.)

> We practice because we want to get any type of advantage over others, be it physical, mental, or spiritual.

To practice with devotion is to remain grateful for being able to practice at all. It is great good fortune to have come across yoga in our lifetime. Many people have never heard about it or are never properly introduced to it; others live in a war-torn country or in economic crisis, both of which make yoga practice difficult.

Again, if our body is crippled or our mind is deranged, yoga will be more difficult. It is good to keep these points in perspective. If none of them applies to us, we are in a fortunate position and need only to sustain a practice and an enthusiastic attitude toward it.

दृष्टानुश्रविकविषयवितृष्णस्य वशीकारसंज्ञा वैराग्यम् ॥ १५ ॥

1.15 Detachment is mastery in not desiring objects seen or heard of.

Having dealt with practice, Patanjali now defines the other aspect of stilling the mind. If one practices but keeps one's desires alive, at some point one will necessarily use the powers acquired in one's practice to fulfill those desires.

In the twentieth century there came to prominence teachers who suggested we should fulfill all our desires as soon as they came to mind. From this satisfaction, it was said, mental stillness would proceed. The problem here is that desires are located in the mind. The heart does not need fulfilment since it is fullness made manifest.

The mind, on the contrary, reacts like a spoiled child. With every demand fulfilled, three new ones pop up. In the end, the entire world is seen just as a giant machine to supply sensory satisfaction and to soothe one's greed.

Happiness is not found in external satisfaction, but only in the stillness of the heart. If we fulfill the desires of the mind, we give two wrong messages:

> We profess that permanent happiness is to be found in fulfilling the desires of the mind, whereas in fact freedom is only within.

> By succumbing to the demands of the mind, we increase its power over us.

The more we realize that we do not depend on the fulfillment of the demands and desires of the mind at all, the freer and happier we are. To be a slave to our desires, like gluttony, has a debilitating effect on our psyche. The realization, on the other hand, that we do not depend on external stimuli for freedom brings incredible strength and mental clarity. This can be seen for example in the lives of Nelson Mandela and Mahatma Gandhi.

Detachment is said to develop in four steps, which can be described as follows:

155

1. Accepting the idea that fulfilling desires does not make us free but creates more desires.

2. Succeeding in letting go of some attachments but not others.

3. Letting go of all attachments on a superficial level. The seed is still there in the mind and could germinate again if the right object is presented.

4. Mastering detachment. It is this level that Patanjali talks about. It is attained gradually.

Detachment is gained from two different types of objects. The first category is objects that are seen. These are the bodies of others, good food, alcohol, drugs, money, real estate, clothes, and all types of wealth and power that we could get attached to.

The second category is objects heard of. These are yogic achievements and all the yogic powers described in the third chapter of the *Yoga Sutra*. Also listed here are achievements in *asana*, achievements in meditation, achievements in *samadhi* and concepts such as enlightenment. So ultimately the desire to achieve *samadhi* will obstruct the path to *samadhi*. To desire means to be in the future with one's mind; *samadhi* means to let go of the concept of future.

तत्परं पुरुषख्यातेर्गुणवैतृष्ण्यम् ॥ १६ ॥

1.16 The highest detachment, which proceeds from knowing consciousness, is to not thirst for the manifestations of the *gunas*.

The highest form of detachment cannot be achieved. It proceeds spontaneously when consciousness (*purusha*) is known. Then all that we were attached to previously appears pale and stale compared to the glory of one's true nature. Everything we know and can know is, according to Samkhya philosophy, manifested by the three qualities (*gunas*) of nature (*prakrti*). The *gunas* in various combinations manifest the visible gross world, the invisible subtle world, our body, mind, ego, and intellect. The only two categories (*tattvas*) of existence that are not produced by the *gunas* are the two unmanifest categories, which are nature or world ground (*prakrti*), out of which everything arises, and consciousness (*purusha*), which witnesses everything.

Like a dancer who appears on stage once the audience is settled, *prakrti* manifests the world through its *gunas* when consciousness looks on. This projecting of the world is called experience, which results in bondage. We become bound because we erroneously believe ourselves to be the projected phenomena whereas in truth we are the eternal consciousness.

In a way we can say that we become what we believe or know to be. Consciousness (*purusha*) is forever free but, because we forget our true nature, we start to believe we are the phenomena (world, body, mind, etc.). This is called bondage, and it leads to suffering. We always try to achieve happiness through permanence, but the phenomena are all transitory. Our partners, friends, and family will die; our own body will break down and fail us; our house and car will disintegrate; all the riches we've accumulated will end up in somebody else's hands one day. Once bondage is experienced for some time (according to some orthodox sources thirty trillion incarnations), we have had enough and realize ourselves as consciousness, which is freedom. From this realization of consciousness all thirst for the phenomena that are manifestations of the *gunas* ceases. This is called the highest detachment.

As hard as we try, we can never produce this form of detachment. It results only from having the mystical experience. Then the *gunas*, with their manifestations, fall off us like boulders falling from a mountaintop, never to return.[10]

वितर्कविचारानन्दास्मितारूपानुगमात्
संप्रज्ञातः ॥ १७ ॥

1.17 Objective *samadhi* (*samprajnata*) is associated with deliberation, reflection, bliss, and I-am-ness (*asmita*).

After Patanjali has pointed out the means to still the mind, he will define now the two types of *samadhi*. In the first sutra (I.1) we learned that the term yoga has the same root as *samadhi* (*yujir samadhau*). Vyasa uses yoga and *samadhi* synonymously, and often talks about *samprajnata yoga* instead of *samprajnata samadhi*.

10. Vyasa on sutra II.27.

In the second sutra, Patanjali defined yoga as suspension (*nirodha*) of thought waves. This means the true state of yoga is the higher objectless *samadhi* (*asamprajnata*), which is also the goal of yoga. The first *samadhi* is the path to the second *samadhi*. Most of Patanjali's sutras deal with the first *samadhi* as a path to the second *samadhi*, which is liberation.

The first *samadhi* is called *samprajnata*. *Sa* means "with"; *prajna* is often translated as "wisdom" or "insight." It is the capacity of the intellect to perceive objects as they really are. In this context *prajna* means cognition, being conscious of an object. The best translation for *samprajnata* is cognitive *samadhi*, but we can also call it *samadhi*-with-object. It means that, in this *samadhi*, the intellect is cognizing. "Cognizing" means the intellect is focused on or aware of objects.

The higher type of *samadhi* is *asamprajnata samadhi* — supercognitive *samadhi* — wherein one is beyond cognition of objects but rests in consciousness alone. We can also call it objectless *samadhi*. Some translations have used the expression "unconscious *samadhi*," which is quite confusing since we are one with consciousness itself in this state. The flower-power generation called this state "cosmic consciousness," which describes it more aptly than "unconscious *samadhi*." Since we will be talking a lot about these two *samadhis*, the constant use of words like "cognitive" and "supercognitive" would be alienating, so I have replaced them with "objective" and "objectless" *samadhi*, which are more congenial. Let us keep in mind, though, the more precise translations.

In this sutra, Patanjali defines objective *samadhi*. In doing so he describes four levels of depth, which can be experienced depending on how superficial or internal the object is on which we meditate.

The first step is called deliberation (*vitarka*), a very modest form of *samadhi*. In fact it is often called *vitarka dhyana* — deliberative meditation. The boundaries of meditation and *samadhi* are not rigid, but flowing. Deliberative *samadhi* means that we are focusing on a physical object, which in yoga is called a gross object. The use of the term "object" can be confusing — everything apart from pure awareness in yoga is called object. Even intelligence and ego are objects. Awareness is not an object because it is the subject, the observer.

Let us say we were to practice deliberative *samadhi* on the moon, which is a gross object. Deliberation means that during the *samadhi* there is a discussion going on concerning all the concepts related to the moon. For example, while we focus on the moon, we think about its silvery light, its image in a lake, its consistency, its surface, its orbit, its influence on the tides and our bodily fluids, and its relation to lunacy. That is all. Patanjali has placed the first bar very low. If our mind has achieved identity (*samapatti*) with the object moon, while it deliberates on concepts relating to the moon only and not on any others, this is technically already *samadhi* in Patanjali's sense.

The next step is taken after the first is achieved. In reflective *samadhi* we focus on subtle objects. These are objects that do not have a physical appearance, such as sound, the lotus of the heart, the light in the head, or an idea. In the first *samadhi* we were deliberating, which means we were practicing a deeply concentrated thought based on one object only. In reflective *samadhi* we are reflecting or contemplating, which is a much deeper, subtler type of activity. It is more like becoming receptive for the true meaning to arise. This type of *samadhi* is used if we want to understand the true meaning behind the concepts of the *Yoga Sutra*. We cannot grab them or force them under our control, but we have to reflect until the true meaning is revealed.

The third type of objective *samadhi* is called blissful (*ananda*) *samadhi*. Once the subtle objects are understood, bliss arises. It arises because with this understanding comes the glimpse of freedom. We could say, here we understand for the first time that one day we will be free. From that arises spontaneous happiness. If we do *samadhi* on that object, on that feeling of happiness, then that is blissful *samadhi*. It is a *samadhi* on experience itself.

The fourth type of objective *samadhi* is on I-am-ness. Who is it that says, "I am experiencing bliss"? It is on that I-am-ness that we concentrate in the fourth type. It may sound strange at first to meditate on I-am-ness, which is a function of egoity. But this does not mean that we meditate "what a wonderfully big ego I have": meditation on egoity means something different. In yoga we first learn to observe the body. Once this observation is established, we know that we are not the body but an observing agent independent of the body. Otherwise we could not observe the body. The next step is that we start observing our thoughts. Eventually, from being established in that observation, we know that we are not our thoughts, since we can detach ourselves and observe them like the thoughts of a stranger. Who are we, then, if we are not the body and not the mind (*manas*, the thinking principle)? The agent that claims ownership of body and mind is called *ahamkara* — ego. Its function, which is the erroneous commingling or mixing of seer (pure consciousness) and seeing (the mind), is called egoity or I-am-ness (*asmita*).

In the last of our objective *samadhi*s, meditation is done on this pure I-am-ness. It needs to be pure: it cannot be mixed with notions like, "I am great" or "I am bad." If *samadhi* can be sustained on the pure notion of I, without any discussion or thought arising on who or what we are, several fundamental revelations will happen. One is that egoity is based on ignorance, not knowing ourselves. If we go deep into egoity, we find that it arises out of intellect/intelligence. Once we have found intelligence, in it will arise discriminative knowledge of what is real and unreal. From this eventually will rise realization of consciousness (*purusha*), which is liberation. This last state is described in the next sutra.

विरामप्रत्ययाभ्यासपूर्वः संस्कारशेषोऽन्यः ॥ १८ ॥

1.18 The other [*asamprajnata samadhi*] results from the practice of stilling the fluctuations of the mind and leaves only residual subconscious imprint.

Now Patanjali defines the second higher *samadhi*, which is referred to in this text as objectless *samadhi* (*asamprajnata samadhi*).

The sutra here picks up the definition of sutra I.2 and elaborates on it. Every time the mind waves are suspended (*nirodha*) for an extended period we are in objectless *samadhi*. On the other hand, if objectless *samadhi* becomes permanent, the mind is permanently suspended, which is liberation.

Only objectless *samadhi* can confer this effect, because as long as the mind rests on an object, as in objective (*samprajnata*) *samadhi*, the mind waves are

focused (*ekagra*) and not suspended (*nirodha*). Objective *samadhi* therefore cannot produce liberation.

Just as a stone thrown into a lake will produce waves that distort the surface, so will an object in the mind produce thought waves that, even if single-pointed (*ekagra*), will ruffle the surface of the lake of the mind. It then cannot be used to reflect on our true nature. It is only objectless *samadhi* that will show us our true nature.

Vyasa says the highest detachment mentioned in sutra I.16 is the means to this *samadhi*. This is a paradox. Sutra I.16 states that this highest detachment results from knowing consciousness. But realizing consciousness itself is only possible through objectless *samadhi*.

About this paradox the following has to be understood.

The mystical experience, which is a temporary objectless *samadhi*, cannot be forced or achieved at all. It is not the case that from doing this and that the mystical experience will result. Since the mystical experience depends heavily on the subconscious conditioning of the seeker, or should we rather say lack thereof, at no point can we be certain what exactly produces the experience in a particular person. This reverberates in the *Yoga Sutra* through the many different suggested techniques. On the other hand the element of unpredictability concerning the mystical experience has led to the belief that it is bestowed through divine grace.

Once the experience is had, one knows that nothing one has ever done in one's life could have produced it. The human being is too small to manifest such magnificence. The only thing we can do is bring ourselves into a position so that the indescribable can happen.

Supreme detachment and practicing the stilling of the mind are aids, but cannot be called the efficient cause. They are, rather, an invitation. Once the guest (*asamprajnata samadhi* or a glimpse thereof) has arrived, consciousness is known. From this knowledge results permanent supreme detachment, leading to permanent abiding in consciousness (liberation).

Before that happens, though, we have to take another look at the mind. As I have pointed out, the mind consists of conscious activity, called fluctuations or thought waves (*vrtti*), and subconscious activity, called subconscious imprint (*samskara*). The subconscious imprints are a result of our thoughts and actions. The mystical experience (a glimpse or short *asamprajnata samadhi*) suspends the mind or results from the suspension of mind, but it does not destroy our subconscious conditioning. That is why, when the *samadhi* is over, the mind will remanifest from the leftover conditioning (*samskaras*).

We should not be disappointed when this happens. It is asking too much that conditioning should be eradicated by an initial one-hour objectless *samadhi*. We have to continue our path with conviction.

When objectless *samadhi* becomes permanent, it will delete the conditioning or destroy what are called the seeds of suffering. From the seeds sprout new ignorant action and thirst for manifestation of the *guna*s, which is thirst for life. Then it is called *nirbija samadhi* — seedless *samadhi*.

More about that later.

भवप्रत्ययो विदेहप्रकृतिलयानाम् ॥ १९ ॥

1.19 Among the bodiless ones and the ones absorbed in *prakrti*, there is the intention of coming into being.

In this and the next sutra, two types of objectless (*asamprajnata*) samadhi are considered. Sutra I.20 describes objectless *samadhi* as preceded by yogic practice and produced with yogic intent, which is liberation.

Liberation does in some way imply leaving or going beyond the realm of manifestation. The *Samkhya Karika* describes the final realization as the notion of *na asmi* — not-I. This does not mean the I gets annihilated or terminated, as is taught in Buddhism. According to Yoga, I and egoism, like mind, are eternal and will never cease. What it means is that once the yogi realizes him- or herself as consciousness (*purusha*), his or her affiliation with I-ness, ego, and mind ceases. Since the ignorant notion of "I" and "I am an individual, isolated identity in this world" is overcome, we cannot say then that "I" am consciousness. We can then only say that consciousness *is*.

But even to say "consciousness is" is partially incorrect, since consciousness contains the notions of existence, nonexistence, neither, and beyond both.

The *Samkhya Karika* therefore says only "not-I." This does not mean that I am annihilated but, rather, I have recognized myself as that which cannot be described anymore in terms of I-ness.

To realize not-I implies that we have gone beyond wanting to remain an isolated, manifested individual. Why would we want to remain a droplet if we could be the entire vast ocean? Only fear and the ignorance of not wanting to lose the shackles of I-ness will stop us.

A true yogi, one who has studied, understood, practiced, and realized yoga, will lose the intention of "coming into being," which is the opposite of not-I. Coming into being means to sustain one's desire for continuation as an isolated individual, although one should know better. In the traditional context, this means that one will continue to be reborn, out of ignorance. The true yogi will let go of this desire, since manifestation impinges on the ecstasy of pure consciousness.

One of many messages encrypted into this sutra is, "Among those who have not practiced yogic methods with yogic intent, there is the desire for future embodiment." Those are then subdivided into two categories, which are the bodiless ones and the ones absorbed in *prakrti*. Both are very advanced mystical states, which can be held for a very long time. But since the subconscious imprints (*samskara*s) are not deleted in these states, and since I-ness is not overcome, the ones experiencing such states will eventually fall back and come again under the grip of mind and ego.

The first category described in this sutra comprises the bodiless ones. They are powerful beings that exist without the need for a physical body. Traditionally they are understood to be, for example, the gods. When the term "gods" is used in India, we should not confuse it with the Christian God or Allah in Islam or the Brahman of the *Upanishad*s, because all those terms are only ever used in the singular: there can only be one God. The gods of vedic India can be more likened to the gods of the Greeks (Zeus, Kronos, Hera, Aphrodite, Apollo, and so on), the gods of the Romans (Jupiter, Saturn, Mars, Venus, Mercury, etc.) or the ancient Germanic gods (Thor, Wotan, Loki, Odin, Freya, etc.).

The vedic gods are representations of forces of

nature. Varuna, like Neptune, represents ocean; Indra, like Thor, represents thunder; Agni, like Loki, represents fire. The vedic gods certainly have an agenda or an intention of coming into being. When we read the ancient creation myths, we realize that the lives of the "gods" were quite human, indeed similar to those led by some of the characters in recent soap operas. Definitely they are very different from God, Allah, or Brahman, which have no agenda, no intention, and need no becoming, since the one is pure existence as such.

According to Patanjali and Vyasa's understanding, the gods are in extremely long-lasting and powerful states of *asamprajnata samadhi*. But since their residual subconscious imprints (*samskaras*) are not deleted, and since they live in a state of long-lasting pleasure, they do not long for freedom. Longing for freedom depends on the right mixture of pleasure and pain being provided, as in the case of a human. Once the merit of the gods is exhausted they will fall back to a less powerful, conditioned state.

The other category mentioned is *prakrtilaya*, which means the ones absorbed in nature (*prakrti*). Again, this is a very advanced mystical state of objectless *samadhi*. *Prakrti* is the unmanifest source of the world, which brings forth this entire vast universe. However, since *prakrti* is not manifest, it is not an object. Expressions such as "I was one with everything," "I was one with the source of everything," and "I was in everything" refer to that state. Some contemporary teachers have had this experience and teach it now, but it will not lead to liberation and it is not traditional yoga.

Liberation comes about by realizing oneself as consciousness, which is completely different from merging with the source of manifestation (*prakrti*). Since *prakrti* is eternal becoming, oneness with it leads to an intention of becoming, in other words an agenda. One needs to detach oneself from that too, and abide in what is eternal, uncreated, unstainable, and unchangeable: consciousness.

We know now that there are different mystical states, and some are dead-end streets. By closely reflecting on and realizing yogic truth, we will stay on the direct road to freedom. The next sutra explains how.

160

श्रद्धावीर्यस्मृतिसमाधिप्रज्ञापूर्वक इतरेषाम् ॥ २० ॥

1.20 In the case of the others [the yogis], it [*asamprajnata samadhi*] is preceded by conviction, enthusiasm, remembrance, *samadhi*, and wisdom (*prajna*).

Asamprajnata (objectless) *samadhi* is divided into two categories. In sutra I.19, Patanjali described those who harbor an intention of becoming (*bhava pratyaya*) and who therefore do not reach liberation but return to conditioned existence. These are not true yogis, and they did not reach this *samadhi* through proper yogic method.

In the present sutra, Patanjali describes those who reach objectless *samadhi* through prescribed effort (*upaya pratyaya*), which is yogic practice. Those are the true yogis. Five steps are described here that need to be combined with supreme detachment, mentioned earlier.

The first step is conviction (*shraddha*). Conviction is gained by analyzing one's own situation and then studying and applying yogic philosophy. Only if one completely understands yogic philosophy intellectually can one be completely convinced. A vague feeling that "It might work" or "It could be the right thing for me" won't suffice. One needs to be able to think, "This is my situation right now. I am bound. I am a slave of my mind. Due to that, I am ignorant and I suffer. Even if I feel okay now, suffering could be around the corner in the form of my death, disease, death of a loved one, unforseen calamities, and so on. Therefore, I must break free and attain liberation. For this purpose, I have to eradicate my conditioning. This is possible by undertaking the steps and limbs of yoga with the right attitude. From practicing those methods I will attain liberation as others have done before me."

If one understands yoga in this way, step by step, this is called conviction. If one is too unclear to think in that way, more study of yogic philosophy such as the *Yoga Sutra* needs to be undertaken.

The second requirement is enthusiasm or energy (*virya*). Even after one has understood yoga, one could still fall victim to a negative attitude, such as, "I do understand but I don't want to put the energy into it." The right attitude for yoga is to be ready to give everything and have no expectation. If we have the right enthusiasm, which the Rishi Vasishta calls "true self-effort," there is no destiny apart from the one that we create. The yogic path does need energy. After all, we have to free ourselves from our conditioning (*samskara* and *vasana*). How much energy did we invest creating it and over what time span? We will need energy and enthusiasm to undo all this.

The third requirement is remembrance. When we have conviction and enthusiasm, we will be able to start the path of yoga. But sometimes we will get lost or run into a dead-end street. In moments of confusion, it is important that we remember what we are doing. What is my purpose? How did I get here? Where do I want to get to from here? How?

Especially as we start to succeed with yoga, we often tend to lose our intention. We might be happy to stick with *asana* or *pranayama* after we get comfortable in it. We might lose interest in yoga because we notice that our teacher and those around us are not sincere. We might get dejected because we did not get an experience of true yoga. In all of these cases, it is important to remember ourselves, our purpose, our goal, and the correct method. This remembrance will make sure that we stay on course.

The fourth requirement is *samadhi*. Here, as in many other places in the *Yoga Sutra*, the term *samadhi* refers to objective (*samprajnata*) *samadhi*. If we have conviction, enthusiasm, and remembrance, we need only to apply the eight limbs of yoga, which culminate in the practice of objective *samadhi*.

Everybody who fulfills the conditions so far will, after due practice, experience at least the lower rungs of objective *samadhi* described in sutra I.17 (*vitarka*). In many ways objective *samadhi* is the main theme of the *Yoga Sutra*. Its various stages will be described later on. Objective *samadhi* is the path to objectless *samadhi*.

The final requirement is wisdom (*prajna*). There is no good English translation for this word. Precisely, it means "complete knowledge pertaining to objects," which means that we see things as they really are, without our mind modifying them. The term *prajna* is contained in *sam-prajna-ta* (objective) *samadhi*, because we are cognizing objects in this *samadhi*. Wisdom (*prajna*), or the ability to clearly

reflect things as they are,[11] is the fruit and result of objective *samadhi*. From *prajna* comes discriminative knowledge. From perceiving objects (including mind, ego, and intellect) as they really are, we learn that we are not these objects. We learn that the self, the consciousness, our true nature, is not contained in anything that we can observe. This is called discriminative knowledge (*viveka khyateh*) or knowledge of the difference between what is eternal and transitory, self and nonself, essential and nonessential, pure and stainable.

These five requirements — conviction, enthusiasm, remembrance, *samadhi*, and wisdom — are necessary to succeed in objectless *samadhi*. Only when objectless *samadhi* is preceded by them does it lead to liberation (*kaivalya*).

तीव्रसंवेगानाम् आसन्नः ॥ २१ ॥
I.21 For those who practice with ardent intensity, *samadhi* is near.

Samadhi might be way off at first, but if we practice intensely, says Patanjali, it is near. Vyasa adds that whoever practices intensely will experience *samadhi* and its fruit, which is liberation. Vijnanabhiksu lends his support by quoting from the *Vishnu Purana*: "One who attains *samadhi* [attains] liberation in that life itself."[12]

So there is no excuse and no time to waste. Orthodox tradition says that we need the gift of the last birth to be liberated in this life. The gift of the last birth can only be acquired though effort in previous lives.

It is not possible for us, however, to determine from the outside what sort of practice someone has done previously. A person's knowledge cannot be ascertained from outside appearances. Some of the greatest masters lived as beggars in outwardly crippled bodies. Others made themselves purposely ugly or behaved in a repulsive fashion so that they could live and practice in peace.

---

11. Sutra I.41.

12. *Yogavarttika of Vijnanabhiksu*, vol. 1, trans. T. S. Rukmani, Munshiram Manoharlal, New Delhi, 1998, p. 122.

मृदुमध्याधिमात्रत्वात् ततोऽपि विशेषः ॥ २२ ॥
1.22 Those ardent ones are again subdivided into mild, moderate, and intense.

We have, altogether, nine subcategories in the order of their intensity and their closeness to *samadhi*. It is an Indian pastime to create categories and divide them into subcategories. Shankara says in his sub-commentary that the purpose of the sutra is to "make clear that [all] yogins, whether slow or not, do attain their aimed-at goal, [so] it should arouse an undepressed spirit in them."[13] There is only a difference in how fast that goal is reached.

ईश्वरप्रणिधानाद् वा ॥ २३ ॥
1.23 Or from devotion to Ishvara.

According to Vyasa, this sutra answers the question whether there are other ways by which *samadhi* can be attained other than by those outlined so far. *Samadhi* can also be attained by devotion to Ishvara, a statement that is repeated several times in the *Yoga Sutra*. "Ishvara" is a general term for the Supreme Being or Lord. No affiliation to any particular religion is implied. Devotees can fill in the name for the divine as they worship it, whether this is God, Jehovah, Vishnu, or whatever else.

It is very interesting that Patanjali mentions devotion to the Supreme Being here. Although the main theme of the *Yoga Sutra* is the technical instruction of the methods of yoga called Raja Yoga and Ashtanga Yoga, the path of surrender (Bhakti Yoga) is also described and tolerated.

In this regard the *Yoga Sutra* is a mirror image of the *Bhagavad Gita*, which deals primarily with Bhakti Yoga but also accepts the path of Ashtanga Yoga. A third path, the path of knowledge (Jnana Yoga), is also accepted by both scriptures. India had a very tolerant multifaceted culture in its golden days, and people noticed that liberation was possible using any of the three paths. This often led to all three being mentioned, even if a scripture such as the *Yoga Sutra* mainly focused on one of them.

13. T. Leggett, *Shankara on the Yoga Sutras*, p. 106.

Permanently meditating on the Supreme Being constitutes the path of devotion. Here all of one's actions and thoughts are to be surrendered and a feeling of intense love for the Supreme Being developed. This intense love (*bhakti*) will attract the grace of the Supreme Being, who will bestow *samadhi* and liberation onto the yogi. There are schools of yoga that accept this path as the only proper way to do yoga. Especially today in India, most schools of yoga espouse *bhakti*, including the Vaishnava and Shaivite schools. (T. Krishnamacharya was a Vaishnava and K. Pattabhi Jois is a Shaivite.) Opposed to these schools are those of Samkhya — Patanjali Yoga and Shankara's Advaita Vedanta — which put more emphasis on the meditation practice and realization of the individual. The *Upanishads* and the *Brahma Sutra* contain both approaches.

Nevertheless, the inclusion of the Supreme Being (Ishvara) is the one point where Patanjali steers away from the Samkhya system. The Samkhya onto which Patanjali grafted the techniques of yoga is a meditation system that describes the entire world in twenty-five categories. Patanjali kept all these categories and added a twenty-sixth, which is Ishvara. Patanjali's system is therefore sometimes referred to as "Samkhya with Ishvara."

Kapila, the founder of Samkhya, is said to have created a system and an analysis of the world that did not rely on Ishvara. It can be noted also that Mahavira, the founder of Jainism, and Buddha were silent in regard to Ishvara.

They are therefore regarded in Western circles as atheists, which they are not. An atheist is somebody who claims that God does not exist. At no point did Samkhya or Mahavira or Buddha make this claim. The original Samkhya grew out of the idea of creating an explanation of the world and a meditation system that steered clear of religion. It has shown that the world can be explained without resorting to God. The Samkhya meditation system enables people to become liberated even if they don't want to resort to a Supreme Being.

Those theistic schools that believe that only surrender to God can lead to liberation have strongly rebuked Samkhya for this reason. They feel that nobody should be allowed the great good fortune of liberation without personally acknowledging the

Supreme Being. The *Bhagavata Purana*,[14] however, states that the Supreme Being manifested itself as the Rishi Kapila to teach the Samkhya. This seems to confirm the fact that the Supreme Being is happy for people to experience *samadhi* by whatever method they choose. After they have realized their own self through *samadhi*, they can go on to realize the Supreme Self through *bhakti*.

There are many ways of achieving *samadhi*. There is not one proper way. It is our good fortune that the founders of our school — Patanjali, the author of the *Yoga Sutra*, and Vyasa, the author of *Bhagavad Gita* — had the wisdom to realize that, just because we have a particular way of experiencing, not everybody else needs to experience in the same way. Bhakti Yoga is the right path for yogis with an emotional constitution. Buddhi Yoga is the path for yogis with an intellectual constitution, and so on. To say that all have to walk the same path is to not care about the welfare of students but only to press one's own agenda to assert the supremacy of one's own opinion. It really is a form of egoism and a failure to realize that the world is too vast to fit into one's own head.

Patanjali accepted all the ideas of Samkhya, but, since the yoga methods can bestow great powers, he felt it necessary to place the yogi under the patronage of the Supreme Being. In this way, the ego of a headstrong yogi is kept in check.

क्लेशकर्मविपाकाशयैरपरामृष्टः पुरुषविशेष ईश्वरः ॥ २४ ॥

1.24 Ishvara is a distinct form of consciousness (*purusha*), which is untouched by the modes of suffering, *karma*, its fruit, and its residue.

If devotion to the Supreme Being truly produces *samadhi*, what is this Supreme Being that it can produce such effects? We enter now a series of sutras in which Patanjali defines the Supreme Being and its function in Yoga. First he says the Supreme Being is a type of consciousness that differs from others. All beings are consciousness, but they differ from the Supreme Being. In what way?

14. *Srimad Bhagavatam*, trans. K. Subramaniam, 7th ed., Bharatiya Vidya Bhavan, Mumbai, 1997, p. 52.

All other beings are touched by ignorance, egoism, desire, aversion, and fear of death. These forms of suffering (*kleshas*) make us act in a certain way, which is conditioned and not free. From these conditioned actions (*karma*) arise certain fruits or results (*vipaka*) — type of birth, life span, and type of experience. In other words, our past actions have created the life that we are leading now.

Apart from the fruit, our past actions have also created residue (*ashaya*). If it is active now, it is called subconscious imprint (*samskara*). This means it is present, and it determines our actions, but we are not aware of it. If it is inactive it is called *karmashaya*, meaning karmic deposit, in which case it will become active only in future lives. This whole vicious circle, which results in bondage and mental slavery, is described in detail in the second chapter (II.3–II.14).

All beings are subject to these forces, and the process of yoga is designed to liberate us from them. The only being that is untouched by any of them is the Supreme Being. Vyasa says there are many beings that have broken free from this cycle of rebirth and bondage, the difference between them and the Supreme Being being that Ishvara was never bound. Where now, Vyasa asks, is the proof of Ishvara's specialness? The answer he gives is: the sacred scriptures. The sacred scriptures are inspired by the Supreme Being and they prove its supremacy. But the next question is, "On what is the authority of the sacred scriptures based?"

Inquiries of this type may appear boring at first, but they are very important. There is always a place for sincere inquiry in Yoga. As yogis we don't have to accept anything at face value, not even the authority of the scriptures. Doubt is good and should be encouraged by the teacher. If the student cannot express doubt, he or she can never arrive at complete conviction. Belief is not enough; we have to know. We have to come to a state of complete conviction and comprehension concerning these questions.

The answer here is: the authority of the scriptures is based on pure intelligence (*sattva*). This means that when the state of *sattva* is reached the authority of the scriptures becomes self-evident. It also means that the scriptures are an expression of the intelligence of the Supreme Being. Let's keep this statement in mind; we will have to verify it later.

The intelligence of the scriptures will of course not be recognized at first. The intellect has to be made predominantly sattvic for it to be able to recognize the *sattva* of the scriptures. This may take a lifetime of practice and study. But, when it is achieved, it will be worth all the effort.

If you don't want to work for such a long time, consider the following train of thought. Have a look at the DNA code, the human brain, the music of J. S. Bach, the millions of life forms, the subtle balance of life on earth, the subtle balance of earth in space, the subtle balance of galaxies circling around each other. Look at the fact that quarks form protons, neutrons, and electrons, while those form atoms. Atoms form compounds, and compounds form amino acids, which somehow mysteriously harbor or manifest life — life that now thinks for itself. If you can say this does not reflect Supreme Intelligence but is a purposeless accident, then a lifetime of practice and study of yoga is probably needed to purify the intellect. Otherwise you will have at least a basic understanding of the intelligence of the Supreme Being, by whatever name you call it.

There are two more ideas that need to be discussed in the context of this sutra. Vyasa says there are many *purusha*s who have attained the state of liberation. This is not annihilation (*nirvana*) and nonexistence as seen in Buddhism, but a state of ecstatic pure consciousness, albeit bodiless. Otherwise he would have said that prior to their liberation they were *purusha*s, whereas he says they still are. This coincides with the yogic notion of reality: that nothing that exists can ever become nonexistent; it can only become unmanifest. This means that a *purusha* that becomes liberated will not manifest a new body in future lives, but will remain unmanifest and free.

The other idea is rather abstract for consideration so early in our study, but interesting for those who practice philosophical inquiry. As we have seen, there are, according to Samkhya, two basic different categories — consciousness (*purusha*) and nature (*prakrti*). Beings are really only consciousness, and all the other twenty-three categories of Samkhya develop or evolve out of *prakrti*, which we can call procreatress for that reason. The first evolute of nature is pure intelligence (*buddhi*). Vyasa says

that the authority of scripture is based on pure intelligence. This pure intelligence is the intelligence of the Supreme Being, the true author of sacred knowledge. Thus the Supreme Being is not only pure consciousness but also pure intelligence.

It differs in that respect from other beings, which are only *purusha*. Since *buddhi* is an evolute of *prakrti* it means that the Supreme Being consists of *purusha* and *prakrti*.[15] Or we could say the Supreme Being straddles the abyss between consciousness and nature. A devotee would respond, "Of course it does," but this is a revolutionary concept for yoga, and the school of Yoga differs here strongly from the school of Samkhya. There are far-reaching implications here that have not been truly contemplated. One can only be in awe of the ancient masters who practiced such deep analysis.

तत्र निरतिशयं सर्वज्ञत्वबीजम् ॥ २५ ॥
1.25 In the One (Ishvara), all knowing is unsurpassed.

All beings have a certain amount of knowledge. Great masters, yogis, and sages may have incredible knowledge. The Supreme Being, says Patanjali, surpasses all those through its all-knowingness.

We cannot perceive the Supreme Being directly — aside from exceptions such as Arjuna, who was, according to the *Bhagavad Gita*, given the celestial eye. Even then he could not handle what he saw, and his hair stood on end. Apart from such exceptions, the Supreme Being can be known from deduction and from the scriptures (*shastra*). Both need intellectual capacity, which can be gained from yoga.

One of the main subjects of Patanjali Yoga is the conversion of mind into intellect. The difference is as follows:

> Mind (*manas*) goes from thought to thought like a crazy monkey that, having drank a bottle of whisky and then got stung by a scorpion, jumps from branch to branch.

> Intellect (*buddhi*) will go straight to the core of a problem just as a stone thrown into a lake will sink straight to the bottom.

15. Compare H. Aranya, *Yoga Philosophy of Patanjali with Bhasvati*, p. 58.

Vyasa states that out of compassion the Supreme Being has given the scriptures for other beings so that they might escape bondage. He gives an interesting example that won't sit well with modern-day Vedantins:

> The Supreme Being, as the great *rishi*, taught the doctrine to Asuri.

We know now from the *Samkhya Karika* that Asuri was the disciple of Kapila, the founder of Samkhya. The divine origin of Samkhya is again stated here (and, surprisingly enough, accepted even by Shankara in his subcommentary *Vivarana*). Just a short excursion into history here: Samkhya, the ancient and most systematic philosophy, is today widely opposed and "refuted" by Vedantins. This was also done by Advaita Vedanta's main proponent, Shankara, and by its founder, Gaudapada. However — and this is what many Westerners cannot understand — Gaudapada wrote a commentary on the *Samkhya Karika* and Shankara, and Vyasa (who is the founder of all schools of Vedanta through his authorship of the *Brahma Sutra*) wrote commentaries on Yoga (which is a brainchild of Samkhya). Why and how?

A mystic who has seen the truth as represented in his school of thought can recognize it in all authentic systems. He also knows that, though a system can look faultless (such as Shankara's Advaita Vedanta), it can never be the truth itself, but only a representation of the truth. A school of thought such as Yoga, Samkhya, or Vedanta does not derive its authority from its rightness or wrongness, for it is bound to be both right and wrong, but rather from its ability to lead people to freedom.

स पूर्वेषाम् अपि गुरुः कालेनानवच्छेदात् ॥ २६ ॥
1.26 The Supreme Being is the teacher of the other teachers, since the One is not limited by time.

We have heard already that the differences between the Supreme Being and liberated masters are that the Supreme Being was never in bondage and that it is all-knowing.

If we look into the past, a teacher of yoga always received his knowledge from his teacher. This teacher received yoga again from his teacher and so

forth, until we reach back to the dawn of time. The first teacher could not get his knowledge from another teacher, because there was no teacher prior to him. Since he could not have accidentally stumbled upon yogic knowledge, it must have been permanently in him without any beginning. This first teacher was, therefore, the Supreme Being. Since the Supreme Being is not limited by time, all knowledge exists in it eternally. It follows that the Supreme Being is at all points in time simultaneously, whether it be remote past, present, or distant future.

तस्य वाचकः प्रणवः ॥ २७ ॥
1.27 The One's expression is the sacred syllable OM.

Shankara links this sutra to I.23, where it is said that *samadhi* can be attained by devotion to the Supreme Being. How is this devotion to be practiced? It is practiced by mentally repeating the syllable OM.

The importance of OM is difficult for Westerners to understand, but in the *Upanishad*s, which are the oldest and most authoritative mystical scriptures of India, OM is the prime means to attain to Brahman (infinite consciousness). Brahman is the impersonal absolute of which Ishvara, the Supreme Being, is a personification.

The *Katha Upanishad* says, in 2.16, "Brahman is known through the sacred syllable OM. Since Brahman is OM, when OM is known, Brahman is known." The *Mundaka Upanishad*, at 2.3–4, puts it this way: OM is like a bow that hurls the individual self or *atman* into the target, which is Brahman, the infinite consciousness.

The *Mundaka* goes on to say (2.6) that to meditate on OM will lead the practitioner into the blazing light of consciousness. The *Mandukya Upanishad* goes as far as to declare that Brahman and this entire universe are OM. "OM is all that is, all that has been and all that will be. Even everything that is beyond the three time modes is also OM."[16]

The *Maitri Upanishad* explains that, just as a spider climbs from a dark enclosure into freedom by way of its thread, so a meditator attains freedom

16. *Mandukya Upanishad* I.1.

165

through OM.[17] Two meditation techniques, it says, will lead to Brahman: sound and silence.

> Brahman as sound, which is OM, is silence made manifest.
>
> Through meditation on OM we can experience the silence of Brahman.

Meditation on OM is done in three steps. First OM is chanted audibly. The vibration of the sound is said to center and still the mind. The second step is to chant OM only mentally. This is more powerful than step 1. It provides a constant focus for the mind and can be done all the time. A good occasion for it is during *pranayama*. The final step is to be silent and to listen only for OM to come back. The goal is to hear the sound, which is uttered by the Supreme Being. OM is the sound from where all other sounds emerge, and all other sounds merge back into OM.

This may all sound like highly abstract matter for the newcomer to yoga, but when one has actually heard OM — heard how all voices together in this world produce this sound — it is one of the most awe-inspiring and shattering experiences possible. One has literally heard the Supreme Being. There is no more selfish "I do believe" or "I do not believe." Belief, although we treasure it so much, has become irrelevant. Then one knows!

तज्जपस्तदर्थभावनम् ॥ २८ ॥
1.28 Repetition of it and contemplation of its meaning should be done.

This is one of the oldest and most important meditation techniques. One chants OM either mentally or aloud and then contemplates its meaning. Its meaning is that it is the utterance of the Supreme Being and the Supreme Being is remembered thereby. In this way, the mind becomes single-pointed on the Supreme Being. This process is Bhakti Yoga, the yoga of devotion.

It is also called *ishvara pranidhana*, which means surrender to the Supreme Being. It is the last of the five observances that form *niyama*, the second limb of yoga.

---

17. *Maitri Upanishad* VI.22.

तत: प्रत्यक्चेतनाधिगमोऽप्यन्तरायाभावश्च ॥ २९ ॥
1.29 From that practice comes knowledge of the inner self and the absence of obstacles.

The study of the self, *svadhyaya*, is the fourth part of the observances (*niyama*s) that will be covered in the second chapter of the *Yoga Sutra*. Self-study has two dimensions: the study of the sacred scriptures and the repetition of OM. To repeat OM and contemplate the Supreme Being leads to knowledge of the Supreme Being. The Supreme Being is consciousness (*purusha*), like us in many ways but differing in the respects described already. Through repeating OM and contemplating its meaning, consciousness is realized, which is our own self.

In sutra I.23 it was stated that surrendering to the Supreme Being could produce objectless (*asamprajnata*) *samadhi*, which bestows self-knowledge if it is experienced extensively. Then again, in sutra II.45, Patanjali says that *samadhi* will arise from perfecting devotion to the Supreme Being. Implied here is not only the act of making the mind single-pointed, which would produce only the lower, objective *samadhi*, but an act of letting go, of giving up control, of handing oneself over to the Supreme Being. After all, we cannot force or achieve the highest *samadhi*. The last and highest step requires the feminine receptivity of the mystic. Who continues to want, will, or conquer obstructs the objectless *samadhi* through ego.

The present sutra then states that meditating on OM also intercepts obstacles. The obstacles are distractions of the mind. By repeating OM the mind becomes single-pointed and then will not succumb to distractions. What the distractions are will be described in the next sutra.

Here ends a sequence of seven sutras that deal with the Supreme Being. Apart from three others that are scattered over the rest of the four chapters of the *Yoga Sutra*, Patanjali will not address the theme again.

This makes altogether ten sutras, forming about 5 percent of the whole *Yoga Sutra*. Although Patanjali felt it necessary to bring a major change to the Samkhya system by adding Ishvara, it is obvious that he understood *bhakti* as an alternative form of practice. In Patanjali Yoga, however, the Supreme Being is not the sole or prime means to freedom as it came to be in the later Shaivite and Vaishnavite schools of Yoga. Ishvara in yoga is not the creator of the world and the beings. He is not the deep underlying reality of all phenomena, what Vedanta calls the Brahman. He is merely the teacher. For this reason India's orthodox authorities said that Patanjali Yoga could lead to self-realization only and not to God realization. They felt he left yogis too much freedom to use alternatives to meditation on Ishvara if they so chose.

Patanjali intended this pluralism. He taught techniques of mysticism, not religion.

व्याधिस्त्यानसंशयप्रमादालस्याविरतिभ्रान्ति-
दर्शनालब्धभूमिकत्वानवस्थितत्वानि
चित्तविक्षेपास्तेऽन्तरायाः ॥ ३० ॥

1.30 The obstacles, which are distractions of the mind, are sickness, rigidity, doubt, negligence, laziness, sense indulgence, false views, failure to attain a state, and inability to stay in that state.

We will discuss them individually, since they all pose threats to our yogic development.

SICKNESS

If the body is out of balance, this will influence our energy levels and freshness of mind. The quality of one's health will impinge on mental capabilities. For this reason *asana* practice was always a prerequisite for the higher meditative forms of yoga. The view of some meditation schools that one can neglect the body and that exercises are unnecessary is a modern one, not born in tradition.

RIGIDITY

This is the pathological holding onto beliefs such as: Women have to be reborn as men to do true yoga. (Some of the greatest minds were women, such as Gargi in the *Brhad Aranyaka Upanishad*.) Foreigners have to be reborn as Indians to be liberated. (Some of the greatest mystics had never been to India, for example Lao Tzu and Chuang Tzu.) Low-caste

people have to be reborn as Brahmins before they can become liberated. (Kabir was of low caste.)

Rigidity means that the mind is overcome by dullness and heaviness (*tamas*). One cannot adapt to a new situation and cannot accept that things change. One may hold on to a view, not realizing that the opposite may also be true.

DOUBT

Doubt is the inability to see the one truth because everything seems to be true and "everything" is relative. The trained intellect has the capacity to think a problem to an end and to come to a conclusion. If the method used is faulty, or conditioning stains the intellect, doubt will arise.

Doubt usually occurs when the *prana* moves in the lunar channel (*ida nadi*), whereas rigidity tends more to develop if *prana* moves in the solar channel (*pingala nadi*). *Asana* combined with *pranayama* is designed to balance the two.

NEGLIGENCE

Yoga is a precious gift that can take us to rare heights. Not many people get the chance to really use it. If we mix various systems to create an eclectic pulp that suits our own limitations, rather than follow an original source, we shouldn't be surprised if the outcome is just gymnastics.

LAZINESS

Some students once asked the Armenian mystic Georg I. Gurdjieff, "Where should we start?" His answer was: "Commit yourself not to die like a scabies-infested dog." These sound like harsh words, but what he meant was that most humans live in an animal-like state. According to his view, there was a certain urgency about rising to a truly human and awake state.

In terms of yoga, we are looking at a lifetime of study and practice for the average seeker. Whether objectless *samadhi* comes after one year or after five decades does not really matter. As Shankara said, all yogis reach their goal in their own time.

SENSE INDULGENCE

This is a big one for us Westerners. Every advertising pamphlet suggests spoiling ourselves, indulging our senses, pampering ourselves, and treating ourselves.

Indulgence is a behavior that is as pathological as asceticism, and Buddha tried both. As a young prince he indulged in his three palaces: he had one for the cold season, one for the hot season, and one for the rainy season. Later on he practiced austerity for six years but found that, like indulgence, it impinged on the equanimity of his mind.

Indulgence, of course, weakens body and mind. The strongest and most powerful leaders were those who realized that they did not rely at all on external stimulation to be happy.

True happiness and freedom are possible only by realizing what a follower of Vedanta would call our own divinity. If we are cut off from this eternal fountain within us, if we do not know ourselves, then terrible pain ensues and a nagging thirst for life manifests. Then we have to squeeze happiness and thrills from life, most of them lasting moments only.

If we read advertising pamphlets, their language suggests that indulgence could produce divine ecstasy. The truth is that both are completely independent of each other. Sensory pleasure is only that; there is nothing mystical about it. The more we depend on it, the less free we become.

Asceticism, on the other hand, is another extreme of the mind. The implication is that the mere contact of the senses with objects is bad. However, from this contact results experience and from experience, in due time, liberation. With liberation, the thirst for experience ceases.

It is debatable whether it makes sense to starve oneself of experience even though the cause of its need, ignorance, is still intact. As Shankara has shown in his *Brahma Sutra Commentary*, knowledge of deep reality (Brahman) cannot be produced by action, whether it be indulgence or asceticism.

False Views

There are many false views, and not every correct view is right for every person. One of the most dangerous false views is materialism, according to which the consciousness of a human being can be reduced to biochemical and bioelectrical impulses. Not only does this pave the way for a materialistic society, in which people are measured against the value of the goods they have collected, it also opens the door to fascism and genocide.

If we deny that all humans have an eternal, spiritual core, which is sometimes called the self or the soul, then only their material aspect is left. Since the material aspect (body, mind, conditioning, etc.) allows us to judge and categorize a person as more valuable or less valuable, we might easily come to the conclusion that some less valuable ones are in the way of those more valuable. Supremacism starts with materialism, which denies human beings their eternal divine aspect.

False views are avoided through proper meditation practice and philosophical inquiry, which together develop the intellect.

Failure to Attain a State and Inability to Retain That State

These are listed as separate obstacles, but I will treat them together since they are habits of the mind. People of a certain personality type, let us call them "explorers," can easily attain new things, but they can lose them as easily. Those of another personality type, "collectors" perhaps, are good at keeping things, but find it difficult to go out and create something new. Both of these characters are based on identifications created through habits.

In yoga, we need to display both of these qualities at various times. Sometimes a breakthrough in our meditation practice is within reach, but we do not attain it because we do not believe we are that type of person. The yogi next door might find it very easy to proceed to advanced mystical states but can soon be caught up in daily mire.

The truth is that everybody with a brain and a nervous system or, in yogic terminology, everybody with an upright spine (including hominids that permanently walk and sit erect, but not pongids, which only occasionally walk upright) qualifies for *samadhi*. It is often only our limiting beliefs about ourselves, such as guilt and shame, that stop us.

These are the nine obstacles, which are distractions of the mind. They completely overpower the types of mind that are called wild (*kshipta*) and infatuated (*mudha*), and they severely disturb the confused, distracted, or oscillating (*vikshipta*) mind. The obstacles are, however, overcome by a practitioner with the one-pointed (*ekagra*) mind, which is the mind of the yogi proper.

दुःखदौर्मनस्याङ्गमेजयत्वश्वासप्रश्वासा
विक्षेपसहभुवः ॥ ३१ ॥

1.31 Suffering and frustration, unsteadiness of body, inhalation, and exhalation result from the distractions.

From those symptoms we can gauge that various obstacles are present. The obstacles don't just stop at intercepting our yoga practice, but they manifest as various forms of suffering and frustration in our day-to-day life.

They also — and this is very important for the physical side of yoga — manifest as unsteadiness of the body and its breathing patterns. The presence of obstacles can be deduced if one has physical difficulties in sitting peacefully in meditation or in performing *pranayama* exercises. Vyasa states that these difficulties are not present in one of concentrated mind (*ekagra chitta*).

The connection between mental obstacles and physical manifestation is mutual. If the mind is distracted, the life force (*prana*) will be scattered, which results in unsteady breathing and posture. Since thoughts and *prana* move together, we can steady the thoughts by smoothing the flow of the *prana* or we can correct the body and breath through meditation.

For many people the first way is much easier, since meditation is difficult if the mind is distracted. The focus on *asana* and *pranayama* (breathing exercises) will, however, not only alleviate the symptoms of a distracted mind, but will also exercise the mind in concentration and, most important, it will make the flow of *prana* even. This in turn will still the mind.

From the yogic viewpoint, it is not helpful for a beginner to start with meditation (*dhyana*). According to Patanjali meditation is higher yoga, and if the mind is not prepared — if it is neither single-pointed (*ekagra*) nor suspended (*nirodha*) — meditation will lead nowhere. If body and mind are prepared through the outer limbs of yoga, meditation will be successful.

Frequently experienced in meditation is the "white-wall effect" — daydreaming and wafting. Such meditation is detrimental, since it increases the grip of *tamas* and *rajas*. In meditation the mind needs to be bright and luminous and the intellect sharp,

otherwise meditation will lead at best to the "body-less" and "absorbed in *prakrti*" states that were discussed in sutra I.19. A Tibetan lama told me once that incorrect meditation could lead to reincarnation as a fish. He also suggested studying the facial expressions of fishes, to recognize those of certain meditators.

K. Pattabhi Jois has stated that meditation, if performed wrongly, cannot be corrected. As the teacher cannot from the outside assess whether the student is meditating correctly or not, the correct performance of *asana* and *pranayama* must be studied first. Since they are visible, external exercises they can be corrected, and correct performance leads to correct meditation, he says.

However some people are by birth or habit in a state of the single-pointed (*ekagra*) mind. (The yogi would say this was a result of effort performed in previous incarnations.) In Shankara's opinion these people would be wasting their time if it were insisted they perform *asana* and *pranayama*.

तत्प्रतिषेधार्थम् एकतत्त्वाभ्यासः ॥ ३२ ॥

1.32 To remove them, there is the practice of one principle (*tattva*).

How can we remove the distractions of the mind and the symptoms that accompany them?

In sutra I.29 Patanjali has stated already that contemplating the meaning of OM, the Supreme Being, can overcome the obstacles. Now he is talking about the situation where the obstacles have arisen and the question is how to counteract them. He says, "If the obstacles did arise then counteract them by sticking to one method." A list of possible methods will be given later.

If the mind is already distracted so that obstacles do arise, we do not want to confuse it by practicing all methods of yoga simultaneously. Rather we focus on one method now and, when the mind has become focused (*ekagra*), we can shift to a more elaborate plan of higher yoga. Otherwise, we would be like the man who wants to dig a well but sticks his spade into the ground in each location only once before going on to another place. A distracted mind will have the tendency to switch quickly from one method of yoga to the next — possibly switching from one style to another and then from Zen to Tibetan Buddhism and on to Sufism and Taoism. Quite likely any of these approaches would get one to the goal; different methods are suitable for different temperaments. But they have one thing in common: in the case of the average person, achieving the aim will take several decades.

On discovering a new method there is often a thrill similar to falling in love with a new partner. If we keep changing methods and partners we might be able to sustain the thrill for several years, but we will never find out what yoga and love are truly about. The purpose of a relationship is to recognize consciousness in the other;[18] the purpose of yoga is to recognize consciousness in ourselves.[19] Both are achieved by sticking to the same partner/same method respectively.

An alternative reading of this sutra was proposed by the ninth-century commentary of Vachaspati Mishra. He makes the bold statement that *eka tattva* — the one principle — can only be the Supreme Being (Ishvara).

The majority of the commentators that have come after him, especially King Bhoja, Vijnanabhikshu, and H. Aranya, rejected this view since it makes little sense in the context of the *Yoga Sutra*. Authors with a strong devotional Vaishnavite background have usually accepted Vachaspati's rendering, but evidence in the coming sutras will show that this view is not supported by the School of Yoga.

मैत्रीकरुणामुदितोपेक्षाणां
सुखदुःखपुण्यापुण्यविषयाणां
भावनातश्चित्तप्रसादनम् ॥ ३३ ॥

I.33 Clarity of mind is produced by meditating on friendliness toward the happy, compassion toward the miserable, joy toward the virtuous, and indifference toward the wicked.

Shankara states that this sutra is one of the practices of one principle (*eka tattva*) to clear the mind. It amounts to opposing Vachaspati's opinion that *eka tattva* is only meditating on the Supreme Being, which raises

a question as to the authenticity of the *Vivarana*, Shankara's subcommentary on the *Yoga Sutra*.

The *Vivarana* was discovered only in 1950 and its colophon states that Bhagavat Shankara, a pupil of Bhagavat Govindapada, authored it, while the colophon of *Yoga Taravali* says it was composed by Shri Shankaracharya, a disciple of Govinda Bhagavatpada. Some scholars have argued that Shankaracharya and Bhagavat Shankara are two people, and that Bhagavatpada lived somewhere during the fourteenth century. If we look at the commentary to this sutra we can clearly see that the author of the *Vivarana* lived prior to the ninth century.

Shankara reveals himself in the *Vivarana* as an extremely battle-ready scholar. As with all his other commentaries, the *Vivarana* has the structure of a dialogue with one or several imagined opponents (*pratipakshin*s). Whenever any realistic or even unrealistic argument against Patanjali's, Vyasa's, or his own position comes to his attention, he attacks and refutes it pre-emptively to avoid future confusion. Sometimes one feels that Shankara is overly cautious and attacks positions that are unrealistic, but he certainly never leaves unattacked a viable position that was held in his day and that he doesn't share.

He states in his commentary that "practice of one principle" refers to the sutras mentioned afterward (I.33–39). In other words, he does not share Vachaspati's opinion that "practice of one principle" refers only to the Supreme Being. If Shankara had known about Vachaspati's position, he would never have let it pass unpunished. It is clear from the positioning of the sutras that Vachaspati does not state Patanjali's view, which Shankara would have pointed out. From this we can deduce that the author of the *Vivarana* (Shankara) lived prior to Vachaspati, who lived in the ninth century.

We arrive then in the eighth century, which is the date usually given for Shankara. Jonathan Bader offers another interesting piece of information in his *Meditation in Shankara's Vedanta*. He suggests that the texts authored by Shankara Bhagavatpada are the ones composed by the original Shankara, whereas some texts attributed to Shankaracharya are composed by the abbots of the four monasteries that Shankara founded and who all carry the title Shankaracharya.

18. *Brhad Aranyaka Upanishad* II.4.5.
19. *Yoga Sutra* I.3.

We return to the sutra to observe that the distracted mind in which obstacles are present will have the tendency to react with envy if somebody is successful. Our modern-day "tall poppy syndrome" exemplifies this phenomenon. If somebody is outstanding in any respect, we tend to look for a way to reduce him or her to average size. Rather than follow that tendency, Patanjali suggests meditating on friendliness when one encounters such people.

If we encounter the downtrodden, on the other hand, the distracted mind has the tendency to ascribe their predicament to their own fault, to the *karma* that they have attracted, or to their thinking or believing the wrong things. Rather than getting lost on this tangent of the distracted mind, Patanjali recommends meditating on compassion.

If we encounter a person who follows a spiritual path with great virtue, we are suddenly reminded that we should be like them whereas in fact we are not. We might then become jealous and look for a way to discredit them. Here Patanjali suggests simply meditating on joy, which would be the natural reaction if our mind was clear.

The last suggestion is probably the most difficult. If we encounter what appear to be bad or even evil people, we have the tendency to hate them. Often we react in this way because they remind us of something in ourselves, only we manage to conceal it better. Rather than going into hatred, which is only a rejection of our own dark side, Patanjali suggests indifference toward those people.

This method of counteracting the aggravations of the mind is a meditation technique for clearing and stilling the mind.

प्रच्छर्दनविधारणाभ्यां वा प्राणस्य ॥ ३४ ॥
1.34 Or from exhalation and retention of breath (*prana*).

Here is another method by which the mind can be cleared from obstacles. It is retaining the breath after exhalation. Whenever the term *prana* is used in scripture we have to keep two connotations in mind: it means both "breath" and "life force."

Vyasa states that the breath needs to be exhaled through the nostrils and then retained. Retaining after inhalation is not appropriate in this context, since it charges the mind and body with energy. It is more a meditation on fullness, whereas the external breath retention is accompanied by meditation on emptiness, in this case emptiness of the mind.

H. Aranya says that a mere external retention would never have the effect of clearing the mind.[20] Rather, one needs to keep the mind vacant or fixed on the void to attain its clarification. Breathing exercises (*pranayama*) without any meditation aid such as a mantra or visualization are regarded as a very inferior type of yoga.

"To say 'I am not the world' is the true inhalation," says Shankara. "To say 'I am nothing but consciousness' is the exhalation. To sustain that thought is the breath retention. This is the true *pranayama*. Dim wits only torture the nose."[21]

विषयवती वा प्रवृत्तिरुत्पन्ना मनसः स्थितिनिबन्धिनी ॥ ३५ ॥
1.35 Also the development of supersensory perception can aid in concentrating the mind.

As Vyasa explains, the knowledge that we gain from the scriptures, through deduction or from a teacher, is not our own until it is realized. Doubt about the yogic teachings can therefore linger in the back of one's mind. To arrive at conviction in the yogic process, Patanjali here suggests concentrating on certain energy points to gain supersensory perception. Once this feat is achieved, we can trust that the other aspects of the practice will also come to fruition. This theme is further developed in the third chapter of the *Yoga Sutra*, where supernatural powers are adduced to prove the validity of yoga.

The concentration on the points mentioned in this sutra has to be sustained for several days. H. Aranya states that the capability will emerge only if one lives in solitude and fasts[22] — in other words if very little in the way of sensory stimulation and external distraction is present.

20. H. Aranya, *Yoga Philosophy of Patanjali with Bhasvati*, p. 78.
21. *Aparokshanubhuti of Sri Shankaracharya*, vv. 119–120, trans. Sw. Vimuktananda.
22. H. Aranya, *Yoga Philosophy of Patanjali with Bhasvati*, p. 82.

The energy points mentioned by Vyasa as examples are:

Tip of the nose — supersensory smell
Tip of the tongue — supersensory taste
Palate — supersensory sight
Middle of the tongue — supersensory touch
Root of the tongue — supersensory hearing

विशोका वा ज्योतिष्मती ॥ ३६ ॥

1.36 Steadiness of mind is also gained from perceiving a radiant light beyond sorrow.

The light talked about here is the light in the heart lotus. Meditating on the light in the heart or the heart sound is one of the main meditation techniques in yoga. The *Yoga Taravali* and the *Hatha Yoga Pradipika* have as their main theme hearing the unstruck sound, the heart sound (*anahata nada*).

In this sutra the light in the heart is mentioned, and the heart is the origin of the mind. As the *Upanishad*s state, mind and intellect are projected out of the heart and will be reabsorbed into it eventually. Sutra III.34 says that contemplating on the heart will lead to the understanding of the mind, while sutra III.33 declares that everything will be known through the rising light of pure intellect. The light of pure intelligence or intellect is situated in the heart lotus. By meditating on this light, steadiness of mind is achieved.

The light is said to be "beyond sorrow" because sorrow arises from the various forms of ignorance (*avidya*). When one sees the light in the heart, which is the effulgence of pure intelligence, this intelligence will dispel ignorance. Eventually it will produce discriminative knowledge, which is the end of suffering. In this sutra, however, only the light beyond suffering is seen, which is a more modest achievement. This means we get only a sneak preview of pure intelligence, enough to make the mind steady.

The other way of meditating on the light in the heart is to meditate on the notion of "I am" (*asmita*). This I-am-ness is produced from pure intelligence. If we reduce all of our thoughts to I am — or, in other words, if we retrace our thoughts to the notion of I am — this also makes the mind steady. All thoughts contain the notion of I am. In the thought process there are the thinker, the thinking, and the object thought about. For thinking to happen, the notion of I am must be there. If we remain aware of this notion, rather than forget ourselves or forget that it is we who think, then the mind becomes steady.

वीतरागविषयं वा चित्तम् ॥ ३७ ॥

1.37 The mind can be made steady by meditating on a person who is desireless.

Just as a stone thrown into a lake creates waves, so an object reflected upon creates ripples in the mind. And just as the nature of the ripples on a lake is determined by the size of the stone, so are the mind waves determined by the type of object that we encounter. Only when the mind is in suspension mode (*nirodha*) will objects not cause thought waves.

One of the best objects to meditate on is the mind of a person who is desireless. Since every object leaves in the mind its imprint, the mind of such a person draws the meditator toward desirelessness. This is the reason why students experience great peace in the presence of a liberated master. This observation has been elaborated by some Indian schools of thought into the doctrine that it is only the grace of the master that leads to freedom. Other mystics have emphasized, on the other hand, that there is no initiation but self-initiation. Of course no other person can make one liberated, as this would imply that the master could manipulate the law of *karma*. It is true as well that there is a great human tendency to mystify others and project great powers onto them — and the wish that others do the hard work for us.

If a master is free and the student is very open to influence, the mind of the student can become still in the presence of the master, and this aids meditation. It is, however, crucial to choose a true teacher, one who has become desireless. If the teacher still has an agenda, it will excite the mind of the student.

The sutra here does not explicitly indicate a living teacher. Since true sages have become rare in our age, it can be recommended that meditation take place on the ancient masters, such as Kapila, Vasishta, Yajnavalkya, Vyasa, Patanjali, and Shankara. If one studies the teachings of the masters closely, one will eventually feel as if one knows them personally.

The ancient masters were great rational thinkers and exercised vigorous reasoning and logic, but it is especially their heartfelt compassion that we can feel even after two or more thousand years. If a student manages through study to connect to the heart of a master, the mind is easily steadied, even though millennia have passed between them and us.

स्वप्ननिद्राज्ञानालम्बनं वा ॥ ३८ ॥

1.38 The mind can also be steadied by meditating on a dream object or on the state of dreamless sleep.

This is an interesting sutra. Knowledge derived through dreams is highly regarded in many cultures including the Australian Aboriginal, the Native American, and the Tibetan. In these cultures, decisions are often taken only if they have been dreamed. The subcommentator Vachaspati Mishra suggests that if one has a divine vision in a dream one can use that vision to meditate upon.

Vijnanabhikshu takes a different view. He says that life is to be looked at as a long dream. Knowledge derived in the waking state is of the nature of dreams, and, since this realization leads to detachment from all that we so fiercely believe in, it stabilizes the mind. This statement is reminiscent of the *Mandukya Karika*,[23] in which both the waking and the dream states are declared unreal. The *Vijnana Bhairava*[24] describes a meditation technique that follows Vijnanabhikshu's recipe. The advice is to dream as if one is awake and to treat waking states as if one is dreaming. In this way reality is suddenly seen — meaning the true reality, which is beyond sleep and waking.

The second part of the sutra deals with dreamless sleep. In this state, the mind is temporarily absorbed into the heart, but there is no awareness: the idea of nonexistence prevails. Since the mind is completely

23. A vedantic text by Acharya Gaudapada.
24. An ancient tantric meditation text.

steady apart from the fluctuation of nonexistence, meditation done on this state steadies the mind. Meditation on deep sleep is done in the following way: if on waking there is a memory in the mind such as "I slept soundly and peacefully," we use this memory as the object of our meditation.

Usually the recollection is only in the short-term memory, but if we remind ourselves of it several times throughout the day it will enter the long-term memory. It will then be available as an object of meditation any time.

यथाभिमतध्यानाद् वा ॥ ३९ ॥

1.39 The mind can also be stabilized by meditating on any suitable object.

This is a grossly misunderstood sutra. If Westerners hear "meditation on any suitable object," they will understand it to mean just any object. Our contemporary world meditates profusely on the dollar symbol and ideas such as "I am the body," while the advertising industry meditates usually on the female form. It is poor choice of meditation objects and not lack of meditation that is the problem of modern society. Any thought that is repeated frequently constitutes meditation on that thought. To make absolutely sure that one does not mistake this sutra as an invitation to meditate on one's real estate, share portfolio, sports car, or wallet, Shankara quotes the *Upanishads*: "Even if one should obtain objects, let him never dwell on them in any way."[25]

In ancient India a suitable meditation object meant any desired object from within the category of sacred or yogic object. Shankara says it must be a proper object for meditation. Vijnanabhikshu says suitable objects are images of the divine. As we know already, images will color the mind. Obviously we will choose only images that color the mind in the direction we want it to develop. The mind needs to be made sattvic. Suitable objects, then, are objects that are highly, or purely, sattvic.

Objects usually consist of various intertwinings of the three strands of qualities of nature, the *guna*s. S. Dasgupta describes the three *guna*s as mass-stuff (*tamas*), energy-stuff (*rajas*), and intelligence-stuff

25. T. Leggett, *Shankara on the Yoga Sutra*, p. 151.

(sattva).[26] Only objects that consist predominantly of intelligence make the mind steady. Tamasic objects make the mind dull and rajasic objects create suffering. Suitable objects so far introduced are the intellect (buddhi), the I-am-ness (asmita), the Supreme Being (Ishvara), the mantra OM, the heart lotus and its sound and light, the mind of liberated ones, and so on. Among other suitable objects are the breath, a mantra, a lotus flower, the OM symbol, a mandala, and yantra (sacred geometry).

Consciousness is not a suitable object, since it is formless and requires a mind that is empty of obstacles.

परमाणु परममहत्त्वान्तोऽस्य वशीकारः ॥ ४० ॥

1.40 Mastery is achieved when the mind can concentrate on any object from the smallest atom to the entire cosmos.

Once the mind is steadied through any of the previously described methods, one chooses more difficult objects. The smallest meditation objects are elementary particles called subtle elements (tanmatras) in yoga. The biggest object to meditate on is the entire universe. Both are difficult and should not be tackled at first. Once one can sustain focus on them, one meditates on both simultaneously, which is hard to sustain over a long period. If it is achieved, that is called mastery of concentration (dharana) and the mind is now steadied (stithi). No further dharana exercises are required then.

Having described the obstacles and how they are overcome through concentration, Patanjali will now elaborate on the various stages of objective samadhi.

क्षीणवृत्तेरभिजातस्येव मणेर्ग्रहीतृग्रहणग्राह्येषु तत्स्थतदञ्जनतासमापत्तिः ॥ ४१ ॥

1.41 When the mind waves are reduced, the mind appears to truthfully reflect any object that it is directed toward like a pristine crystal, whether it be the perceived, the process of perceiving, or the perceiver. This state is called identity (samapatti).[27]

This is one of the most important sutras to understand and, again, it is one of the most misunderstood.

"When the mind waves are reduced" through the practices described in the previous seven sutras, we come to a point where the mind is focused or single-pointed. In this state, we are capable of perceiving things as they really are; in other words, we cognize objects correctly or we gain all knowledge pertaining to the objects.

Let us be clear that this is not the state of self-knowledge, since that would imply the mind waves have ceased completely, which is the state of suspension (nirodha). Basically we describe here an inferior (objective) type of samadhi, different from advanced samadhi, which leads to self-knowledge.

"The mind appears to truthfully reflect..." means that the image of the object created in the mind seems to be identical with the original object. The important word to notice here is "appears." Complete identity is not possible. If we meditate on the entire universe, as suggested in the previous sutra, our mind would not be capable of reproducing it. Even on earth there are many locations, such as some places in the Gobi Desert, where no human being has ever set foot; to believe we could reproduce the entire universe in our mind is megalomania. Nevertheless, the seemingly truthful representation of an object is important. It means that we completely comprehend an object, whereas in daily life we create for ourselves only a vague simulation of an object.

The reason for this lies in how the mind works.

---

26. S. Dasgupta, *A History of Indian Philosophy*, vol. 1, 1st Indian ed., Motilal Banarsidass, Delhi, 1975, p. 244.

27. The terms *samadhi* and *samapatti* are not quite synonymous. *Samapatti* is the state in which the mind is during objective *samadhi*. Objective *samadhi* is the technique practiced while the mind is in *samapatti*. There is no *samapatti* in objectless *samadhi*, since the mind, however refined it might be, can never achieve identity with consciousness.

The mind (*manas*) is an organizer of sensory input. When it receives sensory data from, let's say, the eye, it compares it to the data received from other senses. As we have noted already, when light enters the eye it crosses over in the lens, and images are depicted on the retina upside down. During our infancy, we learn through the tactile sense that objects are upside down in relation to how we see them, and at some point the mind decides to turn all pictures around, in that way reconciling the optical data with the tactile data. This illustrates how the mind manipulates sensory input to arrive at a workable understanding.

Another example: If we hold our left hand in ice-cold water and our right in hot water for a few moments and then place both together into water of room temperature, the left hand will signal warm and the right hand will signal cold. Both signals are wrong, since the temperature is the same for both hands. Sensory data is evaluated by comparison, by using reference points. Compared to the cold water, the temperate water feels warm, and compared to the hot water it seems cold. We see here that the mind is colored by its previous experience and, through that, its ability to authentically duplicate a present condition is compromised.

A third example: Sigmund Freud discovered that the first people we meet in life leave a conditioning in the mind. A female child on experiencing her father receives an imprint, a conditioning. In the future she will have the tendency to relate to males based on that original conditioning. She may be drawn to certain males because they have similarities to her father, or she may reject them for the same reason. The same happens with a male child in respect to his mother, and it also occurs in regard to the same-sex parent. The important thing to understand here is that, because the mind is colored by past experience, it is stained and therefore cannot truthfully reflect or duplicate a new object.

Obviously, we will develop problems in our relationships if we try to relive our relationships with our parents. If we project a parent onto our partner, we will never find out who our partner really is. If we do not let go of the experience that water was cold just a moment ago, we won't be able to authentically experience what temperature it is now.

The reason why mind works this way is that it is a survival instrument. The task of mind is to arrive as fast as possible, with the greatest possible accuracy, at a simulation of truth. Typical challenges of the mind are: Is the object in front of me edible? Does what I see pose a threat, so that I should run away? The mind is not concerned with recognizing the deepest layer of truth of an object — its such-ness, the object-as-such. The facility concerned with that is intellect. While mind jumps constantly from one object to the next, intellect will zoom into one and the same object until it is comprehensively cognized. The traditional definition of intellect is that which can think about the same object for in excess of three hours without distraction. A big part of the yogi's work is converting mind into intellect. We will hear more about that later.

The mind usually projects our past onto the present. Rather than perceiving reality as it truly is, we see a simulation of reality. This equates to our belief as to what reality is and how it relates to us. Reality does not really relate to us according to Patanjali: he says that nature (*prakrti*) is eternally separate from us (*purusha*). How mind relates to reality, however, usually means how can we profit from it or get an advantage.

So a developer driving through a suburb may look at it mainly as a source of income. A sexual predator driving through the same suburb may see it as a possible source of victims. A more gustatorily inclined person may look out for restaurants, whereas an alcoholic will remember the locations of the liquor stores. All four, due to the superimposition of their goals onto their experience, might fail to register essential features while they hasten toward what is our sure destination, death.

Let's say it is spring and the cherry blossoms are out; there is a good chance most of the characters mentioned above would miss them. The observation of the cherry blossoms is an utterly useless business. No monetary or sexual advantage can be had from them; we can't eat them and we can't drink them either. But in some miraculous way they can make us free and peaceful when it is time to die: We die in fear because we hold on to life. We hold on to life because our deepest thirst is not quenched. Our deepest thirst is to have experience, knowledge, or realization of our true nature. A realization of our nature can be had from watching the cherry blossoms. In fact a cherry tree, or a cluster of cherry trees, in full bloom is more breathtaking than the explosion of the Death Star in *Return of the Jedi*.

There are several reasons why we don't notice them as such. One is that we do not have to pay an entry fee and are not expecting for two and a half hours that something incredible will happen. But the main reason is that all of our past experiences conspire to see the cherry tree as: something that needs to be bulldozed to make way for a new retail outlet, in the case of the developer; something under which to have a sensual encounter, in the case of the sexual predator; something to later be eaten (the cherry), in the case of the gustatory person; and something to be imbibed (cherry liquor) eventually, in the case of the alcoholic.

But if I manage to leave behind all of my past, which has covered my instruments of cognition (senses, mind, ego, intellect) with the dust of the ages, and simply see the cherry blossoms, then this utter abundance, this magnificent manifestation of sheer beauty, which is a completely senseless and useless waste, will stun my mind into silence. In this complete silence, I will eventually realize that it is I who watches the cherry blossoms. From "I am watching the cherry blossoms," comes "I am watching," from that comes "I am," from that comes "I," and from that comes "beyond I," which is consciousness. It is only consciousness that can witness total and unbesmirched beauty. That is how the cherry blossoms can lead to freedom.

But for this to happen the mind needs to be able to truthfully reflect objects without us projecting onto them our needs (to get rich, to procreate, to eat, or to drink).

"Any object that it is directed toward like a pristine crystal…" Here again we can see Patanjali does not talk about self-knowledge or knowledge of consciousness but knowledge of objects, which are different from us. The metaphor of a crystal is used here, reminding us of the discussion under sutras I.3–4. If a crystal is absolutely clear and colorless and we place it next to an object, say a red rose, then the crystal clearly reflects the redness of the rose. The purer the crystal, the more authentic will the

reflection be. From a certain angle it will look as if there is no crystal but only the red rose. If there are hazes or clouds in the crystal, or if it has a color of its own, this will affect its ability to reflect an object.

The same can be said about the mind. If we go into a situation carrying our entire past with us, this will prevent a truthful duplication of a new object in our mind. The purer and more unstained the mind is, the more we can learn the truth about an object. If the mind is stained by past experience, we will project that experience onto our meditation object. The mind will deliver now a simulation of the object modified by the data that we have collected in the past. Necessarily this is far from the meditation object as such. It is only when the mind is completely steadied that it will be capable of reproducing an object to the extent that the duplicate is an almost identical copy of the original. Only in this state is the mind capable of learning the truth about objects. Knowledge in that state is called *prajna* — wisdom.

Before it is achieved, the mind and sensory apparatus are not qualified to cognize the truth. To be precise, we would have to alter statements such as "I saw John" into "I saw somebody whom I believed to be John." Such revisions can be highly important in a homicide inquiry, for example. The simple statement "John is a communist" might have to be changed to "The person whom I believe to be John appears to adhere most of the time to a complex belief system that is frequently labeled as communism." If we rephrase our statements in this way we will suddenly find out how little we know. *Prajna* (wisdom) means that we can see the deepest level of an object.

"Whether it be the perceived, the process of perceiving, or the perceiver." These are the three categories into which meditation objects are classified. The perceived are objects that are clearly outside us, such as the world or the body. We would meditate on these objects first. The next and deeper layer is the process of knowing, which includes the senses such as seeing, hearing, and tasting and the mind that organizes sensory data. Altogether they are called organs or instruments of cognition.

The perceiver is here the I-am-ness or egoity (*asmita*), the agency that owns the sensory data. Let's recall that Patanjali lists among the objective *samadhi*s one called *asmita*. This *samadhi* is based on the I-am-ness that owns the cognized phenomena. If we look out of the window and behold a beautiful landscape, there is only for a split second the landscape by itself; then I-am-ness is activated and says "I observe the landscape, now what? What do we do with it?" This is the perceiver.

Some modern authors have bent this sutra to say, "When the fluctuations are reduced then the mind has union of seer, seeing, and seen." This grossly misrepresents Patanjali's philosophy. He says that the union of seer, seeing, and seen constitutes ignorance (sutra II.17) and egoism (sutra II.6). Freedom in his view can only be achieved by realizing the eternal separateness of seer on the one hand and seeing and seen on the other. If I attempt to read vedantic understanding into the *Yoga Sutra*, this means that my mind is clouded so much by my vedantic past that I cannot represent the object (the *Yoga Sutra*) truthfully as it is, but only commingled with my vedantic conditioning. Maybe in the future we will have yogis who try to read yoga into vedantic scriptures, which would be a shame. Both of these magnificent systems deserve better.

"This state is called identity (*samapatti*)." *Samapatti* is a low form of objective *samadhi*. Let us recall that Patanjali enumerated objective (*samprajnata*) *samadhi* to be of four kinds, called deliberation (*vitarka*), reflection (*vichara*), bliss (*ananda*), and I-am-ness (*asmita*). The first two, deliberation and reflection, form the basis of the various types of *samapatti*. This will be explained further in the following sutras.

तत्र शब्दार्थज्ञानविकल्पैः संकीर्णा सवितर्का समापत्तिः ॥ ४२ ॥

1.42 Deliberative (*savitarka*) *samapatti* is that *samadhi* in which words, objects and knowledge are commingled through conceptualization.

This is the lowest form of *samadhi*. Its difference from concentration (*dharana*) is that we do not have to make a willful effort anymore to avoid thoughts that have nothing to do with the object. The difference to meditation (*dhyana*) is that our mind represents the object truthfully already, whereas in meditation there is only a continuous flow of awareness toward the object. But whereas in a deep objective *samadhi* only the object shines forth without any distortion, in this *samadhi* there is still a deliberation or discussion going on.

Compared to other *samadhis* this *samapatti* is somewhat superficial. From the view of meditation (*dhyana*) this is a deep, powerful, and creative state, due to the knowledge and clarity that it creates.

If we base our *samapatti* for example on *Mula Bandha*, then, apart from the authentic duplication of *Mula Bandha* in the mind, the mind at the same time engages in deliberation. The deliberation happens in the form of conceptualization (*vikalpa*). Conceptualization is one of the fluctuations of the mind. We can say therefore that part of the mind is still roaming to a certain extent, while the main part has already achieved identity with the object. The roaming of the mind does not, however, mean that we are thinking of other things. The mind is completely absorbed in *Mula Bandha*, but only on a superficial level.

The conceptualization consists of three aspects that are mixed together. They are the object *Mula Bandha* as we perceive it right now, the word *Mula Bandha*, and the knowledge of *Mula Bandha* that we have accumulated in the past, such as that it forces the *apana* current upward. The important thing to realize here is that the object *Mula Bandha*, the word denoting it, and the knowledge that we have of it are three completely separate things.

The word *Mula Bandha* is a symbol that we agreed on by convention. If for some reason we were to lose the Sanskrit language, we might in the future call it only pelvic lock. The word would change in that case but the object described would be unchanged. Similarly, our knowledge about *Mula Bandha* might be complete or incomplete, correct or incorrect, but the actual object is not touched by the state of our knowledge. Then again we might perform *Mula Bandha* incorrectly, but we will not change the word we use to refer to it.

In deliberative (*savitarka*) *samapatti* there is a mix of word, object, and knowledge, whereas in deeper *samadhi* types only the object will be there. This type of *samapatti* is practiced first: the mind is still in a superficial state and therefore cannot completely merge with the object. Nevertheless, this is an important training stage that should not be belittled. Deliberative *samapatti* is the foundation or first step to higher *samadhi*.

स्मृतिपरिशुद्धौ स्वरूपशून्येवार्थमात्रनिर्भासा निर्वितर्का ॥ ४३ ॥

I.43 When memory is purified, the mind appears to be emptied of its own nature and only the object shines forth. This is superdeliberative (*nirvitarka*) *samapatti*.

Our memory is loaded with data that we have derived from past events, from reading, or from listening to people, or that we have arrived at by inference (deduction).

In the deliberative (*savitarka*) *samapatti*, all of this knowledge, combined with the words referring to it, is mixed up with true *samadhi*. In *nirvitarka samapatti* (without *vitarka*) there is no such deliberation. For this reason we call it superdeliberative *samapatti* — beyond deliberation. Here the purification of memory has happened, which is nothing but making the mind one-pointed. The methods for making the mind steady have been described in sutras I.33–39, and the majority of the second and third chapters of the *Yoga Sutra* deals again with this subject.

Here we need to understand what super-deliberative *samapatti* is and what its effects are. Without this understanding, the practice of Patanjali Yoga cannot succeed. Purification of memory means that the mind is so focused that it does not keep throwing up more aspects, views, or data that it has stored concerning our meditation object. It is the nature of the mind to bring up all of this knowledge so that we can identify the object. But such unrelenting discussion prevents us from going deeper and realizing the deepest core of an object or the object-as-such. As long as this simulation of the object is present, the object-as-such cannot be perceived.

In this latest *samadhi* the mind appears to be emptied of its own nature of constantly projecting stored knowledge onto the present moment. This is called the purification of memory. The memory is called "stained" or "impure," because the past leaves an imprint on it. If I say that memory is purified, that does not mean it is deleted. It means that permanent projection of the past onto the present has become voluntary. Yogis can choose now whether they want to go into *samadhi* or use the memory to arrive at a conclusion. Memory is at our disposal, but if we don't need it, such as in meditation, we are free not to use it. This means that mind appears to be empty of its nature, which is constant shallow chatter.

The effect is that, for the first time, only the meditation object shines forth in the mind. It is visible without being mixed with what we believe it to be. This is important because for the first time we can see an object as it really is. This means to be truly alive. In many ways we had just been walking corpses before this point; we are real for the first time in our lives. Perhaps we had glimpses of pure unadulterated reality before — such glimpses may happen when for the first time we have a strong experience such as falling in love or having a near-death experience.

The second time the experience comes around, the mind knows what is coming, has filed the experience away somewhere, and does not get stunned into silence anymore.

Samadhi is different from such glimpses because it is a conscious process that can be repeated. If the memory is purified and the mind is emptied of its own form, every experience seems to be absolutely new, fresh, and breathtaking. Boredom is impossible. Boredom arises from an unfocused mind: if the mind is free to project our past onto the present, the present will look like the past and therefore be boring.

Let us say we are on the way home from work. It seems boring because we have taken that way many times and believe we know it from the past. But what about the change of sunlight every day, the color of the sky, the smell of the air, the changes in foliage and flowers, the flight of the birds? All these things are completely fresh and new every moment, and it is only because we project yesterday onto today that we don't notice them. For this reason, we follow the little schemes in our heads and do not hear the many wake-up calls life offers us every moment. If we knew we were dying and this was the last time we would drive this way, the situation would be very different: we would suddenly allow ourselves to perceive everything clearly.

The state of *nirvitarka samadhi* can be compared in some ways to the innocence and freshness of a child — in regard to the freshness with which the present is experienced. The difference is that all information stored in the memory is available when required, such as when a survival task is at hand. In many situations, though, memory is detrimental because it curbs our aliveness. Living from memory makes life appear dull, boring, and predictable. In super-deliberative *samapatti* one has the freshness of a child plus the experience of a lifetime when it is required.

Some contemporary movements have suggested that meditation is only about reverting back to a state of childlike innocence. This is not the yogic view. The purpose of superdeliberative *samapatti* is not to stay in a state of childish ignorance when the *samadhi* ceases. In sutra I.20 Patanjali lists memory under the prerequisites of *samadhi*, meaning that after every *samadhi* we have to remember that we are yogis, that we are unfree now, but that we are proceeding toward freedom through the path of yoga and therefore we need to proceed accordingly. This *samadhi* is only a stepping-stone on the path to liberation and not the goal itself. It gives us renewed conviction (*shraddha*) and energy (*virya*) to go toward liberation (*kaivalya*). If we do not integrate this *samapatti* meaningfully (*smrti*), we will stagnate here.

एतयैव सविचारा निर्विचारा च सूक्ष्मविषया व्याख्याता ॥ ४४ ॥

I.44 In this way, reflective (savichara) and super-reflective (nirvichara) sama-patti, which are based on subtle objects, are also explained.

To recall sutra I.17, objective (*samprajnata*) *samadhi* arises first from deliberation (*vitarka*) then from reflection (*vichara*). In yoga, "deliberation" and "reflection" are defined in the following way. Deliberative (*vitarka*) *samadhi* means meditation on a gross object such as the *bandhas*, the *drishtis*, the sequence of postures, the anatomical or outer breath, a lotus flower, the OM symbol, and so on. Gross here means that

the object has a manifest appearance that is perceptible to our senses.

Reflective (*vichara*) *samadhi* means meditation on a subtle object such as the senses, the process of cognition, the mind, the I-am-ness, the *chakras*, the inner-breath (*prana*), the *nadis* such as *sushumna*, the creative force (sometimes called *shakti* or *kundalini*), the intellect (*buddhi*), and so on. "Subtle" here means not perceptible to the senses, but arrived at through inference, such as "From my behavior I can deduce that I do have an ego and a mind." Subtle objects are also arrived at through testimony, such as the statements of Patanjali, Vyasa, and other ancient authorities, and finally through direct perception by the mind's eye in circumnavigating the senses, which is deep objective *samadhi*.

The two previously described *samapatti*s are based on gross objects with (deliberative) and without (superdeliberative) discussion thereof. The two *samapatti*s described now are based on a subtle object. Let us choose the example of I-am-ness or egoity (*ahamkara*, which, directly translated, means I-maker or that which adds the notion of I to the process of cognition). In reflective *samapatti* I have a seemingly precise duplicate of ego in my mind.

Superimposed on this image, my mind still reflects on all it has learned so far about ego, which could be, for example, Freud's or Swami Vivekananda's opinion on ego. Needless to say, this reflection prevents us from going deeply into our *samapatti*.

In the next higher — super-reflective — *samapatti* we directly perceive ego as such, and apart from that the mind is completely still. For this reason we have an infinitely more precise view and understanding of ego. To obtain a super-reflective view of ego is a very advanced and powerful state of yoga. We could almost say we have gone three-quarters of the way to freedom. In Patanjali Yoga there are really only two views higher than that: the view of intellect (*buddhi*) and the view of consciousness (*purusha*). The latter can only be obtained in objectless or super-objective *samadhi*.

Some schools count a third view, which is even higher. This is the view of the Supreme Being (Ishvara) or infinite consciousness (Brahman). Patanjali is silent here, largely because this is the subject of Vedanta and not of Yoga.

सूक्ष्मविषयत्वं चालिङ्गपर्यवसानम् ॥ ४५ ॥
1.45 The hierarchy of subtlety terminates in nature (prakrti).

According to Samkhya philosophy, onto which yoga is grafted, the world arises from an unmanifest, eternal, uncreated, and subtle matrix, which is its material cause — prakrti (nature or procreatress). Prakrti is like the state before the Big Bang: nothing is manifest but there is infinite potential.

According to Samkhya, from prakrti rises cosmic intelligence (mahat or buddhi). From that arises egoity (ahamkara), from that the subtle space, from that the subtle air, from that the subtle fire, from that the subtle water, from that the subtle earth element. This process is called evolution. In it is a down-and-outward movement that leads to ignorance and bondage. The yogi reverses this process and it is then called involution. The movement is in-and-up, and it leads to freedom and ecstasy.

The first subtle objects one would choose for super-reflective samapatti are those low in the hierarchy, such as the subtle earth element. It is called the elementary particle or infra-atomic potential (tanmatra) of earth. Through the samapatti, the elementary particle of earth returns into its source, the elementary particle of water. Through subsequent samapattis we return water into fire, fire into air, air into space, space into egoity (ahamkara), and finally egoity into intellect (buddhi). Intellect is the highest meditation object, and from it comes discriminative knowledge (viveka khyateh).

Let us note that the objects are ordered according to subtlety. This means that we meditate first on the apparent ones and last on those that are difficult to grasp and therefore need a more developed intellect. Intellect is the subtlest object meditated on. Subtler still than intellect is prakrti, but, since subtlety terminates here, prakrti is not chosen as an object. It is the state in which the three qualities (gunas) are in equilibrium, and here the world is unmanifest. The unmanifest state is reached when we recognize our true nature as consciousness. Then the conditioned mind, which is a product of the intertwining gunas, disconnects from us and returns into its source, prakrti. At this point we need to let go of meditation objects and meditate on the subject (consciousness)

instead. If we continue here we will become one with prakrti, the place where subtlety terminates. Identification with prakrti (prakrtilaya) is also a high mystical state, but it does not lead to permanent freedom. As discussed in sutra I.19, it leads to new ignorance, suffering, and embodiment, and must be rejected. The state of prakrti is different from consciousness, and the goal of the yogi is to identify with consciousness and stay clear of prakrti, which carries the intention of becoming opposed to the pure being of consciousness. Consciousness is not mentioned under subtle objects because it is the subject, the true observer or self.

ता एव सबीजः समाधिः ॥ ४६ ॥
1.46 All these are samadhi with seed (sabija).

The seed (bija) is the object on which we meditate. All samapattis are forms of objective samadhi, since they rely on an external object for arising. The term sabija samadhi is synonymous with the term "objective" or "cognitive" samadhi (samprajnata). Cognition means an object is perceived and identified by the mind.

The higher type of samadhi is seedless (nirbija) samadhi, which is objectless. It does not rely for its arising on an object. The term "ultracognitive samadhi" (asamprajnata) is synonymous with objectless (nirbija) samadhi. In it we have gone beyond the need to stabilize our samadhi through objects.

The other reason why objective samadhi is called "samadhi with seed" is that in it the seeds of subliminal imprint (samskaras), which produce conditioning (vasana), are left intact. From those seeds can sprout new ignorance and new action (karma), which is based on the forms of suffering (kleshas) — but in seedless samadhi those seeds are scorched and therefore lose their capacity to germinate. Only through seedless samadhi is liberation therefore possible.

निर्विचारवैशारद्येऽध्यात्मप्रसादः ॥ ४७ ॥

1.47 From the glow of super-reflective (*nirvichara*) *samapatti*, the inner instrument is purified.

Establishment in super-reflective *samapatti* means that one's mind has the ability to gain identity with a subtle object without discussion going on in the background. Then a glow rises, which purifies the inner instrument of cognition — *buddhi*, the intellect.

It is erroneous for modern authors to translate this sutra as "From *nirvichara samapatti* arises clarity of the authentic self." Patanjali and Vyasa have clearly established a nomenclature of *samadhi*s, with seeded or objective *samadhi*s such as our example here referring to objects. Only seedless or objectless *samadhi*s refer to the self (*atman*) or consciousness (*purusha*). The objective *samadhi* mentioned here has not the power to reveal the self, its purpose being to purify the inner instrument of cognition, the intellect.

The term used in this sutra for inner instrument is *adhyatma*, which means belonging to oneself. Vyasa used this term already when he described the three forms of suffering (*adhyatmika, adhibhautika, adhidaivika*). In this context it refers to suffering created by oneself, such as through one's own ignorance. It is clear that suffering cannot be created by one's true self (*atman*). For a start, consciousness (*atman*) is entirely passive and does not influence the world. This understanding is taught by the *Upanishads*, the *Bhagavad Gita*, the *Brahma Sutra*, and the *Yoga Sutra*. The self does not create. Furthermore, abiding in the self is not suffering but ecstasy and freedom. The term *adhyatma* therefore does not relate to the true or divine self but just to oneself, here the inner instrument.

From repeated application of super-reflective *samapatti*, the mind and particularly the intellect gain the capacity to perceive objects as they really are. This type of knowledge is called *prajna*, which means understanding and comprehending objects on the deepest level. Now the mind has become a tool for knowing things, whereas before it was capable only of believing, suspecting, gauging, or considering. Deep knowledge about objects is possible only with a mind that has gained this ability. Then the inner

instruments are said to be purified, which means that wrong notions cannot stick to them anymore. Why this is so important we will learn in the next sutras.

तंभरा तत्र प्रज्ञा ॥ ४८ ॥

1.48 There the wisdom is truthful (*rtambhara*).

The quality of the wisdom (*prajna*) gained in super-reflective *samapatti* is described now. It is said to be truthful (*rtambhara*). *Rta* is an old terminology that had appeared already in the *Rig Veda*. It refers to sacred order. What is meant here is that one sees things at the deepest level in their such-ness and not how we believe or want them to be.

Vyasa explains that *rtambhara* means complete truth, mixed with not even the slightest bit of untruth. He explains that this highest yoga is reached in three steps: studying the sacred scriptures, inference, and constant meditation practice. This echoes the dictum of the *Brhad Aranyaka Upanishad*, according to which consciousness (Brahman) is attained through three steps. Here they are called *shravanna* (repeated listening to the truth), *manana* (reflecting on the truth), and *nidhidhyasana* (realizing or permanently being established in the truth).

श्रुतानुमानप्रज्ञाभ्याम् अन्यविषया विशेषार्थत्वात् ॥ ४९ ॥

1.49 This knowledge is different from the knowledge gained through scripture and inference, since it is of a particular thing.

Our languages are very imprecise. There are millions of particular objects but there are only a few words to describe them. If we really used a different word for every different object, our language would be unmanageable. Since inference and scripture use language, they describe things only in a general way.

Knowledge gained through the senses pertains only to gross objects (things). All important meditation objects, such as mind, ego, intellect, the heart lotus, and the central energy channel, are subtle objects and cannot therefore be perceived by the senses. That is why we need inference and the testimony of the scriptures. But even when the scriptures are understood and the intellect is made sattvic, so that we can correctly infer subtle objects, there is still a difference to directly perceiving them in *samadhi*. Before we are capable of this direct perception, there might still be a lingering doubt about whether the testimony or the inference is correct. But even if there is no doubt, there is still the fact that the knowledge is not really ours but secondhand.

The mystic Georg I. Gurdjieff said that knowledge is of physical nature. What he meant was that theoretical knowledge does not help much. Only when knowledge has become real, as if it is a physical object that we can touch, will it transform us. Before that philosophy is just theory.

It is not correct to say, however, that we need to experience the truth to be free. No experience will ever, ever lead to freedom, as experience itself means bondage. Experience is defined by impermanence: every experience has a beginning and an end. When it ends it is succeeded by a different experience. If we say we have experienced freedom, then we have not experienced the real freedom, freedom being the end of experience. For this reason the ancient masters used terms like "abiding," "realizing," and "knowing." Once consciousness is known or realized, no experience, whether good or bad, can impinge on that fact.

Such knowledge cannot be gained from reading books of course. But equally it cannot be created by actions, such as *asana*, *pranayama*, or meditation. No amount of reading or performing actions will produce direct knowledge, but study and practice can awaken the potential in us to realize knowledge. As Shankara has shown in his *Brahma Sutra* commentary, the consciousness (Brahman) has no cause. It is eternal and uncreated. This means that the state of Brahman within us is not created by study and meditation; or, in other words, study and meditation are not the direct cause of realising ourselves. Nevertheless they make us capable of realizing what we are already (consciousness). They are necessary for most people.

The necessarily vague words of a teacher will never suffice for showing us the truth. All teachings, whether they are scripture, personal teachings, or inference, rely on words. Words funnel reality into a linguistic code, but this code is very different from reality itself. It may be a beautiful description, but it is not reality itself. Reality must be known directly; only then will it truly awaken the yogi. This direct knowing of reality, without the mediation of words, concepts, teachers, or scriptures, is produced in super-reflective *samapatti* (*nirvichara*). In this way it is different: here we see an object in its totality, whereas the words of a teacher or the scriptures will always be a glimpse through their eyes. We need to see ourselves to become free.

तज्जः संस्कारो न्यसंस्कारप्रतिबन्धी ॥ ५० ॥
1.50 The subconscious imprint produced from such knowing reconditions us.

How is it that it does not help if a teacher tells us the truth? Why do we have to see it ourselves?

The words of a teacher leave a new subconscious imprint in the mind — an imprint of freedom, yes, but in a mind that is full of imprints of ignorance and delusion accumulated during the ages. It is necessarily the case that it won't change much unless the student has accumulated already a critical mass of subconscious imprints of freedom; then the added word of a teacher can tilt the entire personality toward freedom. For the average conditioned student this is not possible. In such a student the fluctuations (*vrtti*) of the mind arise due to past conditioning. Mere reading, meditating, or *asana* practice does not change this conditioning.

The special knowledge (*rtambhara*) obtained in super-reflective *samapatti* is, however, so strong that it deletes the subconscious impressions (*samskaras*) of fluctuation of mind and replaces them with impressions of truth, authenticity, and correct knowledge. We could say this is the secret of yoga's success. This process is also called the conversion of mind into intellect. "Mind" is that which believes, doubts, suspects, and so on; "intellect," on the contrary, is that which knows. Mind therefore needs to be converted into intellect by repeatedly placing within it the subconscious imprint of correct knowledge.

Only when the mind achieves identity (*samapatti*) with the object without any discussion (*nirvichara*) going on does there arise a direct realization strong enough to wipe out the age-old conditioning of delusion and mental slavery. When, through repeated application of super-reflective *samapatti*, enough subconscious imprints are deleted and replaced with helpful ones, the mind will tend to gravitate, even in the intervals between *samadhi*s, to a focused and one-pointed state. In such a mind obstacles are present only to a decreasing extent, if at all.

तस्यापि निरोधे सर्वनिरोधान् निर्बीजः समाधिः ॥ ५१ ॥

1.51 After those have ceased too, the entire mind is suspended, and that is objectless (*nirbīja*) samadhi.

Patanjali finishes off the first chapter of the *Yoga Sutra*, which is called "the chapter on *samadhi*," by reminding us that the journey does not end with gaining complete truth through objective *samadhi*. Yoga is only really achieved after liberation arises. Liberation results from objectless *samadhi*.

This final *samadhi*, however, is beyond being achieved. To reach it, the yogi has to go beyond the idea of doing. After complete knowledge pertaining to knowables (objects) is gained, we next have to know the unknowable — the subject (consciousness). This is done in two steps, or some authorities have it as three. The third step is not a step that can actively be done; rather one needs to surrender to it. For this final transformation to occur, the yogi has to let go of the idea of being the doer.

STEP I

From complete knowledge pertaining to knowables (*prajna*), there arises, after due contemplation, an even higher state. It is called "discriminative knowledge" (*viveka khyateh*), and it arises in the intellect (*buddhi*). After the intellect has penetrated all objects in objective *samadhi*, it eventually realizes that awareness and consciousness are not part of itself (the intellect) but form an even deeper — completely independent — layer called the *purusha* or *atman*, the consciousness. This discriminative knowledge can only arise in its full glory when the intellect is

made completely sattvic through the practice of objective *samadhi*. Discriminative knowledge is the realization of the intellect that it is not the knower, the seer, and that it cannot know the seer.

How is it then that we can say this deep realization arises in the intellect and not in the consciousness? The consciousness is forever free, permanent, and all-knowing, whereas the intellect does know or does not know about a certain object. Whenever we are facing knowledge that arises or is produced, we are looking at the intellect. Consciousness (*purusha*) can never forget itself or remember itself, since it is eternal, uncreated, and unchangeable.

STEP II

In the state of discriminative knowledge we know all that we are not but we do not yet abide in our true nature. As a magnet attracts iron, so the intellect and mind gravitate toward knowledge of objects. To realize our true nature we have to let go of "owning" knowledge and phenomena. We have to stop projecting ourselves out, to look for ourselves outside. This stopping or ceasing is rather a passive nondoing and letting go. It is called *para-vairagya* — the supreme detachment. We have to surrender all becoming, all doing, all wanting, all goals, to become one with pure being. Through supreme detachment, through complete letting go, the mind becomes suspended — it ceases to function as an autonomous unity.

Here all subconscious imprints are wiped out, even those of complete knowledge (*prajna*) and single-pointedness (*ekagra*). This state is now called *dharma-megha-samadhi* (cloud-of-characteristics-dispersing *samadhi*), which is supercognitive (objectless) *samadhi*. The mind is now in suspension (*nirodha*), which means that we are no longer slaves to the mind. We will use it when we need it, rather than have it using us.

STEP III

If *dharma-megha-samadhi* is held for an extended period, the intellect detaches from consciousness, the *guna*s return to their source, *prakrti*, and the seer abides permanently in itself. This is liberation (*kaivalya*). It is a state of eternal, unchangeable, superconscious ecstasy and freedom.

Chapter II: On Practice

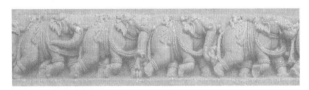

तपःस्वाध्यायेश्वरप्रणिधानानि क्रियायोगः ॥ १ ॥

II.1 The Yoga of Action consists of austerity, self-study, and surrender to the Supreme Being.

After addressing the first chapter of the *Yoga Sutra* to a very advanced student who was capable of focusing the mind, Patanjali addresses the second chapter to a novice student who has a distracted mind and suggests the Yoga of Action (Kriya Yoga). This yoga is called "active" as opposed to the advanced yoga, which appears to be inactive from the outside because it consists mainly of meditation.

In Hatha Yoga the term *kriya* has a different connotation. Here it refers to the *shatkarmas*, the six actions, which are purificatory exercises for the body. In Tantra Yoga *kriya* describes purification exercises for the subtle body, which combine visualization, mantra, and breath.

In Patanjali's yoga, Kriya Yoga consists of austerity, self-study, and surrender to the Supreme Being. The term "austerity" (*tapas*) evokes pictures of people sitting on beds of nails or standing on one leg for ten years. These are extremes. In sutra IV.1 Patanjali lists *tapas* as one of the ways to gain supernatural powers (*siddhis*). If that is the reason *tapas* is practiced, and usually it is, it has to take these extreme forms. Patanjali is critical about the powers: they are considered a distraction in yoga. As well, the *Bhagavad Gita* criticizes *tapas* if it takes the form of self-torture.

In yoga "austerity" means simplicity. Behind the term "simplicity" lies my acceptance of the truth that to be happy I need nothing but to know who I

truly am. By living a simple life without extremes and without constantly yielding to my desires, my mind is concentrated and focused. On the other hand, if I follow the call of this world to "spoil yourself," "treat yourself," and "pamper yourself," I communicate to my mind that I am not in charge of my life. Rather, I cement the belief that a constant stream of external stimulation and sensory satisfaction has to occur for me to keep my mental equilibrium — which means I am not in charge of my life but am a slave to my needs and desires.

To wake up to the truth that I need nothing at all to be internally happy, that in fact constantly following external stimuli separates me from myself, is *tapas*. Austerity will make us strong, whereas gluttony and decadence weaken. The more we believe we need certain things, the more we will be dependent on them. The simpler we can be, the freer we will be. Simplicity makes the body strong and healthy and the mind calm and focused. It is the foundation of self-knowledge, since it means giving up the lie that anything but self-knowledge can make us permanently happy.

A great example of mental focus through austerity was Mahatma Gandhi. By denying himself food and by being imprisoned, his conviction and concentration grew only stronger. Austerity does not mean that we have to live like beggars: some of the greatest yogis of India were emperors and kings. We can enjoy what rightfully belongs to us, after a certain percentage is given to charity, as long as we abide by the ethical rules.

The term *tapas* is formed from the root *tap*, which means to cook. Through simplicity and practice inner heat is generated, which is needed for purification on the physical and mental levels, emotions being a category of mind. Austerity means to be able to perform practice even in adverse situations. The mere fact of performing one's *vinyasa* practice every morning before work is to perform *tapas*.

The second of the three actions (*kriyas*) is *svadhyaya*,

which means self-study or study of the self. Meant here is not self-inquiry as practiced in Jnana Yoga: this highest form of yoga is recommended only to students who have fully developed their intellect. Kriya Yoga, however, is preparatory yoga. A beginner cannot come to the right conclusion regarding the self through direct inquiry. In Kriya Yoga self-study means study of the sacred scriptures. These are divided into *shruti* and *smrti*. *Shruti* means that which has been heard, and it applies to revealed scriptures, namely the *Vedas*[1] and *Upanishads*, which are understood to be of divine origin. *Smrti* means that which has been memorized. The word is applied to scriptures that are based on the revealed scriptures and explain them further, such as the *Bhagavad Gita*, the *Mahabharata*, the *Ramayana*, the *Brahma Sutra,* and the *Yoga Sutra.*

The study of these scriptures aids in removing the veil from the light of knowledge. It achieves that in several ways. First, the repeated hearing of the truth makes one realize that truth in daily life. Second, the contemplation of the heard truth makes the intellect sattvic. Georg Feuerstein says that "the purpose of *svadhyaya* [study of ancient scriptures] is not intellectual learning: it is absorption into ancient wisdom. It is the meditative pondering of truths revealed by seers and sages who have traversed those remote regions where the mind cannot follow and only the heart receives and is changed."[2]

The other traditionally recommended way to meditate on the self is repetition of OM. As the *Upanishads* frequently state, OM is Brahman (infinite consciousness). For more information on OM see sutras I.27–29.

1. The *Vedas* are the oldest type of revealed scriptures. They were considered so sacred that until about 1900 CE they were not written down — this would have, according to tradition, made them impure — but only consigned to memory.

Originally there was only one *Veda*, which had to be memorized by every Brahmin priest. At the outset of the Kali Yuga, the Rishi Vyasa foresaw that, due to the degeneration of human mental capacity, people would no longer be able to memorize the entire *Veda*, so he divided it into four parts — the *Rig, Sama, Yajur,* and *Artharva Veda.*

The *Vedas* contain hymns, rituals, and mantras. Even Western scholars now begin to accept that the early hymns of the *Rig Veda* date back more than eight thousand years. Tradition holds that the *Vedas* are eternal and are "heard" at the outset of each world age.

The *Upanishads* form the concluding portion of the *Vedas.*

2. G. Feuerstein, *The Yoga Tradition,* p. 247.

The third and final aspect of Kriya Yoga is *ishvara pranidhana,* acceptance of the existence of a Supreme Being. One of the problems of yoga is that it bestows great powers. These powers are bound to be abused if, as a yogi, you believe that the world is circulating around you, that it is there to satisfy your whims. Sadly this is exactly what modern society trains us to believe. We are taught that life is about fulfilling our dreams and desires, which consist mainly of consuming, owning, and exercising power. To keep our greed and lust for power under control, Patanjali suggests not placing ourselves in the center of the universe but accepting that this place is taken by the Supreme Being. The yogi then places himself in the service of this Being. To do this, one need not be a member of a particular religion; members of all religions would qualify. This brings us to another question: do I have to believe in the Supreme Being to do yoga?

Any belief, whatever it is, is counterproductive in the context of the practice of yoga. One holds a belief instead of knowing. For example you wouldn't say you believe in your right ear: since you know your ear, no belief is required. Believing always excludes knowing. When *jnana* (supreme knowledge) comes through the practice of yoga, you will know. Do not be satisfied with believing.

Once one has recognized oneself as consciousness, the question whether one believes in God or rebirth has become as meaningless as whether one believes in one's right ear. Patanjali's insistence in the present sutra on accepting the existence of the Supreme Being is not belief. It is a working hypothesis. It is like accepting 0 (zero) when we use mathematics. Arab mathematicians introduced 0, but nobody has ever seen it, nobody can prove its existence. But when we use it, it opens previously unknown horizons to us.

Acceptance is the opposite of skepticism. Skepticism is not the same as doubt. To surrender to the Supreme Being is a condition of entry into higher Yoga. One may practice Samkhya (meditative inquiry into the order of the universe) without *ishvara pranidhana,* since this inquiry does not bestow powers. The powers (*siddhi*s) that come with yoga make it necessary to accept this condition of entry. A Buddhist would call surrendering one's powers to the Supreme Being acting "for the good of all beings."

Without this attitude we will be tempted to use our powers to satisfy our personal egoistic tendencies. This is black magic. The white and the black magician use the same methods and the same powers, but the black magician worships his or her own ego, whereas the white magician serves the Supreme Being. For more information on the role of the Supreme Being in yoga, see sutras I.23–29.

समाधिभावनार्थः क्लेशतनूकरणार्थश्च ॥ २ ॥

II.2 Kriya Yoga is done for the purpose of moving closer toward *samadhi* and for reducing the afflictions (*kleshas*).

Patanjali explains the purpose of Kriya Yoga. The novice is advised to steer away from what is damaging and aspire to what is helpful. Afflictions (*kleshas*) are the forms of suffering. They are unwanted states that surround us and fill us with darkness. There are five forms of suffering, and Patanjali will define them in the following sutras.

One of the problems when we begin yoga is that, while we might have a sincere wish to engage in practice, afflictions in the form of negative habits, addictions, feelings of futility, bad influences, and hindering emotions have such a strong grip on us that we commit negative actions that produce more negative results. This is the vicious circle of *karma*. If somebody is in a downward spiral, it is often not enough to tell them to change their behavior. Their subconscious, which is conditioned by the past, compels them to act in a certain way.

Vyasa, however, writes in his commentary on this sutra that Kriya Yoga, if engaged in properly, will parch the afflictions so that they cannot produce future suffering. Like seeds that have been roasted, they cannot sprout anymore. If Kriya Yoga is done for some time, the modes of suffering will loosen their grip on us, so that at some point we can practice higher yoga.

However, the roasted seeds, although incapable of germinating, continue to exist. It has been observed that many great sages had to go through a lot of suffering before they reached liberation. Some

masters and even deities died violent deaths. Buddha, Milarepa, and Socrates were poisoned; Jesus was crucified; an arrow killed Krishna; Vishnu's head was snapped off while he was leaning on his own bow. J. Krishnamurti, Ramakrishna, Ramana Maharshi and the sixteenth Karmapa died from cancer. Mogallana, one of the two principal students of Buddha, was hacked to death by robbers.

This posed a great problem for Buddhist scholars, who asked, "Why, if he was such a great saint, did he attract such violence?" The answer is simple. Once the afflictions (*kleshas*) have been rendered infertile by the fire of knowledge, they cannot produce new ignorance. However, the *karma* that had been accumulated prior to that and is bearing fruit already (*prarabda karma*) cannot be changed anymore and has to be endured. In Mogallana's case this means the actions that led to him being murdered were performed long before he met the Buddha. But the results of those actions had started to fructify and therefore could not be intercepted anymore, not even by his liberation.

We can learn from this that the setbacks we suffer, although we have practiced for some time, shouldn't dishearten us. They have been caused by actions we performed in the past. Our actions today will determine who we will be in the future.

अविद्यास्मितारागद्वेषाभिनिवेशाः क्लेशाः ॥ ३ ॥

II.3 Ignorance, egoism, desire, aversion, and fear of death are the afflictions.

In sutra II.2 Patanjali suggested the practice of Kriya Yoga to reduce afflictions (*kleshas*). In this sutra he explains what exactly it is that we are reducing. The five different types of affliction are ignorance, egoism, desire, aversion, and fear of death.

Avidya (ignorance) is the opposite of *vidya*, which is true knowledge or science. The term *brahma vidya* means science of Brahman, while *bharata vidya* (science of India) is used to describe all of India's ancient wisdom. *Avidya* has been translated as ignorance, nescience, nonscience, or misapprehension. The term *asmita* we know from the first chapter. It can be called sense-of-I, I-am-ness, or egoism.

Desire (*raga*) and aversion (*dvesha*) are the two

forms of suffering that Buddha recognized. He taught that suffering comes from desiring something that is separate from us (attraction) or rejecting something that is in contact with us (aversion). Both forms of suffering can exist only, he taught, because we do not recognize Mind as space. I write mind with a capital M here to distinguish it from the yogic notion of mind. Buddha took the upanishadic concept of consciousness (Brahman) and renamed it Mind. This idea of mind is very different from the yogic concept, which sees mind either as the thinking agent (*manas*) or as the sum total of thinking agent, ego, and intellect (*chitta*).

According to Buddha, if we recognized Mind (the upanishadic Brahman) as the container that contains the world and all beings, we would realize that we are always united with whatever we desire. At the same time it becomes clear that it is futile to reject anything, because we are connected to everything through Mind.

The last affliction is *abhiniveshah*. It can be translated as fear of death or desire for continuity.

Vyasa says in his commentary that the afflictions are the five forms of wrong cognition (*viparyaya*). Let us recall that wrong cognition is one of five fluctuations of the mind (*chitta vrtti*). Vyasa explains further that the five afflictions, when activated, increase the work of the *guna*s. The *guna*s, the three qualities or strands of nature, increase their activity the more we move away from equilibrium, from the center of the cyclone. They draw us deeper into creation and further away from consciousness. Vyasa continues then by saying that this increase of the *guna*s opens up the current of cause and effect and produces the fruition of *karma*. It is this chain of cause and effect and production of *karma* that our bondage consists of. It will lead to further negative thought, negative action, and mental slavery.

Vachaspati Mishra confirms in his subcommentary that the afflictions should be destroyed because they are the cause of the round of rebirths.[3] In his subcommentary Shankara adds that freedom from the impurity of the *klesha*s comes from the absence of wrong cognition.[4]

3. J. H. Woods, trans., *The Yoga System of Patanjali*, Motilal Banarsidass, Delhi, 1914, p. 106.

4. T. Leggett, *Shankara on the Yoga Sutras*, p. 178.

Concluding, we can say that the five afflictions produce further *karma*, which keeps us from becoming free. They arise out of wrong cognition (*viparyaya*). If this wrong knowledge is replaced with correct knowledge, they will cease and no more *karma* will be produced. The chain of cause and effect will be broken by the knowledge that we are in fact consciousness and not what we identify with.

The next five sutras will describe the individual afflictions, and we will verify Vyasa's claim that they arise out of wrong cognition. These connections are not just dry philosophy; they need to be pondered well. The *shastra*s (sacred scriptures) say that a complete yogi needs to hear about the mechanics of bondage only once to break free. One near completion needs only frequent reflection to realize the truth. Most of us, however, will have to contemplate the subject regularly until clarity is achieved.

अविद्या क्षेत्रम् उत्तरेषां
प्रसुप्ततनुविच्छिन्नोदाराणाम् ॥ ४ ॥

II.4 Ignorance is the origin of the others, whether dormant, attenuated, interrupted, or active.

Vyasa likens ignorance to a field that provides the breeding-ground for the other four afflictions, which are egoism, desire, repulsion, and fear of death. These can occur in four different states: dormant, attenuated (thinned), interrupted, and active. They are described to remind us that, just because we are not fully in the grip of an affliction, it doesn't mean the affliction is not present.

DORMANT STATE

For example, we may not be aware that fear of death is present in us, because we have never had to fear for our life. But if the appropriate stimulus — a life-threatening situation — is presented, the fear will surface. Thus the affliction, fear of death, was in the dormant state. A dormant affliction will awaken once its object is presented. If the affliction does not surface at all, even in a life-threatening situation, it is not present, even in a dormant form.

ATTENUATED (THINNED) STATE

If, for example, we are in a life-threatening situation and we react relatively calmly because, through study of the *Bhagavad Gita*, we have understood that we are not the body, but rather that which cannot be burned by fire, drowned by water, pierced by thorns, or cut by blades, the affliction is said to be attenuated or thinned by Kriya Yoga — in this case through the second aspect of Kriya Yoga, which is *svadhyaya*, the study of sacred scripture.

INTERRUPTED STATE

If an even stronger affliction cancels out a present affliction, that affliction is said to be interrupted. For example, let us say we are committing a bank robbery, and so eager to get our hands on a bag full of dollars that we have no fear of getting harmed. In this case fear is interrupted by greed. It is not that fear is not present, but it is interrupted or suppressed by the stronger notion of greed or desire.

ACTIVE STATE

If the object is presented and we are fully in the grip of the affliction, it is called active. This is the only state in which the effects of the affliction are fully displayed. It is important to realize this: it means that, from our total portfolio of afflictions, only about as much is visible as of the iceberg that sank the *Titanic*.

There is a fifth state of affliction that Patanjali does not count because it occurs only in the yogi. Once the yogi has gained discriminative knowledge (the knowledge that one is not the appearances, but the consciousness in which they appear) then and only then the seeds of the afflictions cannot propagate anymore. The seeds are then said to be roasted in the fire of knowledge, which destroys their potency to sprout. This roasted state is also called the fifth state, which is different from the dormant state of the affliction. If a suitable object is presented, the affliction will not arise.

अनित्याशुचिदुःखानात्मसु
नित्यशुचिसुखात्मख्यातिरविद्या ॥ ५ ॥

II.5 Ignorance is to see the transient as eternal, the impure as pure, pain as pleasure, and the nonself as the self.

Ignorance, which is wrong knowledge, is not only the absence of correct knowledge. It is the opposite of, and prevents perception of, right knowledge. So says Vyasa.

To explain this mechanism, the story of the rope and the snake is often quoted, as it has been already in this text. On his way along a path at dusk a man sees a rope lying on the path and mistakes it for a snake. Afraid, he runs away. The wrong notion of a snake leads to ignorance of the fact that it is a rope. In his village he encounters a man who walked the same path in broad daylight and remembers a rope lying on the ground. He takes him back and wakens him to the fact that the object is actually a rope, not a snake. Once the rope is cognized, the wrong knowledge (*avidya*) is replaced with correct knowledge (*vidya*) and ignorance is gone.

Every human seems to be endowed with a desire to become happy. True happiness, however, can only be had by abiding in the true self (*purusha*). Since we have a vague remembrance of the bliss of consciousness recognizing itself, we cannot be happy in the animalistic, robotlike existence that we live now. We long for recognizing ourselves, but, since we are deluded about our own nature, we constantly reach for secondary satisfactions. These are bound eventually to become stale and fail, for we know deep down that permanent freedom can only be found in what is eternal and pure. Although the blissful state can be found only by recognizing ourselves as consciousness, still we seek to realize ourselves through wealth, power, relationships, sex, drugs, and so on, which are all short-lived.

At the core of ignorance is the idea that my nation, my tribe, my personality, my property, my family, my children, my partner, my emotions, my body, my thoughts is me. But all of that is transitory, even if it lasts for a lifetime or a few lifetimes: all empires fall eventually. The only thing that really is me is the consciousness that contains all those notions, the self that witnesses all that. If I stay with that, ignorance (*avidya*) has been replaced with *vidya*, correct knowledge. Then the afflictions (*klesha*s) no longer have a breeding-ground and will disappear.

The Buddhists recommend staying with the nature of all that arises. What is the true nature of everything that arises in the mind? What is at the core of anger, happiness, hatred, love, fear, boredom, despair, confusion? Not at the surface, but at the very center of it? It is what the Buddhists call *shunyata*, emptiness. The Buddhist technique leads to the same result as the advaitic[5] method of asking who it is that is watching the world, which is the true self. If this true essence is realized, ignorance has come to an end.

How does ignorance lead to the other afflictions? Taking the nonself as the self leads to egoism (*asmita*). Aversion (*dvesha*) is a negative sentiment. Nevertheless those in its grip usually "enjoy" it, are self-righteous about it, and believe it to be a perfectly healthy reaction. If the impure is experienced as pure, desire (*raga*) is produced. Perceiving the impermanent (the body) as permanent (the self) leads to fear of death (*abhiniveshah*).[6]

दृग्दर्शनशक्त्योरेकात्मतेवास्मिता ॥ ६ ॥
II.6 I-am-ness (*asmita*) is to perceive the seer and seeing as one.

Understanding this sutra is of the greatest importance. Here is anticipated what Patanjali says in sutra II.17: The cause of suffering is the false union of the seer with the seen. This is the exact opposite of what the common contemporary misconception (also called New Age philosophy) tells us.

According to this common understanding, the key to happiness is to become completely one with whatever we do or perceive. Another beautiful phrase is: yoga is the union of body, mind, and soul. Phrases like these are easy to sell since they meet the expectations of gullible audiences. But the yogic truth is heartbreakingly different. The sutra says that when the seer, which is consciousness (*purusha*), is identified with seeing, that is egoism (*asmita*). Seeing

here refers to the function of the instruments of cognition. The instruments of cognition are the senses, the mind (*manas*), and intelligence (*buddhi*). They have no awareness of themselves but only reflect the light of consciousness (*purusha*) as the moon reflects the light of the sun. They gather information, process and modify it (that is the problem), and then present it to consciousness (*purusha*) to be seen.

Because of the property of the instruments of cognition to modify what is seen, yogic philosophy does not regard them as being able to perceive the truth. The truth pertaining to knowables (objects) is defined as the essence of an object (*dharmin*) or the object-as-such. Perceiving it is called wisdom (*prajna*). This wisdom can only be perceived in objective *samadhi* (*nirvichara samapatti*), in which the intellect attains identity with the object under circumnavigation of the mind (*manas*) and the senses. The even higher truth pertaining to the knower can only be gained by abiding in consciousness directly, through the mystical state (objectless *samadhi*).

The modification of information through the instruments of cognition was discussed under sutra I.7 using the example of the eye — how the brain converts the inverted image on the retina to an upright image and how it fills in the retinal blind spot. This is how our entire cognition process works. All incoming information is constantly compared with the information already in store. Conflicting data is either deleted or, over time, slowly integrated.

We have thus a constant changing simulation of reality but never a true reproduction of reality in that moment. This makes a great system for navigating a physical body within a space/time continuum, but for experiencing what is called deep reality — the cause of all causes — it leads invariably to sheer nonsense. That is why we have to shortcut the mind in what is called the mystical experience to see reality directly.

Vyasa summarizes the sutra as follows: *Purusha* is pure awareness; *buddhi* (intellect or intelligence) is the perceiving instrument. Taking the two completely separate units for one and the same thing is defined as the affliction I-am-ness or egoism (*asmita*). When the true nature of these separate entities is recognized, that is freedom (*kaivalya*).

5. Referring to the system of Advaita (nondualistic) Vedanta.
6. H. Aranya, *Yoga Philosophy of Patanjali with Bhasvati*, p. 122.

सुखानुशायी रागः ॥ ७ ॥
II.7 Desire (raga) is clinging to pleasure.

This third affliction works in three steps. First there is an experience of pleasure. During this experience a subconscious imprint (samskara) is formed. The pleasurable experience is remembered and a hankering after it develops. Either one tries to repeat it, which calls for constant repetition and sets off an addictive pattern, or one suffers because the repetition is not possible.

The important fact to see here is that the pleasurable experience in itself is not the problem. If we were fulfilled by experiencing it once and could let it go, there would be no desire to repeat it. We could also, whenever the same experience occurred again, enter it with the same innocent freshness as when we had it the first time. This would happen in the case of the jnanin (one who has knowledge). Because a jnanin is fulfilled by abiding in consciousness, there is no void that needs to be filled up with experiences of pleasure. Pleasure-seeking is really engaged in to get an experience of oneself — for example, driving a car at 185 miles per hour, bungie jumping, or any danger sport. Once the light of the self is seen, these activities do not leave any new samskara and therefore do not ask for repetition.

During an experience of pleasure there is an impression of happiness that fills the void left by not knowing oneself. Later, during a moment when there is no strong impression in the mind, this happiness is remembered. One then repeats the experience only to find that it doesn't bring about the same happiness anymore. The happiness was caused by the mind being momentarily overwhelmed by the new experience, and it therefore blanked out for a short time. With the mind blanked out, we noticed the shining sun of the self, possibly only for a second or two.

Because the mind is prepared when the experience is repeated, it will not be overwhelmed anymore, but will wrap up the experience in a nice parcel and interpret it. We then increase the strength of the experience to get to the same state. This is the reason people go to extreme lengths to have an experience of themselves — drug users constantly up the dosage, billionaires build huge business empires, and dictators invade yet another country. The mind can never get enough.

There are two prerequisites for the mechanistic pattern to develop. I call it "mechanistic" here to make clear that it is a robotic behavior, whereas the common sense of our society is that to follow one's desires means to truly become oneself. For desire to develop there needs to be an experience of pleasure and it needs to be had by someone who is inclined to it. There can be various reasons for lack of inclination. If the experiencer knows himself or herself as consciousness, no desire will develop. If the experiencer's inclination is toward hatred or fear, desire cannot develop. In that case the affliction called aversion overpowers or interrupts the one called desire. Characters absorbed in malice are often rather ascetic and not inclined to pleasure. Adolf Hitler fits into this category.

It is important here to realize that desire (raga), and with it all addictions, is a clear form of misapprehension or ignorance (avidya). A drug addict might say, "I just can't help it; I need the drug!" In this statement, the needing of the drug, which is the hankering after a remembered pleasure, is consciously connected with the faculty of I. But the real I, the true self, has no connection whatsoever with the subconscious impression of pleasure, since it is pure awareness without memory. Yoga defines as ignorance the experience of pure awareness or consciousness bound up with experiences like pleasure.

The senses, the mind, and the intellect — in short, the instruments of cognition — produce the experience of pleasure such as the repeating of a drug experience. I, however, am only the onlooking awareness/consciousness, which is completely separate from the experience. I need to permanently deny my true nature as consciousness and insist on identification with the instruments of cognition to be able to say "I need a drug (or wealth, sex, power, fame, or proficiency in asana practice)." That leads us to the conclusion that addiction or any form of desire is a case of egoism/I-am-ness (asmita), since in this statement the "I" is wrongly identified with the instruments of cognition and not with the true self.

Once the self/consciousness is realized, all addiction will drop away by itself, since egoism (asmita) is destroyed and desire will loosen its grip.

To summarize, the affliction called desire (*raga*) creates suffering by producing a craving for repeated pleasure due to subconscious impressions formed when it occurred originally.

दुःखानुशयी द्वेषः ॥ ८ ॥
II.8 The affliction that results from memorized suffering is called aversion (*dvesha*).

In the case of this affliction the same mechanism is working as in the previous one. The only difference is the experience on which it is based. The last affliction was based on past pleasure, this one on past suffering.

If for example we went to the dentist and suffered a lot of pain, the experience would be stored in the form of a subconscious imprint (*samskara*) of pain. Whenever we had to go to the dentist again, the memorized suffering would produce an aversion. We then might go through a period of suffering, possibly only to find that our teeth are okay this time and no new pain will ensue. In this case we would have suffered on the basis of a past experience, whereas the present situation does not hold pain for us. This form of anticipated suffering is called aversion (*dvesha*) in yoga.

Sexism, racism, and nationalism are forms of aversion derived from the same mechanism. We notice some individuals acting in a particular way, which produces aversion in us. From that we infer that the entire group to which the individuals belong will act in the same way. Our aversion is then extended to cover the entire group.

Jealousy is another popular form of aversion. Some people display very strong symptoms of jealousy to the extent that they spy on their partners or do not allow them to leave home after dark, even though they are completely faithful. In this case the jealous partner might have been cheated on in a previous relationship, or might have abandonment issues originating from not getting enough attention from a parent. In both cases the cause is past suffering, erroneously projected onto a present situation.

Aversion, like desire, makes it impossible to experience the present, but lets us act according to a past conditioning. In extreme cases we walk through life like a robot. This is reflected in the term "conditioned existence" (*samsara* — do not mistake this for *samskara*). The opposite of conditioned existence is when we experience every moment with freshness, as if for the first time.

Aversion is a form of wrong cognition (*viparyaya*) — again, like desire. Because I identify the self or pure consciousness as being bound up with subconscious impressions of pain, I can say, "I am jealous." This means I identify myself with the negative emotion; I have become it. If I say instead, "I, the observer, which is pure unstainable, immutable consciousness, cognize a memorized feeling of past neglect," then I do not emote the past but can choose to feel what is present, for example the love for my partner.

Like desire, so also is aversion destroyed by discriminative knowledge (*viveka khyateh*).

स्वरसवाही विदुषोऽपि तथारूढो भिनिवेशः ॥ ९ ॥
II.9 Fear of death (*abhinivesha*), felt even by the wise, arises from the desire to sustain one's existence.

The last affliction is fear — particularly fear of death, which is the root of all fears. Again, it is a form of wrong cognition (*viparyaya*). Because we wrongly perceive the body as the self, fear arises. Knowing the body will come to an end, we take its death to mean our destruction. Abiding in the true self, which is uncreated and therefore indestructible, will end this fear. Or should end it by all means.

But, as Patanjali writes, fear of death is felt even by the wise. Shankara comments on the use of the word "even" thus: "The force of the word even is, that fear of death is logical only in the ignorant, who think of the self as destructible. It is illogical in those of right vision, who think that the self is indestructible."[7] Vyasa points out that this means even people who should know better still think thoughts like "Let me never be nonexistent; may I always live."

The affliction fear of death follows the same mechanism as the previous two. For example we might walk alone along a dark street and get

7. T. Leggett, *Shankara on the Yoga Sutras*, p. 194.

mugged. This triggers in us an immense fear that produces a subconscious imprint of fear. Whenever in the future the appropriate situation is presented, in this case walking in a dark street, the same fear may surface again although no one is threatening us. Again, as with the previous afflictions, it is not the present situation that is the problem (walking down a dark street alone) but the remembrance of a previous condition that makes us act as a programmed robot would.

Vyasa deduces from the fact that all beings are afraid of death that they have experienced death and thus life before. The intensity with which all beings cling to life can only be explained through accepting that we all have experienced death as a process to be avoided at all costs.[8] Shankara elaborates on Vyasa's argument thus: "Unless happiness (pleasure) had been experienced no one would pray for it. Without past experience of pain, there would be no desire to avoid it. Similarly, though the pangs of death have not been (in this life) experienced by a man either directly or by inference, the fact of his lust for life points to experience of death previously, just as there can be no experience of birth unless there has been a birth."[9]

Western science would deny the claim by saying that the urge to sustain one's life is determined by instinct. Yoga rejects this explanation because nobody can explain how instinct works unless (a) it is a form of memory (this is the way yoga explains instinct, and it leads to an inference about past lives, as shown above), or (b) it operates through the existence of a collective mind or subconscious that is independent and located outside the individual. But the latter is also rejected by Western science, which believes that mind is nothing but bioelectrical impulses provoked through external stimuli. To prove their point, scientists argued that individuals would fall asleep if deprived of external stimuli such as sight, hearing, and the force of gravity.

This was proved wrong by the neurologist Dr. John Lilly, who in the 1960s invented the isolation tank. In this device one floats on a strong saline solution, which cancels out any awareness of gravitation. At the same time the isolation tank is sound- and

light-proof, so that one experiences no sensory input whatsoever. Lilly found that, rather than falling asleep, he was lifted into a meditative experience. The isolation tank works like a *pratyahara* (sense withdrawal) device. Once the fuel of the senses is withheld, the mind is stilled and therefore meditation becomes possible.

It is the constant influx of sensory impressions that distracts us from recognizing the underlying deep reality. As sutra I.4 says, "When we cannot perceive our true nature we will identify with the contents of the mind."

ते प्रतिप्रसवहेयाः सूक्ष्माः ॥ १० ॥
II.10 The subtle states of the afflictions are destroyed with the dissolution of the mind.

This sutra is misunderstood in some modern explanations. Often it is interpreted as providing a technique for destruction of the subtle state of the afflictions. The sutra would then suggest destroying the subtle state of the afflictions by destroying one's mind. It is such incorrect interpretations that have given yoga the reputation of being somewhat similar to a bizarre self-annihilation cult. They are invalid for the following reasons:

• To destroy one's mind is a form of violence (*himsa*), which is not acceptable in yoga.

• If the mind nevertheless was destroyed, it would render the practitioner a vegetable. Yoga is, however, a superconscious state and not an unconscious one.

• To destroy and torture one's mind is as wrong as torturing one's body. In the *Bhagavad Gita* Lord Krishna says, "Those who torture the body outrage me, the indweller of the body." The same is to be said for torturing one's mind.

• Mind is eternal, says Vyasa. It is without beginning and end; it is beyond destruction.

• Ramana Maharshi has rightly pointed out that to control one's mind one needs to create a second mind. The same is the case when one tries to destroy the mind: a second mind would be needed to destroy the first mind.

8. H. Aranya, *Yoga Philosophy of Patanjali with Bhasvati*, p. 126.
9. T. Leggett, *Shankara on the Yoga Sutras*, p. 194.

- Torturing the body and destroying the mind will have only one effect: the increase of one's ego.

To get clear about the real content of this sutra we have to look into Vyasa's commentary. He explains that the "subtle state of the affliction" means that state in which the power of the affliction to propagate (its seed) has been parched or scorched. In other words the seed has no power left to make new afflictions sprout.

This means that, once the afflictions have been made subtle, the yogi has to take no further action, since the affliction is sterilized. To settle the matter completely we have to look in Vachaspati Mishra's subcommentary: "That which is in the scope of the exertions of man [the dormant, alienated, interrupted, or fully active state] has been described [in the previous sutras]. But the subtle [the fifth state] is not within the scope of man's exertion that he might escape it."[10]

Shankara says, in his commentary *Vivarana*, "So they [the subtle states of the afflictions] do not need any practice of meditation [since they are scorched already]. No fire is needed for what is already burnt, nor any grinding for what is powdered."[11]

When we take into account this information, the sutra reads as follows: The afflictions, after having reached the subtle state, need no extra meditation technique to destroy them. They are parched already and cannot sprout anymore. They (the subtle ones) will eventually be destroyed with the disappearance of the mind of the yogi.

The disappearance of the mind is beyond the exertions of man (!) It will naturally dissolve into nature (*prakrti*) only when the practitioner dies his or her last death.[12] When yogis have become liberated they do not endeavor to destroy the body, nor do they endeavor to destroy the mind. After the natural span of this last life has come to an end, body and mind and, with them, the seed state of the afflictions will dissolve without any reappearance.

ध्यानहेयास्तद्वृत्तयः ॥ ११ ॥

II.11 Mental processes arising from the afflictions are to be counteracted by meditation.

Vyasa writes in his commentary that the afflictions dealt with in this sutra are those in their manifest form, as opposed to the last sutra, where we were dealing with afflictions in their subtle form. Referring to Vachaspati Mishra's comment for the last sutra, now we are "within the scope of exertions of man." This means that we can and should do something to change the manifest state of the afflictions.

The present sutra recommends counteracting the manifest form of the affliction, also called its gross state, by contemplation and meditation. Let us recall sutra II.4, which states that an affliction can be dormant, attenuated, interrupted, or fully active. All of those four phases, representing the gross state of the afflictions, have to be counteracted by meditation until they have been made subtle. Then no further action is required.

The reduction of afflictions is divided into three stages:

1. Thinning or attenuating by Kriya Yoga.

2. Reduction by meditative insight, which is the stage that this sutra is referring to. The affliction is said to be reduced by meditating on discriminative knowledge (*prasamkhyana*) — the ability to discriminate what is self and what is not self.[13]

3. The third stage of the reduction of the afflictions is their total disappearance, which is covered in the previous sutra. The afflictions will only completely disappear at the moment the mind is dissolved. Within our scope are the first two stages, Kriya Yoga and *prasamkhyana*. About their relationship Vyasa says Kriya Yoga is like removing coarse dirt from a garment by brushing, and meditative insight is like removing finer impurities like a grease stain, which are washed away with care and effort.

What does *prasamkhyana* mean on the practical side? If I experience the affliction fear, for example,

10. J. H. Woods, trans., *The Yoga System of Patanjali*, p. 119.
11. T. Leggett, *Shankara on the Yoga Sutras*, p. 195.
12. Compare *Samkhya Karika*, v. 59.

13. It is difficult to translate *prasamkhyana*. Note that it contains the terms *Samkhya* and *khyateh*. *Prasamkhyana* could be called reasoned knowledge. It means that we use intellect and logic to free ourselves from suffering.

I am to contemplate the source of fear. The source of fear is the wrong notion that the body is the true self, that I am the body. Meditating on discriminative knowledge means meditating on what I am as opposed to what I am not. Fear disappears once correct knowledge is acquired, the knowledge that I am really the self and not the body.

If I experience the affliction aversion, which is clinging to pain, then I am to meditate on the source of aversion. The source of aversion is experiencing one's true self as bound up with the subconscious imprints (samskaras) of pain. The experience of pain is held in the subconscious, which is part of the mind, and neither of them has anything to do with the true self. Meditation here also leads to the insight that, whereas I may have experienced pain in the past, I have only witnessed it, but not become it. The witnessing entity, the consciousness, is completely unstainable; it does not mutate at all in the process of witnessing. This means that pain is a transitory sensation that does not mix with our true nature, which is eternal. Since the consciousness therefore emerges completely pure out of every situation, aversion is not necessary.

क्लेशमूलः कर्माशयो दृष्टादृष्टजन्मवेदनीयः ॥ १२ ॥

II.12 As long as our actions are based on afflictions, karma will sprout from them now and in the future.

This means that the karma, which is stored in the mind, has to be experienced in this life or in future lives, and it is rooted in the afflictions. Whenever we have an experience it will leave imprints in the subconscious (samskaras). When imprints are based on true knowledge or correct perception, they are said to be unafflicted. This means that they do not cause future suffering. Most imprints, however, arise out of ignorance and egoism, such as the notion "I am the body" and the idea that the purpose of life consists in the accumulation of material possessions. Those imprints do pose a problem. Being rooted in afflictions, they will produce karma, which will manifest in the form of new suffering.

There are subconscious imprints of varying intensity. If the intention that has produced the imprint was very strong, it will bear results immediately. So can an act of great villainy result in an immediate repercussion. The same is to be said about an act of great virtue or wisdom — the spontaneous realization of the truth can result in immediate liberation.

Most acts, however, whether vicious or virtuous, are performed with a mellower intention. Even if we do harm others, this was often not our intention, but rather it was lack of care or alertness that was the cause. When we perform good actions, our intention may often be to get more comfortable rather than to break through to a state of pure being. All those acts, which are performed with moderate intensity, will not produce immediate fruition. Rather, they accumulate and build up a store of karma in the mind, called a karmic storehouse or karmic deposit (karmashaya).

If impressions are accumulated in the karmic storehouse, the feeling may arise that they will not bear fruit, since the result is not imminent. The present sutra assures us, however, that all karma will eventually produce results that have to be experienced, whether in this life or in future lives. If the original actions that produced the imprints were based on afflictions (such as ignorance, egoism, desire), then those results will again manifest in afflictive form, meaning they will lead to suffering.

The subconscious imprints (samskaras) produce and crystallize a corresponding mind-set or conditioning (vasana). The difference between subconscious imprints and conditioning is important to understand. Repeated subconscious imprints of the same type will eventually produce a certain conditioning. If I allow myself to react violently and abusively in a certain situation, this will leave an imprint. After the first time I might still have a choice how to react. After repeated imprints my reaction will become more and more automatic. The imprints now enforce each other to produce a tendency called conditioning (vasana). Once an affliction-based conditioning is in place, I will always display a robotic tendency to create more suffering. Although even such a conditioning can be changed, it is much easier to intercept if we are only in the imprint stage.

Every time we become aware that we are acting on the basis of an affliction, such as past egoism, pain, desire, or fear, we need to make a conscious choice to let go of this tendency. This sutra reminds us that all suffering we inflict will return to us eventually.

Shankara explains in his subcommentary why some actions take a long time to yield results while others have their effects immediately. He gives the analogy that in agriculture some seeds sown in the fields germinate quickly, while others take a long time to sprout, depending on the quality and type of seed. Similarly the seed of karmic imprint in the mind will sprout fast or slowly depending on its quality, meaning the intensity of the action that produced it.

सति मूले तद्विपाको जात्यायुर्भोगाः ॥ १३ ॥

II.13 As long as this root of the afflictions, the karmic storehouse, exists, it will bear fruit in the form of types of birth, span of life, and experience [of pleasure and pain].

The root of the afflictions (*kleshamula*) is the store-house of *karma*. As long as this root exists, it will always sprout into new embodiments. The type of *karma* being stored determines our species, class and circumstance of birth, the length of our life span, and the amount and quality of experience therein. Shyam Gosh describes the mechanism of rebirth in the following way: "The situation driving future embodiments must provide necessary opportunity to consume one's *karma* through suitable experiences of pleasure and pain."[14]

Vyasa points out that the seeds of the afflictions will continue to sprout as long as they are not scorched by meditation. Because our meditation did not succeed in our last life, we accumulated new *karma*, which resulted in our present embodiment and its accompanying suffering. It is necessary to point out that the type, span, and experience of our next birth cannot be predicted. It is not dependent on our experience right now but on the predominant type of *karma* in the storehouse. If we have exhausted the good *karma* from our present embodiment, we could have a couple of low births coming up, which makes for a very insecure situation. We must therefore

14. Shyam Gosh, *The Original Yoga*, 2nd rev. ed., Munshiram Manoharlal, New Delhi, 1999, p. 197.

now, in this life, being in the fortunate position that all this knowledge is presented to us, make every effort to break through to freedom. Every life as a human being that is not spent in pursuit of liberation is a waste of a good chance.

According to the scriptures there are many types of rebirths apart from the human kind. Embodied as an animal, one is too unconscious to strive for liberation. Embodiment as a demon or a celestial being is infinitely more powerful than a human one, but they are too absorbed either in their wrath and malice (demons) or in their pleasure and beauty (celestials) to worry too much about freedom. Only human birth provides the right mix of pleasure and pain for the individual to still remain reflective while wanting to break free from enslavement to the mind.

Vyasa also points out another important aspect of karmic deposit (*karmashaya*). *Karma* that has not come to fruition yet can be destroyed before it sprouts. There are certain things in our lives that we cannot change because they fall under the category of *karma* that is bearing fruit already (*prarabda karma*). The seeds of this *karma* have sprouted and must be accepted as ordained and therefore endured, according to Vyasa. However, the entire storehouse of dormant *karma* that is waiting to fructify in some life to come can and must be intercepted now.

In many ways a new embodiment is like a game of dice: one can never predict how it will turn out. Some sages went on to an animal rebirth because, although they had performed great deeds, the strongest idea present in their subconscious at death was coincidentally an animalistic one. On the other hand great evildoers have gone on to become great liberated sages in the same lifetime. In his youth, the Tibetan master Milarepa murdered thirty-five people through black magic, yet went on to become one of the greatest mystics. This became possible because he worked harder on his liberation than possibly any other human being has ever done. Driven by the knowledge of the terrible destiny that awaited him should he die before attaining liberation, he meditated for twenty years naked in a Himalayan cave, without food and surrounded by ice. Such extreme forms of practice are not necessary if we have not been involved in such negative actions.

195

ते ह्लादपरितापफलाः पुण्यापुण्यहेतुत्वात्॥ १४ ॥

II.14 Their fruit is pleasurable or painful, depending on the merit or demerit of their cause.

Here is the reason for strict ethics in yoga. It is not that the masters want to take the fun out of life; it is just that, by our actions yesterday, we created who we are today. Similarly, our actions today will determine who we will be tomorrow. The body will necessarily hurt during morning practice if we become intoxicated the night before. We might not even be able to face practice at all, depending on how intense the indulgence was.

If there is any form of pain in our lives, we need to analyze the cause, which is demeritorious action, and eliminate it. If no cause is apparent, then according to yogic philosophy it is hidden in a past life. Those consequences must be endured, since the cause has been completed and has started to fructify, and for those reasons cannot be changed. Apart from our not taking responsibility for the fact that we have, in the past, brought about today's suffering, there is another dangerous tendency to be looked at in this context.

Often we are too superficial in analyzing the cause of our suffering, which could be faulty practice. We then happily escape into apathy and the feeling that "yoga is meant to hurt," whereas we are actually too lazy to research more deeply or are too stuck in our ways to change.

If we have managed to maneuver ourselves into a fortunate position through meritorious actions in the past, we would do well not to rest on it. The merit will surely become exhausted, and then we'll stand the chance of backsliding. Ideally a pleasant situation will be used for practice and study. In short, this is the time for doing things that will lead to our awakening; they are much harder to tackle when the water is up to our necks. Since the entire world is in constant flux, hard times can be around the next corner, even if it looks as though we have everything under control.

These attitudes will lead to the detachment that will enable us to meet the pain to come. Yoga advises us never to rely on the continuation of pleasure.

You may enjoy it while it lasts as long as there is no attachment to it. If attachment develops, you will depend on the continuation of those particular pleasures to sustain your happiness and freedom. Remember: there is nothing permanent apart from consciousness.

We also need to look at the fact that pleasure and pain are still part of the pair of opposites that Patanjali[15] and the *Bhagavad Gita* suggest we escape from. The Chinese philosopher Lao Tzu says in the *Tao Te Ching*, "Define beauty and you create ugliness. Create right and you define wrong. Better to return into the ocean of Tao." Tao is here the Chinese equivalent of the Brahman.

If we look at this group of sutras that deal with *karma*, we could easily gain the impression that yoga is a simplistic "do good and shun evil" type of spirituality. This is far from the reality. In yoga, liberation is reached through the mystical experience. Ethics are the groundwork, the base camp from which we climb to the summit. They are important because they keep our life simple and straightforward. Without them we would become entangled in the mesh of conditioned existence (*samsara*), so that the mystical experience would become unlikely.

THE IMPORTANCE OF ETHICS

Swami Agehananda Bharati made the attempt to disconnect ethics entirely from liberation.[16] He claimed that the mystical experience was entirely free of value, since it did not lead to a particular code of ethics. The swami overlooked the fact that any malice, any ill will toward a fellow being, comes out of not knowing oneself. If knowledge is gained, one knows one's own self as the self of all beings, and therefore hurting someone else is like hurting oneself.

Furthermore people act unethically for personal gain. When one realizes one's self, one knows oneself not only as the self that shines on one's personal life but as the self that shines light on existence in its entirety. After that, no more personal gain is possible: there is nothing that is separate from one's self any

15. Sutra II.48: "tato dvandva anabigatah" — then there is no attack from the pair of opposites.
16. Sw. Agehananda Bharati, *The Light at the Center*, Ross-Erickson, Santa Barbara, 1976.

more. At this point ethics are not anymore imposed from the outside but come naturally from within.

Ethics are part of the life of a mystic, but, if they are used to replace *samadhi* and mystical practice, they are overemphasized and the system we are looking at is not true yoga anymore. Not only are ethics alone a highly ineffective tool to attain freedom, they can be used to enslave humans further. Placing more and more and stricter rules on people often leads to the rules being grudgingly adhered to and then secretly broken. Or it leads to communicating to practitioners that they can never be good enough however hard they try (a problem for monks in some orders who are expected to adhere to as many as five hundred rules). Some members of the Jain religion drink water and breathe through a filter so as not to ingest and thereby kill micro-organisms; they also constantly sweep the path in front of them to avoid stepping on and killing small insects.

If ethics rule the life of humanity through guilt and shame, they are just another tool used by the mind to increase its tyranny over us. They need to come from inside; then they are liberating. Another great danger with ethics is that those imposing them on others often themselves fail to live up to them. It is interesting how many priests, gurus, and so-called saints in the last fifty years have preached celibacy (*brahmacharya*) and then been found to have had illegitimate sexual relationships, often with children and/or multiple partners.

A strict set of ethics, once mastered, can also be used to boost one's ego and assert one's superiority over others. There was a man who got up every day at 4 AM, was a vegetarian, and neither smoked nor drank. He had no sex. The man claimed to be a messiah, and many believed in him. His name was Adolf Hitler.

Inner freedom can never be attained by following a set of rules, a formula. Freedom is awareness. Any set of rules will be used by the mind and ego to build a new prison. The rejection of all rules, however, is just a new formula. The way out is, rather than through creating yet another set of rules, turning around and becoming aware of that which needs no regulation, that which breathes life into everything and therefore cannot be opposed to life. When that is seen, great compassion for all living beings arises

spontaneously from the heart and does not have to be imposed by the mind. Then we become living ethics, whereas before we tried to simulate life through a dead set of rules.

Ethics can never replace mystical insight, but they clear the way to getting there.

परिणामतापसंस्कारदुःखैर्गुणवृत्तिविरोधाच् च दुःखम् एव सर्वं विवेकिनः ॥ १५ ॥
II.15 To the discerning one, all is but pain due to the conflict of the fluctuating *gunas*, anguish through change, and the pain caused by subconscious impression.

Every experience in which we fall short of realizing our true nature as infinite consciousness leads in the end to suffering. The reason we are not aware of this right now is that, due to our past experience of pain, we have become numb and insensitive.

The apparently pleasurable poses a different problem. Whereas outright pain might drive us to seek for what is eternal (consciousness), pleasure has the tendency to strengthen the bond with what is impermanent (the body). The more pleasure we experience, the more we identify with the vehicle through which we experience — the body, the senses and the mind.

At one point in our lives we realize that the body will fall apart, making pleasure inaccessible, and we react with fear. We start hunting for more pleasure to cover up this fear. Often we expect pleasure and are unhappy because it doesn't come. Or we remember pleasure and can therefore not enjoy what the present moment has to offer. Pleasure tends to draw our thoughts into the past (to pleasure we once had) or into the future (to anticipated pleasure). Both will lead us away from the present.

Please do not understand yoga wrongly here: yoga does not want to spoil your pleasure. But if you are on the quest for freedom (*kaivalya*) and bliss (*ananda*), you have to understand that nothing transitory will get you there. Along with wealth, pleasure has become the god of Western society. Our society had to take on these deities because we have lost all knowledge of our true nature. The Buddha taught that all pleasure is pain, because inevitably we will lose everything pleasant that we have attached ourselves to. Then we will experience pain.

In Western society we are promised that pleasure-seeking is the way to happiness, and we most admire those who are most driven to fulfilling their desires. The Indian idea of happiness is the absence of hankering after enjoyment, which is contentment. Think about it. Giving up the idea that we have to reach out for satisfaction allows us to realize the happiness that is already here. Being deep within us, it doesn't rely on external stimuli. Pleasure-seeking will in fact lead to pain, according to yoga.

This mechanism is realized by the discerning one (*vivekinah*) — a person who discerns between self and not-self. For one who has seen the light of the self, pleasures are no match for abiding in limitless freedom. Once you have seen the ocean, the pond in your backyard is no big deal anymore. The pond in this simile is conditioned existence (*samsara*), the cycle of rebirth. This conditioned existence is painful compared to the ecstasy of becoming one with the ocean of infinite consciousness (Brahman).

What causes this samsaric pain, the pain that occurs in conditioned existence? Patanjali lists three causes of pain the discerning one is aware of, that brought about by subconscious imprint (*samskara*) being the most personal. For example a girl who has had an abusive, violent father will carry subconscious imprints from the experience. These imprints will tend to draw her into relationships with abusive, violent partners when she is grown up. Every experience leaves an imprint that calls for its repetition. Some (but not all) forms of psychotherapy do not reconcile well with yoga, insofar as they embrace the idea that traumas stored deep within should be brought to the surface, relived, and then (so the theory goes) let go. According to yoga, reliving the trauma will strengthen the grip it has on us and actually create new imprints that call forth further traumatic experience.

In other words, the reliving of a trauma makes it less likely that we can let go of it. New Age-like expressions such as "I've had a lot of stuff coming up" or "I'm going through an intense process at the moment" are really a sign of deeper and deeper enmeshing in conditioning, leading to further experience of pain.

An interesting current in contemporary Western culture has it that emotions are somehow closer to the truth than thought. Having suppressed emotion for a long time, we now try to make up for lost time. In yoga, emotions are seen only as another form of mind, no less robotic than thought. Emotions are really only feelings based on past situations. If I am feeling lonely, for example, this feeling relates only to the present moment. If, however, the absence of loved ones triggers in me an overall experience of rejection, cut-off-ness from others, and my inability to communicate, then I should properly say I am "emoting" loneliness. The loneliness is a past experience that "comes up" in present time, a general tendency in the mind that awakens when its object (absence of loved ones) is presented.

Being emotional is therefore opposed to being in the present moment. From the yogic viewpoint it merely amounts to thinking about the past or longing for past sensations. Emotions are clearly not our true nature. The power that is aware of emotions, that presence to which emotions arise, is our true nature (consciousness).

The person who sees this difference is the discerning one (*vivekinah*). To him or her even the opposite of trauma is still pain, since it is a reaction to pain. Only being in the self is one forever free.

After noting subconscious imprinting as the internal cause of pain, Patanjali enumerates two external causes. The first is the constant flux of the qualities (*guna*s) of nature. I use the English term "nature" here for *prakrti*, but let us remember that it has nothing to do with saving the whales or the rainforest, noble causes though these are. *Prakrti* is the origin of the cosmic intelligence that is the blueprint for the DNA code, the structure of molecules and the movement of galaxies around each other. This origin of cosmic intelligence or nature manifests the world through its three strands or qualities: *rajas, tamas,* and *sattva*. They are thought to make up, in different and changing proportions, everything in the world — excluding consciousness, which is not of the world.

Vyasa points out that, since one *guna* cannot make anything of itself, all objects consist of combinations of mass-stuff (*tamas*), energy-stuff (*rajas*), and intelligence-stuff (*sattva*).[17]

The attractiveness and enjoyability of an object will change considerably with perspective, observer, and time. The advertising industry worships the beauty of the female form as the perfect advertising tool, and many consumers are duped, even though we know how the body will change in just a few decades. From a different viewpoint the body might look much less enticing. As one sutra commentator has observed, "The girl that you married at twenty might have looked like an angel to you. At thirty she might look like a demon to you and possibly like an angel to somebody else." This is how the perspective of the observer might change without the object necessarily changing much.

This brings us to the third and last form of suffering, the anguish through constant transformation or change. Our natural tendency is to create system-like relationships: family, homes, circles of friends, company, neighborhoods, clubs, communities, societies, estates, cultures, nations, and empires, which give us a frame in which to settle down and get cosy. But all systems contain entropy, which constantly changes them until they break down.

Entropy manifests in the form of the death of the human body, the break-up of relationships and families, the bankruptcy of companies, the destruction of neighborhoods through racial unrest, terrorist attacks or bombing, the destruction of nations through war and civil war, and the fall of empires through decadence and idiocy. All such changes bring about anguish in the people who experience them. Even if the change doesn't mean we are worse off, the insecurity of having to change engenders fear.

For these three reasons the discerning one looks at the world and experience as painful. We can make this judgment because we know the only state that is not painful. This is the ecstasy and freedom of the natural state, which is the true state of yoga.

17. Terms used by S. Dasgupta in *A History of Indian Philosophy*.

हेयं दुःखम् अनागतम् ॥ १६ ॥

II.16 The pain that is yet to come is to be avoided.

All experiences based on afflictions are painful, says sutra II.15. The affliction-based experiences fill up the karmic storehouse, which leads to new suffering.

We can distinguish three forms of *karma*. First there is the *karma* that we have created in the past and has come to fruition already. This *karma* has produced our current body, with a certain frame of life span, type of birth and death, and type of experience. Within that frame, which we have to accept to a certain extent, there is still a lot we can change. But even if we do everything right we shouldn't be discouraged by setbacks but accept them as results of our own previous ignorance rather than looking to others to take responsibility for them.

The second type is the *karma* that has been created but not yet come to fruition. Its fruition has been intercepted by the *karma* that has given us our present body. We do not know what this *karma* has in store for us, and it must be interrupted. It could be that we have exhausted our good *karma* with this existence and might fall back into lower forms of embodiment. This has to be avoided. The *Yoga Vashishta*, which contains the teachings of the great Rishi Vasishta, claims that any *karma* can be intercepted and there is no karmic destiny for one of true self-effort. Indeed, there is evidence that destiny is modified with an increase in effort. If you believe you can change your destiny, your chances of doing so are improved. Let us make a firm resolve to intercept *karma* that is still in residue mode, *karma* that has not sprouted yet.

The third type is the *karma* we are producing now. This *karma* will, as we have learned already, produce immediate results if it is strong; otherwise it will accumulate in the karmic storehouse. In both cases it will produce new suffering, as shown in the last sutra. The only way to avoid future suffering is to awaken now.

Many people entertain the belief that death will somehow cure all our troubles automatically. Some hope that a deity will transport us to some elusive abode of bliss, whereas the materialists hope death will take care of our problems by switching us off.

However, the belief that death solves our spiritual problems is, according to I. K. Taimni, an absurdity comparable to the belief that night solves our economic problems.[18] Just because it is dark and you can't see the unpaid bills on the table anymore, they don't go away. Similarly, just because the light of your embodiment has been switched off, your karmic responsibilities haven't gone away.

Materialism gave rise to the illusion that we can act according to our liking without the need to feel any responsibility. Many materialists literally behave as if there is no tomorrow. According to their belief, whatever crimes one has committed, at the end of one's life one is simply released into the all-forgetting and all-erasing embrace of death. Why then should one go through all the effort to evolve?

Yoga says we will come back to harvest the fruit of our actions. If we do not want to harvest the fruit of pain, then we are not to sow its seed. The next sutras will explain how future pain is intercepted.

द्रष्टृदृश्ययोः संयोगो हेयहेतुः ॥ १७ ॥
II.17 The cause of that which is to be avoided [pain] is the union of the seer and the seen.

There are many popular misconceptions about yoga, especially in New Age circles. Yoga is called the union of body, mind, and soul, and books suggest to us that happiness lies in the complete union of the doer and the doing. "Become one with all that is" is another popular phrase. Patanjali brushes all of these concepts away with the statement that the cause of suffering is that very union of seer and seen. Exactly the union that contemporary misconception tells us to seek, the ancient teachers identified as the root cause of all suffering.

Vyasa says that, like a treatise on medicine, which is divided in four parts — disease, cause of disease, the healthy state, and the remedy — so also yoga has four parts. The disease is conditioned existence (*samsara*); the cause of the disease is the false union of the seer and the seen, perceived through ignorance; the healthy state is freedom (*kaivalya*), which we can

also translate as transcendental aloneness, because consciousness stands free and untouched by the world. The remedy to reach this healthy state is discriminative knowledge (*viveka khyateh*) or knowledge of the difference between the seer and the seen.

Vyasa also points out that the self/consciousness cannot be acquired and cannot be avoided, which destroys the notion of a spiritual path, because there is nowhere to go. It also destroys the notions of progress and process. Being eternal, uncreated, and immutable, consciousness cannot be attained. It observes, sheds light on the attempt to attain it, but does not change in the process.

The system that deals with this realization is the Vedanta. It is the most direct path to freedom, but many people cannot understand that they are free already. The yoga system is designed for those who are somewhat more ignorant. They need the illusion of going somewhere in order eventually to awaken to the realization that they never were separate from their goal. In other words it is a very down-to-earth, forgiving approach compared to the lofty heights of Vedanta, which is an intellectually more advanced way.

In the previous sutras Patanjali explained the five afflictions, concluding with the statement that, to the discerning one, all conditioned existence is pain. Conditioned existence is described here as the first part of the medical system, the disease. Now he focuses on the second aspect of medicine, its cause. His diagnosis is that the cause is the false union of the seer and the seen. The seer is consciousness (*purusha*), which is awareness. The seen is not only the entire world of objects but also the inner instrument (*antahkarana*), consisting of intellect, mind, and ego.

Imagine sitting in front of a screen and watching a horror movie. If you identify with the characters on the screen, if you are sucked into the film, suffering the horror will become real. You may start to sweat and your heart may beat faster. The way out of this suffering is to realize that it is not your life that is being enacted on the screen: you are just observing it. In the same way yoga says that we — consciousness — are not the agent, not the acting principle in the world. Rather, we are the pure awareness to which body, mind, ego arise. The egoic body/mind

18. I. K. Taimni, trans. and comm., *The Science of Yoga*, The Theosophical Publishing House, Adyar, 1961, p. 168.

is seen as part of the environment (*prakrti*) and not as our true nature (*purusha*). The same idea is stated in the *Bhagavad Gita* at stanza II.27: "Actions are done in all cases by the *gunas* of *prakrti*. He whose mind is deluded through egoism thinks, I am the doer."[19]

Let us recall that in sutra II.6 Patanjali defines egoism as combining the two powers of seer and seeing into a single entity. Here, in II.17, he gives a more universal statement, with the seen also encompassing seeing, which is the cognitive principle. The two sutras state that we are neither the seeing (mind) nor the seen (world), but the consciousness. To identify our self (which is pure, content-less, limit-less, quality-less, infinite consciousness) with our mind, our ego or its contents is defined here as the cause of suffering.

प्रकाशक्रियास्थितिशीलं भूतेन्द्रियात्मकं
भोगापवर्गार्थं दृश्यम् ॥ १८ ॥

II.18 The seen is made up of the qualities light, action, and inertia, and of the elements and sense organs. It exists for the purpose of experience and liberation.

Patanjali describes here the seen, the world. He uses the terms *prakasha, kriya,* and *sthiti,* but their meaning is exactly the same as the Samkhya words *sattva* (light/wisdom), *rajas* (movement/activity), and *tamas* (dullness/inertia), the three strands of nature (*prakrti*) that form, in various intertwinings, all phenomena.

The objects of the macrocosm (world) exist in the form of the five elements: ether, air, fire, water, and earth. In the microcosm (the human being) they exist in the form of the inner instrument, which consists of intellect, ego, and mind, and the outer instrument (body), which consists of the five sense functions and the five functions of action. The *gunas*, the elements and the inner and outer instrument together form the seen. Different from that is the seer, consciousness (*purusha*).

Important here is that, according to Patanjali, the seen does not operate without a purpose. Rather it

acts to provide us with an opportunity to experience and then to liberate ourselves. The world, according to Yoga, is like a stage on which will be enacted the lessons that we need in order to realize ourselves as consciousness. These lessons — we call them experiences — are not predominantly pleasant, but they have the right mixture of pleasure and pain to help us eventually to go beyond both. According to Patanjali, the world does not exist out of itself but only for the need to realize consciousness. In *Samkhya Karika* V.58 it is said that, even as people engage in actions for the sake of desires, so also does *prakrti* manifest itself for the sake of *purusha*.

This manifesting for the sake of consciousness results in experience and liberation. Experience means experience of pleasure and pain, which is also called bondage. After we have had a certain amount of experience, we recognize we are different from all that is experienced and therefore transitory. We then recognize ourselves as the only category of existence that is eternal and unchangeable, the consciousness.

The relationship between consciousness and the world can be likened to that between the sun and a flower. When the sun rises, the flower turns toward it and opens. When the sun describes its path in the sky, the flower traces its movement. When finally the sun sets, the flower closes. Throughout this entire process the sun is completely unchanged. It would perform exactly the same movement if no flower were present. The flower, on the other hand, is completely dependent on the sun. Without the light of the sun the flower cannot exist.

As the flower needs the sun, so the world needs the consciousness. When the consciousness shines its light of awareness, the flower of *prakrti* turns toward it and opens. The world follows the path of the sun of consciousness until it sets, when the end of a world age has come and the world becomes unmanifest. As the sun is completely unchanged during the night, so also the sun of consciousness does not undergo any change whatsoever during the manifold transformations of the world. Like the sun, the consciousness is completely free, existing only out of itself. Like the flower, the world is dependent on the light of consciousness.

19. *Srimad Bhagavad Gita*, trans. Sw. Viresvarananda, Sri Ramakrishna Math, Madras p. 79.

विशेषाविशेषलिङ्गमात्रालिङ्गानि गुणपर्वाणि ॥ १९ ॥

11.19 The *gunas* have four states: gross, subtle, manifest, and unmanifest.

Before the world arises, the three *gunas* are in equilibrium, and nature (*prakrti*) exists only in its unmanifest form. This can be likened to the state of the universe before the Big Bang. You could say it didn't exist, but really it did exist as a potential, as a seed state. Vyasa explains that the unmanifest (*alinga*) state of *prakrti* is neither existing nor nonexisting, neither real nor unreal. We can understand this only if we leave behind the tenets of Aristotelian logic, which formed the bedrock of Greek philosophy and all Western philosophy after it. Western logic says that if A is right and B is wrong, A cannot be equal to B. This is the logic of the mind.

Eastern or paradox logic we can call the logic of consciousness. Consciousness is the container that brings forth all possibilities. All possibilities therefore need to be included in the logic of consciousness. According to paradox logic, if A is right and B is wrong, then A and B can be identical, nonidentical, both identical and nonidentical at the same time, or neither of the two. All these possibilities appear in consciousness, but they do not appear to the limited simplistic human mind.

The second state of the *gunas* is the manifest state. According to the Rishi Vyasa, cosmic intellect or intelligence arises out of the unmanifest *prakrti*. Intellect is for this reason called the first evolute of *prakrti*. When we practice meditation (involute), intellect then obviously is the last thing to become unmanifest. Out of the manifest arises the subtle state of the *gunas*. This produces ego and the subtle essences (*tanmatras*). First ego emerges; then ego or cosmic I-maker (*ahamkara*) casts the notion of I on whatever the intelligence perceives. Ego owns phenomena; without ego no world could arise. After ego arise the five subtle essences of the elements, which have also been called infra-atomic potentials. We have to understand them as the deep essences or physical laws of the elements according to which all phenomena and occurrences develop. They are essences of sound, touch, form, taste, and smell.

The last state of the *gunas* lets the sixteen gross categories arise. From the five subtle essences

(*tanmatras*) arise the five gross elements (*mahabhutas*). From essence of sound arises space. From essence of touch arises air, from essence of form arises fire, essence of taste produces water, and essence of smell produces the element earth. The difficulty in understanding these concepts lies in the difficulty of translating the terms into English. They are only properly understood once they are seen in meditation.

From ego then arises the group of eleven. This comprises the five sense functions (hearing, touching, seeing, tasting, smelling) and the five functions of action (speech, grasping, locomotion, excretion, procreation). The eleventh and last is the mind (*manas*).

It is interesting to see that the three constituents or divisions of the inner instrument (*chitta*) emerge over three transmutations of the *gunas*. This might explain why they have such extremely different functions. The manifest *gunas* produce the intellect; the *gunas* in their subtle state develop ego; finally, from the *gunas* in their gross state emerges mind. The process of the *gunas* moving from unmanifest to gross is called evolution. In this process the world is projected out. The process of the *gunas* moving from gross to unmanifest is called involution. This is the process of yoga, and here spiritual ecstasy and freedom are attained.

The term "evolution" in Western thinking includes the notion of progress. In Indian philosophy there is no progress, since infinite consciousness (Brahman) is beyond time. Nothing is created; everything is eternal. Evolution therefore means a movement down and outward, from intelligence toward the earth element. The process of yoga is called involution, which is inward and up toward consciousness.

द्रष्टा दृशिमात्रः शुद्धोऽपि प्रत्ययानुपश्यः ॥ २० ॥

11.20 The seer is pure consciousness. Although it appears to take on the forms of the phenomena that it merely observes, it really stays unaffected.

Vyasa explains that the intellect (*buddhi*) is changeable in the way that it either knows or does not know about an object. The seer (*purusha*) is unchangeable because it is ever aware of what the intellect presents. It cannot look away and ignore it. Therefore it is immutable awareness. If we remember the space nature of consciousness, we know that all phenomena arise within it. Consciousness cannot decide to exclude and reject certain objects and it cannot hanker after or desire others because by nature it forever contains everything. Whoever has understood, contemplated, and experienced this is a knower, and forever free.

The difference between intellect and consciousness is that the intellect cognizes and interprets sensory input pretty much in the way that a computer does. Like a computer it is totally unconscious. On the other hand the seer — the consciousness — does not modify sensory input at all: it merely witnesses. The Rishi Panchasikha explains that the seer (consciousness) follows the modifications of the intellect.[20] On the one hand this makes the intellect appear to be conscious; on the other hand consciousness appears to modify sensory input.

When we start on the path of meditation we need first to choose gross objects because they are easy to contemplate. In the Ashtanga Vinyasa system we start by meditating on the moving human body, which is a gross object. It includes also the outer or anatomical breath. This stage is called *asana*. Once we have achieved that, without losing our focus during the practice we start focusing on the movement of the inner breath (*prana*), which is a subtle object. This stage is called *pranayama*.

After we are firmly established in our subtle focus, we start contemplating the senses, the process of perception, which is yet subtler. This stage is called *pratyahara*. Subtilizing our focus even more, we contemplate the mind, which is the master sense and collector of sensory input. This is *dharana*. Once we can hold our focus there, we start to meditate on pure I-sense, *dhyana*. The highest form of meditation is to meditate on the difference between the intellect (*buddhi*) and consciousness (*purusha*). This is objective (*samprajnata*) *samadhi*. After one has established the difference and abides in consciousness, it is called objectless (*asamprajnata*) *samadhi*.

In this state of right knowledge the false appearance, according to which the seer takes on the forms of the phenomena, which it only observes, is dispersed. Then the self is rightfully seen as unaffected.

The Armenian mystic Georg I. Gurdjieff called this "self-remembrance," a term that is infinitely more elegant than "self-realization." The self has always been real; we haven't. The self, as the Rishi Ramana affirms, is reality itself; in fact he goes so far as to say it is the only reality.[21] We, having attributed the light of consciousness to our mind, accepted the changing content of the mind as our nature. For this reason we have to remember ourselves as our self, the unchangeable, infinite consciousness.

तदर्थ एव दृश्यस्यात्मा ॥ २१ ॥

II.21 By its very nature the seen exists only for the purpose of the seer.

This statement is in accordance with the *Samkhya Karika*, which says the world is brought forth by *prakrti* for the purpose of liberation of *purusha*.[22] It has no other purpose than to provide experience for consciousness (*purusha*), which will eventually lead to liberation.

Consciousness is forever inactive; it only witnesses. One of the few words we can use to describe consciousness is awareness. Shankara in his subcommentary rightly points out, however, that it is only aware as long as an object is presented.[23] That means the quality of awareness pertains to the relationship between the subject consciousness and the object presented to it to be aware of. This is crucial to our understanding, as it offers the reason for the arising of the world. It takes the arising of the world for consciousness to display awareness.

For the practitioner of physical yoga it is important to remember that the human body is not an end in itself. Its only reason to exist is to be a vehicle of action for consciousness. We need not get too attached, therefore, to performing hundreds of fancy postures, which are of little use by themselves. They perform a purpose only if they point toward liberation, which they do if done in the right context. They are an obstacle to true yoga if they are engaged in to boost the ego or for the purpose of self-gratification.

20. H. Aranya, *Yoga Philosophy of Patanjali with Bhasvati*, p. 180.

21. David Godman, ed., *Be As You Are — The Teachings of Ramana Maharshi*, Penguin Books India, New Delhi, 1985.
22. V. 56.
23. T. Leggett, *Sankara on the Yoga Sutra*, p. 244.

Since by nature the seen exists only for the purpose of consciousness, once this purpose is fulfilled it rightfully ceases to be manifest. The purpose of the world is to provide experience and liberation; once this is achieved, the world and the body cease to be manifest.

This cessation, though, is not complete. It only means that the *guna*s fold back from the gross, through the subtle and manifest, into the unmanifest (*alinga*) state of nature (*prakrti*). Why is this the case? Why does *prakrti* not cease altogether? The next sutra will explain.

कृतार्थं प्रति नष्टम् अप्यनष्टं
तदन्यसाधारणत्वात् ॥ २२ ॥

II.22 Although the seen ceases to be manifest as far as a liberated *purusha* is concerned, it may continue to manifest for others, which are still in bondage.

Let us look at the Shaivite[24] universe of creation. Brahman, the infinite consciousness, here has two poles. They are Shiva, which represents the Samkhya principle of consciousness, and Shakti, which represents Samkhya's nature. Shiva rests in the crown *chakra*, which is represented on earth by Mount Kailash. Shakti condenses and crystallizes through void, intellect, ego, ether, air, fire, water, and earth, and eventually rests as the serpent power (variously called Shakti or *kundalini*) coiled in the base *chakra*.

The important fact is that when Shakti rests in the base *chakra* self-awareness is lost and the world arises. This is the process of evolution. When we start the process of yoga we help Shakti to subtilize and re-ascend through the *chakra*s and elements until she is reunited with her lover consciousness, Shiva. At this point self-consciousness is gained and awareness of the world ceases. The system here described is *Kashmir Shaivism*, created by the Masters Vasugupta and Abhinavagupta. Their work formed the foundation of tantric philosophy.

Tantric schools use the same categories as Patanjali

and the original Samkhya. The difference is that they personalize them and clothe them in a sexual metaphor, the unification of Shiva and Shakti. At the time of the rise of Tantra, many people experienced the older schools as too intellectually abstract. Giving the Samkhya categories a human face and sexual identity proved successful. It also provided a beautiful explanation for why the world loses any relevance for an awakened one. We have to remember, though, that it is not something entirely new but a reinterpretation of ancient wisdom.

Shaivism is a devotional path with personal deities, and yet it comes to the same conclusion as the analytical Samkhya approach. Advaitic[25] sages such as Ramana Maharshi also testify that awareness of the world ceases for one who sees the light of the self.

There is an important misunderstanding here to be aware of. Some modern authors, often inspired by Vedanta and Buddhism, have described yoga as a cult of self-annihilation. This view shows a lack of understanding of Patanjali's system. The sutra here clearly states that, for the liberated yogi, awareness of the world ceases and not awareness of the true self. This means that, after freedom is achieved, we are permanently established in awareness of consciousness. This is a state entirely different from annihilation; it is, rather, limitless freedom and ecstasy. That which could limit — the world of appearances — is lost out of sight, since it has served its purpose.

However, although the world has lost any significance for the liberated one, it continues to provide its service for those who still need it. Luckily so: otherwise each world would provide service only for one liberated individual. But since nature performs her service "selflessly"[26] for the sake of all *purusha*s, she continues to work for all others. We see here already the motherly quality of nature, which was later elaborated into the concept of the mother goddess Shakti.

When we compare such different approaches as Patanjali's Yoga of Concentration, the Advaita (nondualistic) approach of reflection, and the Bhakti approach of surrender, we notice that they sometimes differ very much in terms of philosophy.

24. A system in which Shiva is the Supreme Being.

25. Referring to the system of Advaita (nondualistic) Vedanta.
26. *Samkhya Karika*, v. 60.

For a scholar it makes a big difference whether a system is dualistic or monistic, qualified monistic, or unqualified monistic. For the mystic these categories are of no importance: the systems are different roads to the same place. One road might go along the beach, another over the mountains, a third through the jungle. Which road one takes is only a matter of individual preference; it's not that one is better than the other. All systems are but simulations of reality, each one better suited to a particular type of personality. None of them can be a complete representation of reality, since they are creations of the mind and by nature the mind is incapable of reproducing reality as it truly is.

The millennia-old squabble of scholars about who has the better system merely amounts to discussing who has the right personality. Since all the philosophical systems based on the *Upanishad*s describe the path to the mystical experience for different personality types, each of them works for that particular personality. It might not work for another. All of them therefore exist in their own right only as far as they are capable of leading people to liberation. If a system is logically more sound than another, but cannot free people, it is worthless and must be discarded.

On the path to liberation one must also free oneself from the categories of the mind such as logic. After all, reality itself is paradoxical and all-including, not logical, analytical, and exclusive. The mind is only a tool that we use like a muscle. If the mind gets control of us and uses us, it is called bondage. The result of the tyranny of the mind can be seen in five thousand years of warfare and atrocities.

To illustrate the conflict between systems, let us look at the Samkhya concept of *purusha* (consciousness), of which Samkhya says there are many. This seems to be opposed to the Vedanta concept of *atman*, of which there is only one. A similar conflict existed in physics when light was described as either being a particle or a wave. There was supporting evidence for both views, and each view excluded the other and proved the other wrong. But both schools of thought were helpful if applied in certain situations. Eventually physicists agreed to say that under certain circumstances light displays wave characteristics and under different circumstances it has particle characteristics. After the opponents got over who was right or wrong, they managed to find a description that could help all.

The same is the case with consciousness. It is neither Samkhyite nor Vedantic nor Buddhist. Under certain circumstances it behaves like Samkhya's *purusha*, and to use the *purusha* concept will help us then to understand what consciousness is. In a different situation, from another viewpoint, it behaves like the vedantic *atman*, and then this view is helpful. In a third situation it will be more helpful to work with the Buddhist notion of emptiness (*shunyata*). We will then realize that consciousness is (a) many, (b) one, (c) both and, (d) none of them. This is necessarily so, since consciousness contains everything. If we were to observe something that does not embrace (a)–(d), then that by definition could not be consciousness.

We must use the upanishadic systems to realize ourselves as consciousness without getting attached to one of them. Otherwise we will develop an agenda, which means we'll attempt to stake out intellectual territory. The focus is then on not whether I abide in truth but whether I'm right and somebody else is wrong. Then we have fallen again into the traps of the mind, taking a concept for reality. The systems are important because they can help us become ourselves. But after that, when deep reality (Brahman) is seen, they have no more importance.

स्वस्वामिशक्त्योः स्वरूपोपलब्धिहेतुः संयोगः ॥ २३ ॥

II.23 The meeting [of the seer and seen] causes the understanding of the nature of the two powers of owner and the owned.

Patanjali describes an important paradox here. Why, scholars have asked, does consciousness entangle itself in the world? Why does it become bound only to be liberated again? Why does it not remain pure consciousness in the first place, without letting a world come into being?

These are typical useless questions of the mind. To become preoccupied with answering them will lead to an increase of the rule of the mind over us.

The world is here and we are part of it. Or more precisely we are the containing matrix in which it arises. And since this matrix is all-encompassing, every world that can arise will arise in it. This matrix, Brahman, is the womb of everything and has unlimited potential. Just as a mother, when the time has come to give birth, can't run away and refuse to have it happen, so consciousness has to be aware of whatever is presented to it. To make a judgment is not within the capacity of consciousness, since it is formless.

The sutra says that the meeting of subject and object brings about understanding of the nature of the two. If the meeting did not happen, the subject would never become a seer or owner because there would be nothing to see. Consciousness would never be realized as limitless space, since space is only significant when objects and sentient beings occur within it. In other words it takes the occurrence of the world, the seen, to bring out the space nature of consciousness. It takes the arising of the seen for the seer to experience itself as the seer. In other words, if the seer doesn't see anything, he or she is not a seer after all. Consciousness that is not presented with objects (the world) to be aware of cannot develop its quality of awareness.

Shankara uses the metaphor of a mirror and a face reflected in it. Only through the meeting of both and the subsequent depiction of one in the other can the nature of both be apprehended. Consciousness works in a very similar way to the mirror. The nature of both can only be experienced when objects are presented. In both cases one will be drawn first to enjoy and perceive the objects arising in them. After consecutive representations of objects, one is then drawn to the mirror/consciousness quality of faithfully representing what appears in them without interfering or modifying it at all. This is the quality of consciousness: it does not act.

The mind can be likened to an artist who paints our image. The painter will represent his perspective, his impression of us, and his mood; in fact his entire past will collaborate to produce his representation of us. This might possibly be much more flattering than looking in the mirror, but, as Patanjali says in sutra II.20, "The seer only sees, having no intention at all." And this is exactly how the mirror sees:

without any intention of making things more beautiful or more ugly. Presenting an object causes no change in the mirror (well, unless it's a hammer or brick presented with great force). Looking at this quality, we can understand the immutability of consciousness, which is untouched by any occurrence.

Vyasa explains in his commentary that the seer meets the seen for the purpose of seeing. From that seeing arises knowledge of the nature of the world, which is called experience or bondage. After enough bondage is experienced, there arises from it knowledge of the nature of the seer, which is liberation. This is the yogic view in a nutshell. But, continues Vyasa, experience of the world is not the cause of liberation, since liberation is the end or absence of bondage. Bondage is caused by misapprehension, whereas liberation is caused by discrimination. It appears that we have to go through a process of misapprehension before we can discriminate. This process is called *samsara*, conditioned existence.

तस्य हेतुरविद्या ॥ २४ ॥
II.24 The cause of this meeting is ignorance.

Ignorance (*avidya*), the master affliction, has already been described in sutra II.5. Ignorance is the belief system that results from false knowledge (*viparyaya*).

This false knowledge makes us believe that we are the body, that we are our emotions and thoughts. *Viparyaya* is defined in sutra I.8 as wrong knowledge without foundation in reality. Reality is that which is permanent. Returning to the metaphor of the TV screen, we can note that, however many pictures are displayed on the screen, none will ever stick to it. New pictures will always replace them. Once the film is over, the screen will be empty. The only thing permanent here is the screen, which means the screen is the reality, whereas the pictures are only fleeting images superimposed on the screen. Although there exists a certain proximity between screen and image, both will remain forever separate. The screen won't take on the qualities of the images, nor will it alter them.

Similar is the case with the seer and the seen. There is a certain proximity between our true nature as the immutable consciousness and the constantly changing seen, which is the body, emotions, thoughts, and so on. However, in reality they touch as little as do a screen and the images displayed on it. This wrong knowledge, according to which we are body and mind, results in subconscious imprints (*samskaras*) in which we appear to be bound up with external, constantly changing things. These imprints eventually densify to a field that is called conditioning (*vasana*). In this case the imprints born from wrong perception (*viparyaya*) lead to the conditioning of ignorance. From this ignorance sprout all the afflictions, the different forms of suffering.

The concept of ignorance (*avidya*) as the cause of the commingling of consciousness and world developed in later centuries into the elaborate concept of *maya*, the veil of illusion.

तदभावात् संयोगाभावो हानं । तद्दृशेः
कैवल्यम् ॥ २५ ॥

II.25 From the absence of ignorance the commingling of the seer and the seen ceases. This state is called liberation (kaivalya), the independence from the seen.

The state of *kaivalya*, which is the goal of yoga, is described here. In the four steps of the medical system, *kaivalya* represents the healthy state. It is therefore also called the natural state. For yoga does not create through exertion some remote aloof paradise for the few: it merely re-establishes us in the truth of who we are, which is the natural state to be in.

Unfortunately the natural state is not normal anymore. *Kaivalya* can be translated as independence, freedom, aloneness, or "transcendental aloneness."[27] It can also mean liberation, since it is the opposite of bondage or mental slavery.

It is interesting to look at what the word "aloneness" means. It is somewhat similar to loneliness but yet entirely different. Loneliness is the state in which one yearns or longs for the company of another but is deprived of it. It is a lack of something that makes it impossible to enjoy the mere absence of company.

The blues singer Janis Joplin said, "On stage I give love for 50,000 people but at home Mr. Loneliness awaits me." She died soon afterward from an overdose of drugs. It is interesting that she described loneliness as the absence of love. Also significant is her attempt to fill the gap left by this absence through the intake of an enormous amount of drugs.

Aloneness is the exact opposite of that. It is the drawing together of the words all-one-ness. To be aware of all-one-ness is to see Brahman, which is deep reality or truth. On the deepest level everything is an expression of the one reality, infinite consciousness.

One who has realized this is alone or all-one: all-one because once one has seen the space nature of consciousness one knows that one is forever united with all living things. The very same consciousness contains us all. The very one self is looking out through all creatures' eyes. According to the *Bhagavad Gita*, "He who sees the supreme Lord abiding equally in all beings, ... he sees indeed."[28] All-one-ness means to have recognized that at the deepest level all sentient beings are one consciousness. Such a person is called alone since one has found in one's heart the heart of all beings. No external contact like company is needed to experience happiness. In that state the deep wound called loneliness is healed. In fact company cannot heal loneliness because it cannot be ongoing: one day we, or our friends before us, will die. Then the wound — which has only been covered up — will break open again.

The wound is healed only when one has found in one's heart the self, which is the self of all beings. This self the *Gita* calls the Supreme Lord, the *Upanishads* call Brahman, and Buddha calls *nirvana*. Once this self is found, one does not approach others anymore out of need but because one wants to give. Because the mystic does not need others, but can choose freely to be with others, he or she is said to be alone. It is a state of freedom. If one is lonely, one needs to seek others. In truth, however, one is not interested in them but only in their capacity to soothe one's loneliness. There is no choice: one has to go about seeking others to relieve one's pain.

For this reason the mystic is called the true

---

27. Leggett uses this term in his *Shankara on the Yoga Sutra*.

28. *Bhagavad Gita* 13.27, trans. Sw. Vireswarananda, p. 271.

friend. Since the mystic has realized him- or herself as the container that contains the world and all beings, mystics have no further agenda in this world. They have no point to prove. They do not need others for company, entertainment, or pain relief, but see in others that reality they have found in themselves. That person is our real friend who truly sees our innermost self, which is free, independent, uncreated, unstained, and free of all that changes and becomes.

Because this true meaning of the word "aloneness" has been lost, the term "transcendental aloneness" has been introduced to translate *kaivalya*. But why did Patanjali use the word "aloneness" to describe what is called in most scriptures liberation (*moksha*)?

Bondage is created by the illusory commingling of self and world. Although this togetherness of the eternal separate entities is based on wrong perception, it nevertheless is taken to be true and creates suffering. When, through correct perception, the eternally untouchable, unstainable nature of the self is recognized (which like the mirror can reflect so many objects though they never stick to it), that is called the independence or aloneness of the self.

If we remove an object after the mirror has reflected it, no trace of object-ness is left in the mirror. Similarly, whatever thought, emotion, or memory is witnessed by our consciousness cannot leave a stain on it, cannot be bound up with it. Because consciousness/self is forever untouched by the seen, it is said to be alone.

Ignorance makes it appear as if impressions of past identification, pleasure, pain, anger, or fear are bound up with the screen on which they appear. Ignorance commingles the phenomena with the awareness to which they arise. When ignorance ceases, awareness is seen as standing alone. Awareness is the only thing that never changes. It simply observes, witnesses, without ever taking on the constantly fluctuating qualities of the observed object, the world.

विवेकख्यातिरविप्लवा हानोपायः ॥ २६ ॥
II.26 The means to liberation is permanent discriminative knowledge.

After having described the forms of suffering, their causes, and the healthy state, Patanjali now describes the remedy. This is the permanent ability to discriminate between what is eternal, pure, free, and essential on the one hand and transitory, impure, bound, and nonessential on the other.

Let us go back to looking at consciousness/self as the TV screen on which all images are displayed — or, better, the containing space/time matrix in which the phenomena appear. The matrix is more realistic since it is four-dimensional; the TV screen is easier to understand because we can see it. The pictures on the screen in the course of an evening will constantly change while the screen remains the same. Likewise the self is permanent, and body, mind, and all objects superimposed on it are transitory.

Since subconscious imprints, formed through past experience, will be bound up with and stick to body, mind, and objects, they are called impure. When we watch a movie we realize that in its course our impression of its characters changes as they are stained or tainted by the action. In a similar way, all produced objects are stained by our subconscious imprints, which are based on ignorance, egoism, desire, pain, and fear. The only pure unstained thing at the end of the movie is the screen to which impression attaches. Likewise the self is said to be pure and the phenomena are impure.

During a movie we realize that all the characters act according to previous set conditions. Western psychology attributes this conditioning to early childhood; Eastern mysticism attributes it to previous incarnations. Whichever way, the characters on the screen don't act freely but in a conditioned way. They are bound by their past. The only free "object" is consciousness, which appears beyond space/time; in fact space/time occurs within it. No image or phenomenon can leave a conditioning imprint on consciousness. Body, mind, and objects are said to be bound and consciousness is said to be free.

When we spend an evening watching TV we may see the news, advertisements, a comedy, a thriller, a documentary, and a movie about animals. During that evening no single element would have appeared in all the movies; nothing would have been essential but the screen. Likewise the objects displayed to the self are nonessential, and the self is essential.

The ability to discern between the real and unreal or essential and nonessential is called discriminative knowledge. This knowledge needs to be there permanently; only then will it provide the means for liberation. We may attain a partial knowledge with relapses into ignorance, or the discriminative knowledge may appear in glimpses only. This is not sufficient: it needs to be permanent. Let us remember the story of the snake and the rope. The wrong perception of a piece of rope lying on the path at dusk led to the wrong cognition of a snake. This illusory knowledge (*viparyaya*) led to the right knowledge (*pramana*) not being cognized. After being shown the rope, the observer gains right knowledge, after which the wrong knowledge is destroyed.

This discriminative knowledge between real and unreal, between rope and snake, between self and nonself, needs to be permanent. Otherwise we will again hallucinate a snake in the darkness when we see a rope — or experience ourselves as the changing body / mind when in reality we are the eternal, immutable self.

तस्य सप्तधा प्रान्तभूमिः प्रज्ञा ॥ २७ ॥
II.27 For him who is gaining discriminative knowledge, this ultimate insight comes in seven stages.

This sutra cannot be understood without consulting Vyasa's commentary. He explains the seven stages as follows:

1. The yogi gains insight of what is painful, what is suffering, and therefore what needs to be avoided.

2. The light of knowledge destroys the accumulated *karma*, and the afflictions (*klesha*s) are dried up.

3. *Samapatti*, the state of mind during objective *samadhi*, has been experienced, the mind is stilled and the desire to attain further insight ceases. This is an important step. All desire to penetrate more deeply into the mystery from this point on is an obstacle.

4. Discriminative knowledge is acquired, and one lets go of all effort to become more proficient in yoga. All that can become more proficient in yoga is by definition body, mind, and ego. The consciousness / self, since it is by nature eternal and unchangeable, cannot ever become more proficient or less proficient. Consciousness is the permanent and true state of yoga. Once we have realized the difference between self and nonself, we know that all that grows, develops, deepens, matures, and becomes more proficient is impermanent and therefore not the self. At this point practice can become a means to bolster one's ego and may be discarded. Any unnatural effort has to cease.

These first four stages are called "freedom from doing." Once they are completed, the remaining steps cannot be performed or achieved; doing can get one only up to here. From this point surrender, nondoing, cessation, and grace continue the process.

There is an important tantric Buddhist treatise about this experience called *The Song of Mahamudra*, composed by the Siddha Tilopa. In it Tilopa addresses his student Naropa, who later became the author of the *Six Yogas of Naropa*, some of which Krishnamacharya learned from his master Ramamohan Brahmachary in Tibet.

In his song Tilopa says, "Without making an effort, but remaining loose and natural, one can break the yoke thus gaining liberation."[29] The abandoning of effort is explained here to be a necessary prerequisite of freedom. A little further along Tilopa says, "For if the mind when filled with some desire should seek a goal, it only hides the light."[30] Tilopa tells Naropa here that, at this stage of his education, he has even to give up the desire for liberation because this, like any desire, clouds the mind.

Contemporary teachers have frequently commented on *The Song of Mahamudra* and some have suggested following Tilopa's advice without the student practicing beforehand. They fail to mention that the student Naropa, when he heard these words, had already undergone one of the severest

29. G. C. C. Chang, trans., *Teachings and Practice of Tibetan Tantra*, Dover Publications, Mineola, New York, 2004, p. 25.
30. Ibid., p. 27.

twenty-year-long trainings ever suffered at the hand of a master. Only after such training was completed was the student deemed ready to hear the highest truth. In fact treatises revealing the highest truth were kept secret over centuries, being confined to the memory of just a few masters. They would be recited only when the student was ready to handle their truth.

In the *Yoga Vashishta*, for example, it is said that deities were only created for those who cannot worship their own consciousness/self directly, but to disclose this information to the uninitiated attracted the death penalty in the old days. Those teachings were kept absolutely secret because it was understood that only one steeped in practice and discipline could handle them. Today we can download all this information from the Internet. Spiritual life has not become easier through that, possibly more difficult. Often we encounter such a hodge-podge of teachings and half-realized untruths that they become completely unintelligible and do more harm than good. Again, if one mixes several systems, one might be seduced into combining the aspects that suit one's limitations and omit the challenging elements.

Tilopa suggested to Naropa, after the latter had practiced fiercely under his guidance for twenty years, that he now discard all practice and become spontaneous, relaxed, and natural. Of course it was only after Naropa had mastered all previous stages that the time had come for him to become free from doing. Some modern teachers have used Tilopa's advice to suggest to their students that they discard practice and discipline altogether and live according to their whims right from the beginning. Such a message will obviously sell really well. It is what human society has done all along; what is new is that it is sold to us as being "spiritual."

Students who have a tendency to spontaneity and find discipline difficult will jump at the suggestion that they stop practicing. Spontaneity based on a subconscious tendency is really only avoidance, reflecting an inability to keep the mind focused. Some students become bored after having done the Primary Series a thousand or two thousand times. However, any sign of boredom tells us only that the mind is not resting in the present moment. Simply

sitting and watching one's breath is, from the standpoint of the mind, boring. If, however, one surrenders into the experience, it can reveal a majestic beauty that is difficult to rival by any sensory input.

Yes, the practice may be discarded one day by one who has attained discriminative knowledge, but not before. It is this knowledge that lets one know whether the discarding is just another trick of the mind or is born from the stillness of the heart.

As the first four steps of the sevenfold insight are called freedom from doing, so are the next three steps called "freedom from the mind."

5. The mind and its constituent cause, the ego or I-principle, having fulfilled their purpose, are released and return to their causal state.[31] Shankara's phrase "returning to the causal state" has created some confusion. It does not mean they cease to exist: it means they lose their grip on the yogi and are consulted only when necessary. Just as one uses one's hands when driving a car, but at other times they may rest in the lap, so the mind should only work when necessary. A muscle that does not cease effort when no action is to be performed is said to be in spasm; similarly we may say the human condition is to suffer from mental spasm. If the mind goes on simulating reality even if there is absolutely no reason for it to do so, then it is in control of its owner rather than vice versa.

6. One gives up one's conditioning. Once it has been given up, and has released its grip on the observer, it will never again return. The observer now spontaneously rests in the present moment, without any limiting past conditioning. This spontaneous freedom, though, has nothing of the randomness that ego and mind in their normal states attribute to it.

7. The self is finally shown to be self-illuminated. As the sun is self-illuminated and the moon only reflects the light of the sun, so the self shines forth the sun of awareness and the intellect only reflects it onto objects. In this stage the *gunas*, the qualities or strands of creation, detach themselves or, better, appear to detach themselves from the self, which really is eternally untouched and pure. It is only our illusory identification with the impermanent that makes us seem attached to phenomena. With this

31. T. Leggett, *Shankara on the Yoga Sutra*, p. 256.

insight of the untouchability of consciousness, the self finally is seen as standing alone. This is the insight of freedom (*kaivalya*), which still falls short of *kaivalya* itself. *Kaivalya* goes beyond any insight and wisdom, and is inexpressible.

योगाङ्गानुष्ठानाद् अशुद्धिक्षये
ज्ञानदीप्तिराविवेकख्यातेः ॥ २८ ॥

II.28 From practicing the various limbs of yoga the impurities are removed, uncovering the light of knowledge and discernment.

This is the pivotal stanza in the entire *Yoga Sutra*. Up to this point Patanjali has explained why we practice and defined all the terms involved. First he described *samadhi* to create an interest in the practitioner. Then he showed that we shouldn't be satisfied with our present situation, since it is suffering and darkness. After that he showed how the suffering comes to be and, finally, what removes it.

The bulk of the remaining sutras Patanjali dedicates to the methods and techniques of yoga. And it is here that his Yoga earns its claim of being an independent system of philosophy (*darshana*). While its cosmology is 95 percent identical with Samkhya's, and its goal can hardly be distinguished from that of Vedanta, its methods are absolutely unique. Samkhya and Vedanta rely principally on reflection, contemplation, and intellectual analysis; Yoga, however, has a far more comprehensive catalogue of methods and techniques.

It is suggested that all limbs be practiced in some form, starting with the lower ones to ensure harmonious development. The first four limbs provide a solid base and firmly establish one for what is to come. To ignore them and go straight to advanced meditation practice can lead, in an extreme case, to schizophrenia. A schizophrenic person, from the yogic viewpoint, is not mad, but sees too much and cannot integrate it. On an energetic level that means one or all of the three higher *chakras* are open, while one or all of the four lower *chakras* are closed (excluding the base *chakra*, which deals with survival: closing it leads to death).

Especially the opening of the sixth (third eye) and

the seventh (crown) *chakras* can lead to perception of things so powerful that it can be like the opening of Pandora's box. To stay on the safe side we first have to become a fully integrated and mature human being, which is achieved by opening *chakras* two, three, and four. Especially opening the fourth, the heart *chakra*, enables us to relate to others and ourselves from a position of love. Not to open these *chakras* is like building the walls and roof of a house without putting in the foundations first. It is prescribed therefore that one does the groundwork first, establishing oneself in the lower four limbs, which has a solidifying effect.

There are certain problems associated with the other end of the ladder, though. For example the practice of *asana* bestows certain powers, which can lead to an increase of I-am-ness or ego (*ahamkara*). Practicing to look good in the postures, to be better than others, to increase self worth, or to gain the approval of the teacher are all egoic reasons. Egoity (*asmita*) increases by maintaining identification with the body. In due time egoity must be reduced by practice of the higher limbs, which has a transcending effect. In other words they teach that I am not the body and the ego. If one develops a powerful practice of *asana* and *pranayama* only, one can easily, seduced by the arising powers, become an egomaniac and even more deeply enmeshed in conditioned existence. To counteract this egoic tendency, the higher limbs need to be included from a certain point onward. The combined practice of all the limbs will remove the impurities, and all shortfalls like schizophrenia and egomania will be avoided.

What are the impurities? They are chiefly the afflictions, which are ignorance, egoism, desire, aversion, and fear. Removed together with them are subconscious imprints, their resulting conditioning, wrong perception of reality, and *karma* resulting from past actions. These impurities cover the light of knowledge, and once they are removed it shines like a lamp that was previously covered by a veil. The highest expression of the light of knowledge is discernment (*viveka*): the ability to discern between what is real and unreal, self and nonself, permanent and transitory.

Patanjali has thus explained the entire whys of the practice. He will now turn to the hows.

211

यमनियमासनप्राणायामप्रत्याहारधारणाध्यान-
समाधयोऽष्टाव अङ्गानि ॥ २९ ॥

II.29 Restraints, observances, postures, control of the inner breath, sense withdrawal, concentration, meditation, and samadhi are the eight limbs.

Patanjali lists eight limbs. The Rishis Vyasa (*Mahabharata*), Yajnavalkya (*Yoga Yajnavalkya*), and Vasishta (*Vasishta Samhita*) mention the same number. Some sources, for example the Saptanga Yoga of Rishi Gheranda, note six or seven limbs.[32] These numbers have been reached by omitting the first two limbs, the ethics. Since we are asked to practice ethics in all life situations, later teachers argued that they were not exclusive to yoga and for this reason did not need to be mentioned as a limb of yoga.

Another argument brought forward was that the ethics shouldn't be included since they do not directly contribute to *samadhi*. However, in sutra II.45 Patanjali states that *samadhi* is produced by surrender to the Supreme Being. Since surrender to the Supreme Being (*ishvara pranidhana*) is the last of the ten ethical rules, it is established that ethics not only contribute to *samadhi* but are also one of its fundamental tributaries.

It is mainly the medieval Hatha texts that abolished the ethics. This coincided with a general relaxation of ethical standards, which led to the situation that women were not allowed to leave their homes without applying the red dot to their third eye. Yogis had been using their accumulated power to hypnotize women and obtain sexual favors. Hypnotism targets the third eye (*Ajna chakra*), and the red dot was thought to shield one from such attacks. By the end of the eighteenth century lawlessness among yogis was so widespread that in many rural areas of India the terms "yogi" and "scoundrel" had become interchangeable. Some orthodox circles in India still reject yogis today as people who are seeking occult powers, although historically this is degeneration. Sadly enough it is often this nonauthentic side of yoga that attracts Westerners.

The eight limbs are to be practiced by beginners sequentially, so one starts with *yama* and not

32. *The Gheranda Samhita*, trans. R.B.S. Chandra Vasu, Sri Satguru Publications, Delhi, 1986.

with *samadhi*. Eventually, as one matures in the various forms of practice, the limbs are practiced simultaneously.

अहिंसासत्यास्तेयब्रह्मचर्यापरिग्रहा यमाः ॥ ३० ॥

II.30 Nonviolence, truthfulness, nonstealing, sexual restraint, and nongreed are the restraints.

We are now looking at the five forms of restraint. *Himsa* means violence, *ahimsa* is nonviolence. It is the first and foremost of all *yama*s. The Buddhists suggest counteracting any urge to viciousness by contemplating the fact that the cycle of rebirths has gone on for such a long time that all beings at one point have been our mothers. For this reason we need to appreciate all others and not harm anybody. If we recognize that it is the same consciousness that looks out of every eye, we understand that, with every person we harm, we really hurt only ourselves. Every being is on a quest for happiness of some form or another; others are not so different from us that we need to violate them. The wish to hurt is usually born from not acknowledging that what we see in them is ourselves.

The idea of restraint is to enable us to live in harmony with the community around us. If we do not stick to those rules we create conflict. In an atmosphere of conflict it is difficult to practice yoga. Not only are harmful actions toward others based on afflictions such as ignorance, egoism, and aversion, but they also produce new subconscious imprints of violence. For example, if we abuse somebody once, it becomes easier for us to do it again. The hurdle for repetition has been lowered. If we have initiated a domestic fight with our partner, we have laid, via imprint, the foundation for its repetition. It is more likely now that it will happen again. A serial killer, having gotten away with murder once, is likely to repeat the action in decreasing time intervals.

To violate others is based on wrong perception (*viparyaya*). We violate others in an effort to dominate them. We try to dominate because we believe that, in their subdued state, others pose no threat to our security. We feel our security is at risk because we are in conflict with ourselves. We identify with the notion of conflict because we believe we have to become somebody, to get somewhere, to develop, to follow a path, to complete a search. In short, conflict arises out of the desire to become, rather than accepting what is now.

That which becomes, gets somewhere, grows, and develops is body, mind, ego, intellect. These are all part of creation (*prakrti*). It may sound strange, but the notion of a spiritual path creates conflict. To see oneself as that which is at peace already — the immutable, eternal, and infinite consciousness — is correct perception (*pramana*). Once this is accepted and reflected upon, the need for conflict drops away and the quest for security is surrendered. Security cannot be attained as long as we hold the belief that we are transitory. Once we know ourselves, fear will drop away and with it the urge to dominate others. Violence is of no use anymore. This is the reason behind accounts of animals abandoning all hostility in the presence of a *jnanin* (one who has knowledge of the self). Since a *jnanin* has found peace within, animals feel completely unthreatened.

The second *yama* is *satya* (truthfulness). The yogi needs to be truthful in word, thought, and action. There is an important reason for truthfulness being mentioned after nonviolence, and that is that our truth should not compromise our nonviolence. In other words, nonviolence overrides truth. We should never use truthfulness to harm or violate others.

In this context, though, we come across one of the most tragic misunderstandings in the history of Indian thought. The *Chandogya Upanishad* states, "A truth uttered should never harm." This has been misinterpreted to mean, "A truth uttered should never be unpleasant," which encourages flattery and sweet talk. The result is still observable in India today. When we ask for directions in the street, people who hesitate to utter the truth ("Sorry, I don't know"), because that would be unpleasant, often send us in the wrong direction. We find out the truth ten minutes later when we arrive in the wrong place. This is much more unpleasant.

At the core of the problem is a famous passage in the *Mahabharata* epic. Yudishthira, the rightful emperor of India, is deprived of his empire by his evil cousin Duryodhana in a deceitful game of dice.

Although he has many opportunities to talk straight with his cousin, he does not do so because he is the mythical son of Lord Dharma, the God of right action. He believes it is not right to be unpleasant to Duryodhana and tell him the truth of what sort of a person he is. In the course of the game of dice Yudishthira loses also his wife, the empress of India, Draupadi, a very passionate woman. Brothers of the evil Duryodhana drag Draupadi by her hair as a slave before the assembled court and attempt to disrobe and dishonor her. Yudishthira and his brothers do not interfere, because they believe it would be unpleasant to tell Duryodhana what every truthful husband would tell anybody who dragged his wife by her hair and attempted to disrobe her.

But, because the unpleasant truth is not uttered, the greatest catastrophe in Indian history takes its course, one from which India has never recovered. It weakened its defenses so much that it was eventually taken over by Buddhists, Muslims, and Christians, after which it broke into pieces.

Observing the scene of Draupadi's dishonoring are the spiritual elders, the preceptors Bhishma and Drona. Although they dislike Duryodhana, neither of them steps in and utters the unpleasant truth about his character. Bhishma and Drona are held in high regard, and when they remain silent everybody assumes that Duryodhana is right in what he does. Duryodhana sentences Yudishthira and his brothers and Draupadi to twelve years of exile. They have to live like beggars for twelve years in the forest and a thirteenth year in disguise. After thirteen years they will have the right to get everything back. However, as we can imagine, after thirteen years Duryodhana has become comfortable in his wealth and power, and laughs at the five brothers when they demand their empire back.

Again, the five brothers find it unpleasant to confront Duryodhana, who is untruthful. At this point Draupadi cannot bear it any longer. Screaming and cursing, she breaks down and exposes the untruthfulness of the five brothers, who have done nothing to save her honor. We can assume the situation would have been very unpleasant for our five heroes.

But the unpleasantness doesn't end there. Draupadi's best friend, or maybe her only friend, incidentally is the Supreme Being, manifested in the form of Lord Krishna, who by chance is also present. Krishna, in place of the five brothers, takes the terrible oath that he will destroy everybody who was present on that fateful day and did not intervene when Draupadi was dragged before the court by her hair. And not only that, he vows to destroy anybody who takes the side of the evildoers.

The remaining chapters of the *Mahabharata* let us witness how Krishna keeps his promise. The greatest military force ever assembled arrives on the battlefield and a total of 2.5 million warriors enter the crushing jaws of death. In fact almost the entire Indian warrior caste and aristocracy were eradicated during those days, with the effect that India could not defend herself anymore and became easy prey for foreign invaders. The foreign invasions into India destroyed arguably the richest cultural heritage in the world. The Nalanda University alone, which had probably the biggest library on the planet, was destroyed during the Mogul invasion. It burned for eight months until it was reduced to rubble.

All of that happened just because a handful of people had a wrong notion of truth having to be pleasant. If Yudishthira, Bhishma, and Drona had honestly communicated to Duryodhana what they thought of him, he would have had an unpleasant time at first, but possibly he would have seen his shortcomings and changed his course of action. Most likely the majority of Duryodhana's supporters, such as his weak father, the King Drtharashtra, would have fallen away from him and only the diehards such as his best friend Karna would have remained loyal. Without Drtharashtra they would not have been strong enough to create so much havoc, and the entire course of Indian history would have been different.

The idea that truth needs to be pleasant is wrong perception, and needs to be abandoned. The original idea is that truthfulness should not be used to harm and violate others, but to withhold the truth just because it is unpleasant can be even more harmful, as we have seen in Duryodhana's case. Honest feedback might be unpleasant at first, and even invoke a crisis, but then it can give rise to healing.

For example if a child is torturing animals or other children, we expect the parents to correct the

actions of their child. This correction may be unpleasant for the child, but it is better for the animals, the surrounding community, and in the long run for the child also. Negative actions will leave subconscious imprints (*samskara*s), which fill the karmic storehouse (*karmashaya*) of the child and lead to more suffering and more negative actions. The truth must be spoken in such a way as to avoid harm, but it is bound to be unpleasant sometimes.

The third *yama* is nonstealing (*asteya*). This means not only refraining from taking what belongs to others, but also not desiring their wealth. Desiring somebody else's property is another result of not realizing the space nature of consciousness. Since we are the container in which objects appear, we can neither reject nor accumulate any of them.

The fourth *yama* is sexual restraint (*brahmacharya*). The Rishi Vasishta explains: "Sexual restraint for householders means to have intercourse only with their lawful partners."[33] Householders are people who live in society and typically have a job and a family. Opposed to them are monks and recluses, for whom is prescribed no sex at all. The majority of yogis always had families and participated in society. An Imperial Census for India in 1931 revealed that more than a million yogis lived in India.[34] Almost half of them were women and many had family. This should also dispel the myth that only males practiced yoga.

When K. Pattabhi Jois was asked for the meaning of *brahmacharya*, he used to say it means to have one partner only. The yogic view of a relationship is not to consume another person like an object but to recognize divinity in one's partner.

The Rishi Yajnavalkya expresses it in the *Brhad Aranyaka Upanishad* thus: "The husband is not to be seen as the physical form, but as the immortal consciousness (*atman*). The wife is not to be looked at as the body, but to be recognized as the immortal consciousness." Partnership is used in yoga to recognize the inherent divinity in the other. This does exclude casual sex. The problem here is that usually one of the partners (often the female) looks for more than just sex. This partner will be hurt

---

33. *Vasishta Samhita* I.44.
34. G. W. Briggs, *Gorakhnath and the Kanpatha Yogis*, 1st Indian ed., Motilal Banarsidass, Delhi, 1938, pp. 4–6.

when being abandoned. Casual sex in this case is a form of violence.

Let us look at the case of two consenting partners engaging in casual sex. There is no violence involved here, one may say. The following, however, must be considered: Sexual intercourse is in many scriptures described as *karma mudra*, the seal of *karma*. It seals a strong karmic bond between the partners, even if we have become so desensitized that we can't feel that anymore. This karmic bond is formed through a connection of the subtle bodies of the two partners. In popular language we call this connection "heartstrings." It can be felt even long after two partners have separated. When this connection is formed we have a certain karmic duty toward the other, especially in nurturing and supporting them emotionally and making them feel loved. Swami Shivananda went as far as to say that, for every affair we have, we will be reborn to satisfy that person throughout a marital life. Whether that's true or not, if we keep "breaking hearts" it will get back to us sooner or later.

In the *Upanishad*s the term *brahmacharya* has a different connotation. According to the *Mundaka Upanishad*, "The true self is attained only through truth, discipline, knowledge and *brahmacharya*." Contemporary orthodox authors want to read celibacy into this passage, but this does not hold up, since the most self-attained people in India's history, the ancient *rishi*s, often had several wives and in some cases more than a hundred children. *Brahmacharya* in the upanishadic context means absorption in Brahman (consciousness). It is this absorption that leads to attainment of the self. We know, however, that Patanjali does not use the word *brahmacharya* with this meaning since he, as a true Samkhyite, never uses the word "Brahman" to mean consciousness.

The last *yama* is nongreed. Our focus should not be on accumulating things. Others should not suffer shortage through our accumulations. One should not be dependent on objects. We can enjoy what is rightfully ours, but should not get attached to our belongings. If through some misfortune we lose what we have — let's say the share market drops — we shouldn't hanker after it, but let it go. We should not accept any gifts that are given to manipulate us, such as bribes.

जातिदेशकालसमयानवच्छिन्नाः सार्वभौमा महाव्रतम् ॥ ३१ ॥

II.31 The five restraints practiced universally, uncompromised by type of birth, place, time, and circumstance, constitute the great vow.

Many people observe the restraints in a compromised form. Somebody who is born into a tribe or family of hunters or farmers might observe nonviolence but still kill animals related to their profession. This is referred to as compromised through type of birth. If somebody refrains from killing or lying or stealing as long as they are in a sacred location like a church, then the *yama* is said to be compromised by type of place. If a person refrains from beating his or her children only because it is Christmas or Easter, but not on other days, then the restraint is said to be compromised by time. If somebody adheres to nonviolence, but compromises this stance for example during war or acts of terrorism, the restraint is said to be compromised by circumstance.

The commentator H. Aranya gives us an example of nonviolence compromised by duty.[35] Arjuna, the hero of the *Bhagavad Gita*, had the duty to fight, since he was a member of the warrior caste. Aranya points out that yogis practice noninjury everywhere and always, and therefore discounts Arjuna's status as a yogi.

Patanjali states that if the five restraints are practiced uncompromisingly, meaning universally in all situations, then and only then do they constitute the great vow (*maha vrata*). It has been mentioned before that Yoga never went as far with nonviolence as Jainism, with its extreme concern for the lives of tiny creatures.

We know that the lymphocytes of our immune system continuously massacre millions of organisms that try to invade our body. The pus in a wound is nothing but dead lymphocytes, which died by "heroically" defending their mother country (our body). There is no way to be absolutely nonviolent as long as we are alive. Even to commit suicide — which would be the only way to stop constantly killing other organisms — is seen as the absolute act

35. H. Aranya, *Yoga Philosophy of Patanjali*, p. 213.

of violence and an insult to God. Nonviolence in many ways is a privilege of the rich, as with certain saints who have servants to sweep the path in front of them. A farmer will kill millions of organisms while plowing a field, but without his work we all would starve. A shoemaker is regarded as a low-life in India since his hands touch leather, which is taken from a cow. At the same time, everybody uses his services and, ironically, they can touch their leather shoes because, it is believed, the shoemaker has absorbed the impurity.

Milk is considered the purest food in India, and the cow gives it freely without us having to harm her. But she has to have a calf to give milk, and 50 percent of the calves are bull calves. These are sold by Brahmins to supposedly "impure" Muslims, outcasts, and Christians, who slaughter and eat them and therefore become impure through violence. The Brahmin who has cashed in on the bull calf stays pure because impurity can't transfer through money! Sadly enough, philosophy is used here to distribute demerit from the educated and privileged (the Brahmins) to the uninformed and poor (the low castes). We are to remember here that Yoga needs to be a tool in the service of humankind and not vice versa. Yoga started by promising that it can reduce human suffering; if it cannot deliver on the promise, we had better look for something else.

Let us note, however, that Patanjali does accept certain compromises of the great vow. For example, he does not hesitate to compromise truth if it would hurt somebody. So also the great vow is a relative one.

शौचसंतोषतपःस्वाध्यायेश्वरप्रणिधानानि
नियमाः ॥ ३२ ॥

II.32 Cleanliness, contentment, austerity, self-study, and devotion to the Supreme Being are the observances.

While the restraints are directed outward and create harmony with our surroundings, the observances (niyamas) are directed inward and form the bedrock of practice. Cleanliness (shaucha) refers to cleanliness of body and mind. Cleanliness of the body is achieved through hygiene, eating of pure, natural food, and abstaining from intoxication. Cleanliness of the mind is practiced through abstaining from thoughts and emotions of greed, jealousy, envy, hatred, anger, and so on, and to know what such thoughts lead to.

Contentment (santosha), the second observance, is a very interesting concept. In contemporary use in India, the term santosha is synonymous with happiness. Millennia of education have deeply engrained in the Indian mind the notion that happiness is the opposite of desire, and only when one lets go of all hankering and is utterly content can happiness enter.

How different this is from the Western concept. We are taught to visualize our dreams, which usually involve a yacht, a private plane, a sports-car collection, several mansions in different climatic zones, designer dresses worth $50,000, and so on and on. All of that is imagined as being washed down with an endless stream of champagne. After this process of visualizing our dreams is complete, we are supposed to motivate ourselves. Yes, we do have the will and the power to change. Yes, we have the capacity and the intelligence and the capability to do whatever it takes. And nothing can stop us.

After this process of motivation is activated, we create a plan for how the goal is to be achieved. Then we swing into action with such zeal that everything between us and our goal gets bullied out of the way or bulldozed over, whether opponents, competitors, rival companies, foreign governments and cultures, indigenous tribes, untouched landscapes, or rare species of plants and animals.

It is exactly this attitude that has enabled our Western culture to overrun and vandalize almost every country in the world and gobble it up. Have we become happy in the process? Hardly: rather, more greedy. If we were to recognize that all the happiness we are looking for is already in our hearts, we wouldn't have to search and destroy the entire world for it. Peace starts with contentment. Only if we are content with the now can we become silent enough to hear what needs doing. Otherwise this silent voice is overpowered by the yelling and shouting of our exaggerated and imagined needs.

The following three observances have been mentioned already under the heading Kriya Yoga, the

216

yoga of action. As they have been described in sutra II.1, a brief outline will suffice here. Austerity (*tapas*) is the ability to face adversity. Even when facing hardship in our practice, we are asked not to give up. Successful practitioners might enter into periods of hardship that can last for years. It is in the face of such hardship that a real researcher of yoga arises or one remains a shallow good-weather practitioner. We need to ask ourselves at this point what we are ready to give to become free. We have to expect that, when we practice, certain things will happen that will test us. The purificatory effects of the practice can be temporarily unpleasant, depending on our past actions.

The fourth observance is self-study (*svadhyaya*), which according to Vyasa is chanting the sacred syllable OM. It is chanted first aloud and then silently, then it is heard. The other aspect of self-study, according to Vyasa, is study of *moksha shastra*, scripture dealing with liberation. Principally this means the *Upanishads* and all systems stemming from them, such as Samkhya, Yoga, and Vedanta.

The last observance is devotion to the Supreme Being (*ishvara pranidhana*). Whether we devote ourselves to formless infinite consciousness (*nirguna brahman*) or to a form such as Krishna, the Christian God, or the Mother Goddess (*saguna brahman*) depends on the personality of the practitioner. All forms and the formless are valid. Devotion means that one surrenders all one's actions to the Supreme Being. That this surrender is not an unimportant ancillary technique is attested in sutra I.29, where Patanjali says that from surrender to the Supreme Being come *samadhi* and the nonarising of the nine obstacles of yoga.

वितर्कबाधने प्रतिपक्षभावनम् ॥ ३३ ॥

II.33 If conflicting thought obstructs those restraints and observances, the opposite should be contemplated.

If one feels plagued by thoughts of hatred, for example, it is suggested that we think of what such thoughts will lead to. After all, we carry this brain, we feed it, we protect it, we keep it warm, we rest it, so we should be entitled to tell it what to think. We own the brain and not vice versa.

If we allow ourselves thoughts of hatred, in due time they can turn into violent behavior. This will produce a karmic backlash and more violent thoughts. Once the community around us wants to pay us back for our negative actions, it will be difficult to practice. We need to understand that those thoughts and actions will be detrimental to us in the long run.

Through the method of contemplating the opposite, further harm is avoided for now. But once we are established in practice and have recognized that our neighbors are expressions of the same infinite consciousness as we are, it doesn't make any sense to be at their throats. Once we have gained knowledge (*jnana*) we will be compassionate toward others. Until then we should adhere to the code of ethics; otherwise we will enmesh ourselves further in conditioned existence, which in turn will make *jnana* even more inaccessible. The theme is further elaborated in the next sutra.

वितर्का हिंसादयः कृतकारितानुमोदिता लोभक्रोधमोहपूर्वका मृदुमध्याधिमात्रा दुःखाज्ञानानन्तफला इति प्रतिपक्षभावनम् ॥ ३४ ॥

II.34 Obstructing thoughts like violence and others, done, caused, or approved of, stemming from greed, anger, or infatuation, whether they are mild, moderate, or intense, will result in more pain and ignorance. For to realize that is to cultivate the opposite.

Obstructing thoughts in this case are all those that pose an obstacle to adhering to the restraints and observances of yoga. They cloud our perception of truth and therefore result in ignorance. For this reason they will produce suffering in the future. In reality those obstructing thoughts, although we sometimes may think they are an expression of our spontaneity, freedom, individuality, or creativity, stem from nothing but greed, anger, or infatuation.

For example we wake up one day and say, "Today I'm not going to practice." To practice daily, even if it is sometimes hard to do so, is *tapas* (austerity), the third *niyama*. But instead of realizing that we are violating the observance, we confuse our-selves into believing that not to practice is an expression of our freedom, spontaneity, individuality, and creativity. But this belief is nothing but infatuation. Being infatuated with our ego and our grandeur, we believe that abstaining from practice shows our freedom and the slavery of those who practice daily. If we really are free, then we are free to practice rather than being slaves to the mind, which supplies us with reasons not to practice.

Another cause of failing to sustain *tapas* is anger. We may experience anger and frustration in our lives due to our constant habit of identifying with what is impermanent. Instead of becoming free by letting go of the anger, we carry it into our practice, making practice difficult. Then we claim that practice is hard and no fun, and therefore we don't want to do it. The practice in itself is free, spontaneous, individual, and creative; it is we who make it a chore and a drag.

Especially when we are motivated by greed, if we want to get through the practice, get better, get powerful, get impressive, get recognition, then the practice can become an arduous duty rather than an exhilarating journey into freedom. In the *Bhagavad Gita*, Lord Krishna suggests surrendering the fruit of one's actions. In our case that means we forget about the gain, the goal, and the benefit and do the practice just because it is there, we are there, and the mat is there. Just because the world exists, we live. Just because we live, we practice. No further reason is required. This is to practice with an empty heart.

Another reason we may find for violating our *tapas* is boredom. We claim that the practice is boring us, but what is underlying boredom is nothing but anger. Because we fail to acknowledge our anger and let it go, we cannot tell ourselves the truth. Failing to tell the truth to ourselves (which brings us back in the present moment), our attention has to wander now into the past or the future. With our attention straying from the present moment, we are no longer present in our practice, which becomes boring. In this way anger leads to boredom. Whenever we are bored in our life and practice, we have to look where the anger is hiding. Every second of our existence, even if we are merely breathing, can be a revelation of beauty. Boredom merely shows that we don't allow ourselves to be present.

We know now how thoughts that obstruct the *yamas* and *niyamas* arise from greed, anger, and infatuation. These thoughts will lead to future suffering and ignorance. In this context it is not significant whether violence or thoughts of violence are mild, moderate, or intense. In any case they will bear fruit. Also whether we commit such thoughts or actions ourselves, cause others to do them, or approve of them is of no significance. They will still bear the same fruit.

In this context it is interesting to look at another popular misconception about nonviolence. Eggs are sneered at as food in India. Although they are not fertilized and therefore are not alive, to eat them is considered violence. Different is the case with milk, which we looked at in sutra II.31. As Patanjali points out, acts of violence will cause pain and ignorance whether carried out, caused, or approved of. The Hindu notion of milk-drinking being nonviolent is therefore discredited.

Nevertheless we have to let go of the idea that complete nonviolence is possible. A Hare Krishna community that kept its own dairy cows found this out the hard way. After they realized their bull calves would be slaughtered if they sold them, they decided to keep them. This way their *ahimsa* (nonviolence) would stay intact. Following the principle "What can go wrong will go wrong," the cows of the community gave birth to eleven bull calves in a row. We might suspect Lord Krishna had a helping hand there, to make his point.

The community then decided not only to keep the growing bulls but also not to have them castrated, which also would constitute violence. For this reason the eleven bulls could be put to no practical use whatsoever, because bulls are too aggressive to pull carts or to plow. Oxen are used for this. Furthermore the eleven bulls had to be kept in eleven rather large individual paddocks so they did not kill each other. When the author visited the community in 1995 it had given up its milk production and turned into a bull sanatorium. Milk was purchased on the commercial market, tainted by violence, but better than no milk at all.

Having become realistic about how far we can take nonviolence, it is still important that we adhere to the ethics as much as possible. If we do not do our best, we will indeed experience suffering and ignorance in the future. To accept the thought that violating ethics will cause future suffering constitutes meditation on the opposite — so claim Vachaspati Mishra and Shankaracharya in their respective subcommentaries.

अहिंसाप्रतिष्ठायां तत्सन्निधौ वैरत्यागः ॥ ३५ ॥
II.35 In the presence of one established in nonviolence, all hostility ceases.

In the next eleven sutras Patanjali describes the effects that the restraints and observances have when mastered. In this sutra Patanjali says that those firmly established in nonviolence are so nonthreatening that man and beast alike can in their presence let their defenses down and become peaceful. Aggression is often based on fear and can be relinquished once we see there is no reason to fear.

This insight reverberates in the story of Buddha and Angulimala. On his wanderings, the Buddha once came to a village that formed the entrance to a vast forest. When he entered the village begging for alms, people advised him not to go any farther. Living in the forest was a serial killer who had vowed to slay a hundred people, cut their fingers off, and wear them as a necklace. His name, Angulimala, in fact meant finger necklace. He had already killed ninety-nine people and was waiting for his last victim in order to fulfill his oath. Buddha was not disturbed by the story and told the villagers there was nothing that could stop him from walking his path. If he was supposed to serve as the hundredth victim in this way, at least he would relieve Angulimala of his terrible oath. He was not concerned at all. After much crying and despair, the villagers eventually had to let Buddha go into the forest.

After he had walked for some time he encountered Angulimala sitting in a clearing, easily recognizable by his necklace of fingers. "What are you doing here?," he shouted. "Don't you know this is my forest? I am Angulimala." It did not escape his eye that there was something special about the Buddha. The grace with which he strode and the atmosphere of peace that surrounded him presented a completely new experience. Buddha now stood right in front of him.

Angulimala saw the stillness and the serenity in his eyes: this was a man such as he had never encountered before. He was touched by the stranger and didn't want to kill him, but had to uphold his reputation. "Go back to where you came from," he said. "I can't let you through. I have taken a vow to kill a hundred people and wear their fingers around my neck. If you don't turn around you force me to kill you." Buddha replied, "Nothing can turn me away from my path, not even death. I have decided to take this path and nothing can change my decision. If that is unacceptable to you, you may kill me."

Angulimala couldn't believe this. The entire world was in fear of him, and here was a man who didn't care a bit. "I will kill you in a moment, but let me ask you one thing. Are you not afraid?" Buddha just shook his head and stood there in complete surrender. At the same time Angulimala saw in his eyes that this man had come home, that he had found something that he, Angulimala, could not take from him whatever he did — he had found peace and did not know fear.

Angulimala knew then that he had found his teacher. He broke down crying and asked to be initiated as his student.

This story beautifully illustrates how complete harmlessness can instill a similar feeling in others. This does not mean, however, that nonviolence ensues in all situations. The Buddha himself was poisoned by a man who disliked the community of monks; Milarepa was poisoned for a similar reason; robbers chopped to death Buddha's greatest student, Mogallana. When Jesus Christ was sentenced to death, the Roman magistrate Pontius Pilate, like Angulimala, realized the man before him was a saint. He did not want to be responsible for killing him, so he ruled that the people of Jerusalem could ask for one person to receive amnesty. What did they do? They asked for the murderer Barabbas to be released and Jesus to be killed. If there was anybody firmly established in nonviolence, that person was Jesus.

Robbers looting his ashram beat up the Indian saint Ramana Maharshi. Shams I. Tabriz, the master of the Sufi poet Rumi, was murdered by people who were jealous of his influence on Rumi. The two main protagonists of nonviolence in the twentieth century, Mahatma Gandhi and Martin Luther King, were both assassinated. The Indian epics *Ramayana* and *Mahabharata* are full of stories of saints being harassed by demons. Most prominent is the Rishi Vishvamitra, who couldn't complete a sacrifice because the sacred location was constantly being desecrated. There are even demons in the epics that openly admit they get more pleasure by devouring pious, righteous people than sinners. When the Mogul army invaded India, the inhabitants of several Buddhist cities left their homes and lay down in front of the approaching army. This was meant to stop the invaders from raiding the town. But the Mogul commanders let their army ride over the peaceful protesters and killed them all.

There is anecdotal evidence suggesting that through our nonviolence we can make others peaceful, but at the same time other evidence suggests the opposite. Why does Patanjali then generalize that "all hostility ceases" if we are established in nonviolence? He does it to incite us to practice. It is a common trait of Indian masters to overstate the effects of the practice to make sure that students take it up. We know from Vyasa and Shankaracharya that it is the responsibility of the teacher to explain the practice in such a way that we take it up and stick to it. Some aspects described in an idealized way can help in that regard.

सत्यप्रतिष्ठायां क्रियाफलाश्रयत्वम् ॥ ३६ ॥
11.36 When one is established in truthfulness, actions and their fruit will correspond with one's words.

This sutra refers to another great power that was acquired by the ancient *rishi*s. Through their intense austerity (*tapas*) they acquired the ability to change the course of events with their words. Since they were completely truthful, the future had to change, if necessary, to accommodate their words. They used this power mainly through their weapon, the curse. In a curse, the *rishi* made a certain statement about the future and, since he was never untruthful, the future had to unfold according to his words. This change of the future, though, used up a lot of the merit he had accumulated through long *tapas*. It made him vulnerable.

According to mythology, gods and demons sometimes used third persons to provoke the wrath of a *rishi*. The subsequent curse would then use up his power and weaken him. Indra, the king of heaven, used heavenly nymphs (*apsara*s) to reduce the accumulated *tapas* of the Rishi Vishvamitra.

As Patanjali will explain later, such powers form an obstacle on the path of yoga. They are dangled there like a carrot in front of us to convince us to practice. Later we are asked to abandon these powers, since they prevent *samadhi*. Let us abandon the quest for power right from the outset, since it is a dead-end street. This is in accordance with the *Bhagavad Gita*, where we are asked simply to act without asking for profit.

अस्तेयप्रतिष्ठायां सर्वरत्नोपस्थानम् ॥ ३७ ॥
11.37 When established in nonstealing, all is but jewels.

We are asked here to look at a piece of gold in the same way as a lump of clay. If we give up our preconceived ideas about appearances, suddenly the preciousness of every moment reveals itself. By looking at the world without seeking to benefit or profit from it, all its beauty is revealed. From wanting to get something out of every situation, we close ourselves to the many gifts that we receive every moment.

The traditional understanding of the sutra is that if one does not care at all about riches, they will start to care about us. According to popular belief the celestial diamond-spewing mongoose will appear before us and shower us with jewels once we are established in nonstealing.

For the modern practitioner it is important to realize that the road to riches might lead over stock-tracking software or real-estate seminars but not over meditation. Time spent meditating is completely wasted if you are in the pursuit of wealth. To become rich, one needs an urge for wealth and a strong competitive edge. Meditation reduces such urges, and it is detrimental to one's competitive edge. If you meditate you might find you can't be bothered any more to run after money beyond what's necessary — especially if meditation has led you to recognize the space nature of consciousness, according to which things can be neither gained nor lost. No material gain whatsoever ensues from the mystical experience. Many mystics lived in poverty, though this is not a requirement.

ब्रह्मचर्यप्रतिष्ठायां वीर्यलाभः ॥ ३८ ॥

11.38 When established in sexual restraint, vitality is gained.

The Indian idea is that the energy usually wasted through sex is transformed and can be used for higher purposes. Sexual energy is seen as capital that can lift us into the divine dominion if used properly. Sexual restraint is thought to increase intelligence and memory function.

True sexual restraint is rare, however. It is said that in each age there can be only one who masters it. That one was Hanuman in the Treta Yuga (the age in which Rama appeared) and Bhishma, Arjuna's foster grandfather, in the Dvapara Yuga (the age in which Krishna appeared). The ancient *rishi*s did not practice complete sexual restraint: they all fathered many children.

The ability to transform and use is the key. If sexual energy is simply suppressed and bottled up, it can turn into hatred and become very dangerous. Some political leaders have known about this and used their knowledge to further their aims. That is how the Nazis managed to unleash a terrible force, as Wilhelm Reich explains in his book *The Mass Psychology in Fascism*. The mere suppression of sexuality does not lead anywhere if one does not know what to do with the energy.

अपरिग्रहस्थैर्ये जन्मकथंतासंबोधः ॥ ३९ ॥

11.39 One established in nongreed attains knowledge of past and future births.

Greed arises through attachment and identification with the body and all objects that it enjoys. Once we know the eternal self, we continue to respect the body as the vehicle to liberation and tend to its needs, but we are not preoccupied by its needs anymore. We realize that the objects of enjoyment cannot

liberate us; they have, rather, a peculiar tendency to bind us, although this tendency lies in our subconscious conditioning and not in the objects themselves. For one that is permanently established in self knowledge, the objects of enjoyment have lost any grip. That does not mean such a person has to live like an ascetic. In fact the fanatical avoidance of pleasure by an ascetic shows that he is still under the spell of pleasure.

The *jnanin* (knower) is indifferent. "If pleasure comes, good; if no pleasure comes, also good." This attitude is *aparigraha* — nongreed. One does not hanker after any objects whatsoever. How can it be that such a person knows about past and future?

The person who is firmly established in the self exists beyond time, since the self is timeless and permanent. Whereas the body, the mind, the ego, and the intellect exist within time, time exists within the self. In other words, time appears on the screen of the self. All phenomena that exist within time, whether past, present, or future, are witnessed by the self. Since the quality of the self is awareness, it cannot do any other than witness; and since it is permanent it is aware of everything that occurs within time. Therefore the self is aware of our entire evolutionary past, beginning with the microbe and ending with the great dissolution (*pralaya*). As well, the self is witness to the ever-unfolding world ages (*kalpa*s). Beyond that, the self is witness to the deep reality that never unfolded, that never dissolves — the reality that gives birth to all appearance without ever being affected (Brahman).

One established in nongreed can therefore download knowledge of past and future. Many great masters, however, have shunned the notion of doing so. From the perspective of the self, attachment to knowledge about one's past and future is as insignificant as attachment to sense objects. It is a power that one can use to impress others, but the things one sees in the past and future are as significant as things seen on the TV screen. Sages usually did not bother to develop this power.

A man once came to the Buddha and asked, "How often do I have to be reborn?" The Buddha looked up to the sky and said, "As many as the stars in the sky, that often will you be reborn!" The man went away in horror, because his life was a drag. Another man asked Buddha, "How often will I come back?" The Buddha pointed to a huge banyan tree and said, "As many as the leaves on that tree, that often will you be reborn!" The man jumped up and danced around in great happiness because he really loved his life — and he became liberated on the spot. Since the man became liberated we can assume he did not come back for future embodiments. Did the Buddha err, then, when he predicted that his questioner would come back as many times as there were leaves on the banyan?

No, he saw the potential of this person to have that many more lives. But the man took the opportunity we all have in every second of our lives — to become free right now. The future lives that the Buddha saw do still exist, but they don't exist anymore in regard to that man. He dis-identified with and liberated himself from his own future. For a true *jnanin* all residual *karma* is interrupted. Residual *karma* is *karma* that has not come to fruition yet; its interruption produces freedom. For that reason any look into the future is uninteresting. The future that is foreseeable is the future we want to become free of.

The orthodox Indian idea is that all beings go through a cycle of thirty trillion lives and then become liberated. Yoga does not accept this destiny but attempts to liberate us now. As the Rishi Vasishta said, "For one of true self-effort there is no destiny."

शौचात् स्वाङ्गजुगुप्सा परैरसंसर्गः ॥ ४० ॥
II.40 From cleanliness arises protection for one's own body and noncontamination by others.

Cleanliness of body and mind creates a protective shield around the body. Although hygiene protects the body from infectious disease, the cleanliness referred to here is predominantly abstention from thoughts of hatred, greed, and infatuation. Such thoughts will manifest as actions of hatred and the like, and these will lead to damaging of the body. Another implication of negative action needs to be considered. In the early stages of yoga practice students may be quite fragile and easily distracted from their path.

During those early days it is important to protect one's enthusiasm and interest in the practice.

There is a physical law that energy always flows from the higher to the lower potential. A novice student can easily lose the yogic merit he or she has accumulated, through keeping bad company. One can readily pick up negative attitudes and emotions from others, especially when one is open to them. Such contamination is said to be counteracted through cleanliness. With the use of the term "noncontamination" I am following Georg Feuerstein, who says that Patanjali's term *jugupsa* "conveys the idea of being on one's guard with respect to the body, of having a detached attitude towards our mortal frame."[36]

This use of "noncontamination" is opposed to the unfortunate term "disgust," which some commentators use. Some religious authorities, Christian and Hindu, view the body as disgusting. Materialistic people, on the other hand, are completely absorbed by the body and its needs. Yoga takes a neutral stance here. The body is seen as potentially that by which the spirit is bound,[37] but on the other hand it is acknowledged as a tool for achieving liberation.[38]

However, the feeling of disgust toward one's own or anyone else's body creates nothing but a new obstacle to yoga. Disgust falls into the category of repulsion (*dvesha*), which is one of the five afflictions (sutra II.8).

Repulsion is based on a negative imprint (*samskara*) that will condition one's actions and lead to future suffering and ignorance. As we have learned in sutra II.8, it is a form of wrong cognition (*viparyaya*) in which one erroneously perceives one's consciousness as being bound up with egoic notions such as disgust. The body cannot disgust the self, since the self does not judge at all. The ego can, however, and will happily do so, since it will trigger the previously described mechanism and thus an increase of ego. To look at one's body with disgust is therefore not a yogic teaching at all.

36. Georg Feuerstein, *Yoga Sutra of Patanjali*, p. 87.
37. *Shvetashvatara Upanishad* 5.10
38. *Shvetashvatara Upanishad* 5.12.

सत्त्वशुद्धिसौमनस्यैकाग्र्येन्द्रियजयात्मदर्शन-
योग्यत्वानि च ॥ ४१ ॥

II.41 From purification of the mind arise joy, one-pointedness, mastery of the senses, and readiness for knowing the self.

Now the effects of mental cleanliness are discussed. Mental cleanliness means to cease to identify with thoughts or emotions of hatred, greed, envy, jealousy, pride, and so on. Once these are abandoned, the original *sattva* quality of the intellect shines forth, which is joy. Out of this joy develops one-pointedness, according to Vyasa. This is easy to understand: how can the mind be one-pointed if it is still distracted by misery, malice, and its own problems? All these take energy away from our contemplation.

Once we are established in mental cleanliness, we experience joy because we know that freedom is near. The joy that develops gives us the freedom to devote ourselves exclusively to our discipline (*sadhana*). This is called one-pointedness. From one-pointedness develops mastery of the senses.

So far our happiness has depended on external stimulation. To remain happy we require an endless supply of power, money, sex, drugs, excitement, and consumption. First, the senses reach out to these stimuli. They draw the mind after them to organize the impressions collected. Then the ego reaches out to own them, and finally the intellect gets clouded and we lose sight of our true nature. This development is intercepted by mastery of the senses. This means that the next time an object of desire floats past we stop the senses from reaching out and embracing it. Then things will just be as they are, without us clinging to them.

From mastery of the senses we necessarily become ready for self-knowledge. As long as we constantly reach out for happiness we cannot see that it is already there, inside. First we have to abandon the attempt to "go for what we want." Only then can awareness turn around and find that everything is there already. This is readiness for knowing the self.

संतोषाद् अनुत्तमः सुखलाभः ॥ ४२ ॥

II.42 From contentment results unsurpassed joy.

Vyasa explains by quoting from the *Puranas*: whatever joy there can be through sexual pleasure, whatever joy there can be had in heaven, is not even a sixteenth of the joy that is experienced when one's desires cease.

When in the process of evolution we forget our true nature as infinite consciousness, we still have a faint memory of the fulfillment we once had — fulfillment we experienced through the love affair with our own heart,[39] the first and foremost of all loves. Expelled from the Garden of Eden, we wander through life and project our longing onto the outer world. We are disappointed over and over again, however, because the joys of heaven and earth taste stale compared to recognizing ourselves as consciousness. What we call joy is nothing but a temporary covering of the disappointment, a soothing of the pain created by us losing ourselves in the jungle of conditioned existence. We cover the wound by experiencing some short-lived joy, which wears off quickly. Feeling the pain again, we need stimulus.

We have to realize that the wound will not heal unless we accept the medicine. The medicine is letting go of the idea that any form of external stimulus will help. With the letting go of this idea comes contentment. For the first time we can just sit and be, and not try to do something to get better. Out of sitting and being eventually arises the joy of pure being, which surpasses any joy dependent on the presentation of earthly or heavenly objects.

कायेन्द्रियसिद्धिरशुद्धिक्षयात् तपसः ॥ ४३ ॥

II.43 Austerity (*tapas*) destroys the impurities and thus brings perfection of the body and the sense organs.

Tapas, like yoga, is a system of psycho-technology, but it is even older than yoga. It developed out of shamanism. The *tapasvin* practices extreme forms of asceticism to achieve supernatural powers (*siddhi*s),

---

39. In line with Indian terminology, heart (*hrdaya*) is used here not to mean romantic love but our core, the self.

which are also called perfections. Perfections of the body are abilities like traveling through space and time and walking on water. Perfections of the senses are clairvoyance, the ability to read other people's thoughts, the divine ear, the magic touch, and so on. We are told here that the practice of *tapas* will produce such powers.

For the yogi, however, the powers are not an end in themselves, as is the case also for many *tapasvin*s (those who exclusively practice *tapas* and not yoga). After the veil of the impurities (greed, envy, hatred, and so on) has been removed, the yogi uses the strength gained to obtain self-knowledge and thus become liberated from bondage. To desire superpowers will lead to bondage just as does the desire for wealth, status, and the like.

In yoga, *tapas* has not the same connotation as when it is practiced exclusively, outside of the yogic context. In yoga, it refers to the ability to sustain our practice in the face of hardship. From this ability great power arises. This is especially true in the case of the Ashtanga Vinyasa method. However, we need to be careful how we use this power. From a yogic viewpoint the reason to practice *tapas* is only to remove the veil of the impurities to prepare us for the revelation of the light of the self. Any attachment to powers would cover the light with a new veil of ignorance.

स्वाध्यायाद् इष्टदेवतासंप्रयोगः ॥ ४४ ॥
II.44 From establishment in self-study (svadhyaya) results communion with one's chosen deity.

Svadhyaya means study of sacred texts. These texts contain the testimonies of the ancient masters. Since the intellectual condition of humankind has progressively worsened with the advance of time, testimonies of contemporaries are to be viewed with suspicion. In the present dark age (Kali Yuga), teachers who are not corrupted are extremely rare. We have therefore to rely on the study of the ancient scriptures such as the *Upanishads*. *Svadhyaya* also refers to repetition of a mantra, such as the sacred syllable OM. To one established in these practices, one's chosen deity or meditation deity is revealed.

Which deity that is is not specified. The practice of yoga is open to all faiths. According to yogic teachings, all deities are but representations of the one Supreme Being. Because there is only one, they cannot be representations of somebody else. The Supreme Being is a projection of the formless absolute. Because that is difficult to comprehend, it is acceptable to project an image onto the Supreme Being. This image is one's *ishtadevata*, one's meditation deity. The meditation deity will enable us to develop a close personal relationship with the Supreme Being. However, as the *Bhagavad Gita* states, "Whatever deity you worship, you always worship me."

It has been common in the past to judge others because we think our *ishtadevata* is superior to theirs. This has given rise to hatred, warfare, and genocide. An attitude of tolerance is important. Even if we do not understand what our neighbour worships, we should not allow that to produce feelings of superiority because we think ours is a better God.

समाधिसिद्धिरीश्वरप्रणिधानात् ॥ ४५ ॥
II.45 From devotion to the Supreme Being comes the attainment of samadhi.

Patanjali has been criticized by theistic philosophers such as Ramanuja for underestimating the importance of the Supreme Being. On the other side, Samkhya teachers like Ishavarakrishna do not mention the Supreme Being. Like the Buddha, they accepted worship of the gods and maintenance of temples and customs, but they denied that this contributes to our liberation. The masters Ramanuja and Madhva, on the other hand, taught that we can do nothing whatsoever toward our liberation but to ask for the grace of the Supreme Being.

Patanjali treads the middle ground. He includes the path of action, which means doing the work ourselves, but he also includes the path of surrender to the Supreme Being. From the mystic's point of view, the *samadhi* of the different schools is the same, and it doesn't matter which technique we employ. This is very much Patanjali's position.

Whether we approach the Supreme Being, which is nothing but infinite consciousness, from an emotional Bhakti angle or from an analytical Advaita perspective is only a question of individual constitution. The subcommentator Vachaspati Mishra explains that the other seven limbs (those other than *samadhi*) are there to support devotion to the Supreme Being, which according to him is the only way of attaining *samadhi*. That Patanjali wanted to describe devotion as the only path to *samadhi* appears inconclusive from the context of the *Yoga Sutra*: in other passages of the sutra he appears to be very open to other possibilities.

Krishnamacharya, as a follower of Ramanuja, taught that the *Yoga Sutra* accommodates three levels of practitioners: beginning, intermediate, and advanced yogis. On all three levels, however, surrender to the Supreme Being needs to be practiced.

According to Krishnamacharya, sutra II.1 prescribes surrender to the Supreme Being for beginners (*kriya* yogis), sutra II.32 prescribes it for intermediate yogis (*ashtanga* yogis), while the present sutra (II.45) enshrines it for advanced yogis (called simply yogis). According to Krishnamacharya, a true yogi is one who can surrender directly. From this surrender, *samadhi* proceeds without any detraction due to inferior forms of practice.

स्थिरसुखम् आसनम् ॥ ४६ ॥
II.46 Posture must have the two qualities of firmness and ease.

With the effects of the restraints (*yamas*) and observances (*niyamas*) given, Patanjali concludes his description of the first two limbs. He has described these two limbs only briefly. His descriptions of the first five limbs are in fact very concise, hinting at the fact that the *Yoga Sutra* addresses the more or less established student.

He will now cover the third limb, *asana*, in three stanzas. That doesn't mean posture is unimportant. Had that been the case, Patanjali would not have declared *asana* to be one of the eight major aspects of yoga. He will cover *pranayama* in only five stanzas and *pratyahara* in just two.

Most of the *Yoga Sutra* deals with *samadhi* and its effects. It is here that Patanjali's main interest lies. Teachers such as Svatmarama and Gheranda devoted themselves almost exclusively to the first four or five limbs, which does not mean they regarded *samadhi* as an inessential form of practice.

Patanjali uses two qualities that are diametrically opposed to describe posture: firmness and ease. If the posture is to be firm, effort will be required — contraction of muscles that will arrest the body in space without wavering. Ease on the other hand implies relaxation, softness, and no effort. Patanjali shows here already that posture cannot be achieved unless we simultaneously reach into these opposing directions. These directions are firmness, which is inner strength, and the direction of ease, which brings relaxedness.

Vyasa gives a list of postures in his commentary to show that yogic posture (*yogasana*) according to yoga *shastra* (scripture) is meant here, and not just keeping one's spine, neck, and head in one line. He also says that the postures become yoga *asanas* only when they can be held comfortably. Before that they are only attempts at yoga *asana*.

Shankara elaborates further to say that, in yoga *asana*, mind and body become firm and no pain is experienced. The firmness is needed to block out distractions since, after *asana* has been perfected, we want to go on to *pranayama*, concentration, and so on.

Mention of the absence of pain is interesting. If the field of perception is filled with pain, the mind will be distracted. Patanjali's definition of posture as ease automatically eliminates that which causes pain. If you are in a posture and experience pain you will not be at ease.

The widespread tendency in modern yoga to practice the postures in such a way that they hurt leads to being preoccupied with the body. This is by defi-nition not yoga *asana*.

According to scripture, in *asana* the limbs have to be placed in a pleasant and steady positioning so as not to interfere with the yogi's concentration. The inner breath (*prana*) is then arrested and moved into the central channel (*sushumna*). *Sushumna* will eat time, and the fluctuations (*vrtti*) of the mind will be arrested. Meditation on Brahman will then arise.

Asana is thus a preparation for *samadhi*, whereas practices that lead to pain will increase the bond between the phenomenal self (*jiva*) and the body, which in itself is the yogic definition of suffering. Those practices might be gymnastics, they possibly

225

could even be healthy, but they are not yoga, which is recognizing the false union (*samyoga*) of the seer (*drashtar*) and the seen (*drshyam*).[40]

प्रयत्नशैथिल्यानन्तसमापत्तिभ्याम् ॥ ४७ ॥
II.47 Posture is then when effort ceases and meditation on infinity occurs.

The sutra is similar to verse 114 in Shankaracharya's *Aparokshanubhuti*: "True posture is that which leads to meditation on Brahman spontaneously and ceaselessly and not what leads to suffering."[41] Here again it is implied that as long as we are involved in effort we are not in the true posture. It is the preparatory stage to the posture that is signified by effort and discomfort. When, through training of proprioceptive awareness, the limbs arrive in the correct position, effort suddenly ceases.

The cessation of effort has already been described in sutra II.27. Freedom from doing is there listed as a prerequisite to higher yoga. All effort and intent are finally surrendered in complete detachment (*paravairagya*), described in sutra I.16. The *prana* then flows calmly and the disturbing movements of the mind cease. Then occurs meditation on infinity, in which body and mind are experienced as emptiness. This meditation will happen spontaneously, as Shankara says, without any further artificial effort. This is because, once the emptiness nature of body and mind is perceived, the obstacle to meditation on infinity (*ananta*) is removed.

How do we practice meditation on emptiness? Patanjali does not talk about the infinity of space here, which is an unrewarding meditation object. The infinity of space can be understood through mental reflection; meditation is not required. Patanjali suggests here to meditate on the infinity of consciousness. The *Taittiriya Upanishad* states, "satyam jnanam anantam brahma"[42] — Brahman is reality, knowledge, and infinity. Infinity is here listed as an attribute of Brahman. Patanjali does not use the term "Brahman," because it implies reducing his separate

categories *purusha* and *prakrti* to one. However, he uses *ananta* to refer to the infinity of consciousness, against which the infinity of space is insignificant. He will state exactly this in sutra IV.31.

It is significant, though, that Patanjali uses the term *ananta* instead of Brahman, which is Shankara's choice, to denote infinity. Ananta is another name for the divine serpent Adishesha, which is invoked in the "Vande gurunam" chant. One of Ananta's duties was to provide a bed on which Lord Vishnu could sleep. The Lord had a very weighty appearance at times. When he vanquished the demon king Bali he assumed a form so huge that he strode across the three worlds in three steps (*trivikrama*). With the third he pushed Bali back into the nether world.

In the *Bhagavad Gita*,[43] the revelation of the universal form of Vishnu (*Vishvarupa*) is described thus: "Then the son of Pandu [Arjuna] saw the entire universe with its manifold divisions united there, in the body of the God of gods."[44] Three stanzas later Arjuna exclaims, "I see you with many eyes, hands, bellies, mouths, possessing infinite forms on every side; O Lord of the universe, O you of universal form, I see, however, neither your end nor your middle nor your beginning."[45]

Vishnu is described as the God of infinity and vastness. As we have seen, when it was time to provide a sofa for his sleep, Ananta, the personified infinity, was called. The sofa needed to have two opposing qualities: it needed to be infinitely firm to uphold the vastness of the Lord; on the other hand it needed to be infinitely soft to provide the best of all beds for Vishnu. For this reason Ananta is seen as the ideal yogi, uniting the opposing qualities of firmness (*sthira*) and softness (*sukham*), which makes all of his movements true posture.

One may think this a steep call for the third limb only, but Vyasa affirms, "When the mind is in *samadhi* on the infinite, then the posture is perfected." We need also to understand that the Lord Vishnu is nobody but our own self, as the *Yoga Vashishta* states. Whereas then the mythological serpent of infinity provides a perfect bed for the God who represents

40. Sutra II.17

41. *Aparokshanubhuti of Sri Sankaracharya*, trans. Sw. Vimuktananda, Advaita Ashrama, Kolkata, 1938.

42. II.1.1.

43. XI.13.

44. *Srimad Bhagavad Gita*, trans. Sw. Vireswarananda, Sri Ramakrishna Math, Madras, p. 226.

45. Ibid., p. 228.

our innermost self, on an individual level, if our body is held in perfect posture, embracing the qualities of softness and firmness, then we see that very self effortless and spontaneous. In this way *asana*, although much sneered at by scholars, is an expression of the divine if practiced from such a high perspective. Otherwise it is sport only.

The view that Patanjali gives of *asana* is that of a frame or base for the two highest yogic practices, which are complete surrender (*paravairagya*) and objectless (*asamprajnata*) *samadhi*. *Asana* is engaged in to create a frame for these practices, its purpose being fulfilled only when we abide in these states. On the other hand, surrender and *samadhi* occur within *asana*. As we progress we don't abandon the lower limbs, but they occur naturally and spontaneously to provide the base for the higher limbs.

तततो द्वन्द्वानभिघातः ॥ ४८ ॥
II.48 In *asana* there is no assault from the pairs of opposites.

This stanza refers to the state where true posture is achieved and not the preparatory stage where effort and discomfort prevail.

The first pair of opposites we encountered was firmness versus ease. By simultaneously integrating both extremes, we rest, effortless and free in the core. Then meditation on Brahman is possible. Now Patanjali defines true posture as that in which we rest free from any assault of opposites. The opposites are the extremes to which the mind tries to attach itself. For example, before I meditate I need to gain mastery over hundreds of different yoga postures. This is an extreme, and the mind might claim it in order to understand yoga, which by definition the mind is not capable of doing.

The opposite is the attitude that meditation needs no preparation whatsoever. Here the mind dupes us into believing that no posture and no level of proficiency are necessary for meditation. In between these extremes is the state of pure being, where one just exists unaffected by the chatter of the mind. The mind is constantly trying to figure out what is going on out there. It develops a model of reality and then presents it to the path of cognition — ego, intelligence,

consciousness. If we reach out and identify ourselves with any of those models that are here called "extremes" or "pairs of opposites," then we are returning to conditioned existence and are strictly speaking only attempting yoga. Seeing that we are practicing yoga, the mind gets interested in understanding what yoga is. It might say Ashtanga is the right way; other styles are wrong. Or it might say Mysore-style classes are right; talk-through classes are wrong. It also likes to come up with notions such as Hindus are good, Christians and Muslims are bad, or vice versa.

Nowhere is this principle better explored than in the posture itself. We might be in a handstand and the mind might say handstand means pushing the floor away from you. Having attached ourselves to one pair of the opposite we fail to own the other side, which is to reach down into the floor and to draw the heart down into the floor. We have been struck by the assault of the opposites, which means to fall for one extreme and thereby lose our center.

Let us take backbending as an example: The mind says backbending means contracting the back of the body. But if we ignore the mind and stay unassailed by the extremes, we realize that we have to lengthen the back, because a shortened back cannot arch. If we are in *Pashimottanasana* the mind might first grasp this posture as "thrusting the head to the knee." A year later the mind might have modified this to "pulling the heart to the feet" — which is much better but still an extreme. Then eventually we stop listening to the mind and arrive there, where every cell of the body awakens and participates in the posture.

If we are then asked, "What is *Pashimottanasana*?" we really couldn't say anymore. Any new concept would be just another set of opposites and extremes. Instead of reaching out and becoming one with concepts and extremes, we abide at the core and spontaneously just exist.

Some commentators erroneously claim that Patanjali is speaking here about a type of anesthesia, a numbness that arises if we have endured the pain of the posture long enough. This numbness will surely arrive if one promotes it, and in fact many yogis have gone down that avenue. Yoga, however, is a path to pure being that leads to greater sensitivity rather than numbness.

In his commentary on sutra II.15, Vyasa explains

that the *vivekinah*, the discerning one, is like an eyeball sensitive even to the touch of a cobweb, whereas the average person is like any other part of the body, which is numb to the cobweb. The *vivekinah* is therefore more sensitive to pain and not numb. Nevertheless he stays free, since he knows he is not the pain: he only witnesses it.

Identifying yoga with numbness is a sad development. It robs us of such pristine moments as when we observe the sun rising and the first rays of light piercing a crystal-clear dewdrop on a leaf, and for the first time we observe pure being revealing itself without it being commented upon by our mentation. Then we know that the sun of knowledge has risen within — and no amount of anesthetic will make that happen.

तस्मिन् सति श्वासप्रश्वासयोर्गतिविच्छेदः
प्राणायामः ॥ ४९ ॥

II.49 When posture is accomplished, *pranayama* is then practiced, which is removing agitation from inhalation and exhalation.

The Sanskrit "tasmin sati" means when the previous limb (*asana*) has been accomplished. Vyasa affirms that mastery of *asana* is necessary before *pranayama* is practiced, as does the *Hatha Yoga Pradipika* also.[46] But it is nowhere stated what exactly "accomplished" or "mastery" means. Contemporary India seems to have a rather laidback attitude toward what perfection of *asana* means — but definitely not gymnastic or contortionist performance. And the yoga master T. Krishnamacharya is known to have taught *pranayama* to students who were too sick to practice *asana*.

Pranayama is a compound noun consisting of *prana* and *ayama*. On the subtle plane it refers to extension or expansion of vital force. In sutra I.31 the disturbed inhalation and exhalation that accompany obstacles of the mind are mentioned. In this context — on the gross plane — *pranayama* is understood to be regulation of the breathing process. Both definitions have in common the notion that a calm flow of *prana* and a smooth and even flow of anatomical breath are necessary as a prerequisite for meditation.

A third meaning is described in A. G. Mohan's translation of *Yoga Yajnavalkya*.[47] Here *prana* is said to extend twelve *angulas* (finger widths) over the surface of the body, which corresponds to a scattered state of mind. Yajnavalkya teaches the drawing in of *prana* to the body to make the pranic body and gross body equal in size. This corresponds to a calm mind. In this context we can call *pranayama* contraction or concentration of *prana*. A contraction is also described in the *Hatha Yoga Pradipika*, which suggests forcing *prana* into the central energy channel, said to be one-thousandth of a hair's breadth.

Patanjali will give yet another definition of *pranayama* in the next sutra, were it is taken to mean breath retention (*kumbhaka*). This is an advanced stage of *pranayama*, undertaken only after the present stage, the calming of the flow of *prana*, is achieved. This first stage is practiced through simple techniques such as *Ujjayi* and alternate nostril breathing (*nadi shodana*) without *kumbhaka*.

Usually the term *pranayama* implies that we are working with the *pranamaya kosha*, the subtle sheet or subtle body. By directing the movements of the outer or anatomical breath, we influence the movements of *prana*, the inner breath or life force. The movements of *prana* are parallel with the movements of *vrtti*, which are the fluctuations or modifications of the mind. Thus, if the movement of *prana* can be calmed and smoothed, the same will apply to the mind's fluctuations.

In Western circles *pranayama* consists mainly of simple breathing exercises. However, when I studied *pranayama* in India, I was asked after a few months of introduction to spend a considerable part of the day in retention (*kumbhaka*). This is based on the following idea: small animals that breathe quickly have a short life span; animals with a medium breath count have a medium life span; the animal that breathes the slowest, the maritime turtle, lives up to eight hundred years. To breathe fast means to accelerate time; to breathe slowly means to slow down the passage of time. When no breath at all is there, such as in *kumbhaka*, time for the yogi stands still. All time spent in *kumbhaka* is, according to yogic teaching, added on to one's life expectancy as predetermined by one's *karma*. The *pranayama* practice

---

46. Stanza II.1.

47. p. 10.

that was suggested to me consisted of eighty *kum-bhaka*s with a duration of sixty-four *matra*s each (approximately sixty-four seconds) four times a day. This adds up to 5.7 hours per day spent in *kumbhaka*, during which time one doesn't age. Thus, following this regime on a daily basis would add an additional 25 percent to the remainder of one's life span.

A word of caution. The medieval texts abound in warnings of the dangers of *pranayama*. This is not to be taken lightly. *Pranayama* can be learned only from a teacher and never unsupervised from books. *Pranayama* tends to heat and compress the mind to make it concentrated. A tendency to short temper can be increased through *pranayama*, and the outcome can be an angry personality.[48]

There have also been cases of yogis cracking their skulls open or even dying from increased pressure in the head.[49]

Whereas *asana*, meditation, and self-inquiry can be practiced with an agitated mind, the practice of *pranayama* will rather worsen this condition. It is difficult to fit into a Western fast-paced lifestyle. One can hardly throw in a *pranayama* session between the board meeting and picking up the kids from day care.

If, nevertheless, engagement with *pranayama* is desired, it is advisable to do short breath retentions (*kumbhaka*s) only. If we want to practice the typical retentions that are taught in India, which are in excess of a minute, we need to modify our lifestyle.

A possible way of integrating intense *pranayama* with a Western lifestyle is to practice it intensely on vacations and retreats in the countryside. Traditionally these intense *kumbhaka*s were not practiced in cities, but outside human habitations. Increased population density can have an adverse effect on intense *pranayama* due to the accumulated tension of millions of minds packed tightly together in a metropolis. Big cities can have a Faraday-cage-like effect, where mystical insight is distorted or intercepted through the closeness of many agitated minds. *Pranayama* practiced in polluted metropolitan air is not as beneficial as if it is practiced in clean air. Intense *kumbhaka*s might be better performed where clean air is available.

The hand position used in *pranayama* is called *Shanka* (conch) *Mudra*. In it the right thumb is used to block the right nostril (*pingala*), while the ring finger and little finger are used to block the left nostril (*ida*). The pointing and middle finger are folded.

The significance of the *shanka mudra* is as follows. The thumb represents supreme spirit (Brahman). The pointing finger, which represents self (*atman*), and middle finger, which represents intelligence (*buddhi*), are passive, since *pranayama* does not deal with them. They are folded toward the thumb, symbolizing that they are bowing to supreme spirit. The ring finger, which represents mind (*manas*), and little finger, which represents body (*kaya*), have an active role, since *pranayama* facilitates purification of body and mind.

बाह्याभ्यन्तरस्तम्भवृत्तिः देशकालसंख्याभिः परिदृष्टो दीर्घसूक्ष्मः ॥ ५० ॥

II.50 There are external retention, internal retention, and midway suspension. By observing space, time, and count, the breath becomes long and subtle.

Patanjali mentions three different ways in which the breath can be retained. Some later scriptures mention many more, but we have to understand that *pranayama* plays a much greater role in Hatha Yoga, where the focus is to make the body immortal. In Patanjali's eight-limbed yoga, *pranayama* is used as a tool to facilitate concentration and meditation, nothing more.

The term *pranayama* is often used synonymously with *kumbhaka*. The *Hatha Yoga Pradipika* states that "*Kumbhaka*s are of eight kinds," and then lists the names of the *pranayama* techniques.[50]

The three techniques mentioned in this stanza are all forms of retention — not inhalation, exhalation, and retention as many modern commentators erroneously claim. Vyasa clearly says in his commentary, "There the external is that which is the cessation of movement after expiration; the internal is the

---

48. For a case study compare Sangharakshita, *The Thousand-Petalled Lotus: The Indian Journey of an English Buddhist*, Sutton Pub. Ltd., 1988.

49. Ram Das, *Miracle of Love*, Munshiram Manoharlal, New Delhi, 1999.

50. *Hatha Yoga Pradipika*, II.44.

cessation of movement after inspiration; the third is the confined operation where the cessation of both takes place by a single effort."[51]

In other words the first technique mentioned is to exhale and then arrest the breath, which is known as external (*bahya*) *kumbhaka*. Patanjali has mentioned it already in sutra I.34, where the ability to clarify the mind is ascribed to it.

The second method is inhaling and then arresting the breath, which is called internal (*antara*) *kumbhaka* in the Hatha texts. This technique is mainly used to increase vitality through storing *prana*.

The commentators disagree about the third method. According to Vyasa the cessation of both inhalation and exhalation takes place through a single effort, and it is then called midway suspension. According to H. Aranya,[52] Vyasa's single effort means the simultaneous application of all *bandhas*, which in Hatha Yoga is called *Mahabandha Mudra*. *Mahavedha Mudra* and *Khechari Mudra* are similar methods. The *mudra*s are not much mentioned in the yoga sutras as their use was secret, to be learned only personally from a teacher.

Patanjali further says that by these three techniques the breath will become long and subtle if space, time, and count are observed. Space refers to the area where the breath ends or begins or the place up to where *prana* is felt. The inhalation is usually felt to begin at the navel (*Nabhi chakra*), but with training it can be felt to rise from the base of the spine (*Muladhara chakra*). The exhalation usually ends in a place called *dvadashanta*, twelve finger widths (*angulas*) from the nostrils. It is to this place that the pranic body extends.

Time is the length of time one spends in inhalation, exhalation, and retention. It is measured in *matras*. In a typical *pranayama* one would spend for example sixteen *matra*s in *puraka* (inhalation), sixty-four *matra*s in *kumbhaka* (retention), and thirty-two *matras* in *rechaka* (exhalation). One *matra* is the time that one needs to circle one's knee with one's hand once, or clap one's hand twice, or blink one's eye three times. In other words one *matra* is roughly equivalent to a second. However, the reason why those very

subjective parameters are given is that they can and should change with our condition and the condition of our surroundings on that day. On a humid and hot day there is less oxygen available.

The same applies at a great altitude. If we are tired or weak we cannot utilize oxygen and *prana* as effectively. In all these cases we will automatically speed up our *matra* count, and it is meant to be that way.

If challenging *pranayama*s are performed with the stop-clock and we rigidly keep identifying a *matra* with a second, then damage of lung tissue can occur. Also *rajas* and *tamas* will then rise in our mind. However, as the *Hatha Yoga Pradipika* states, "Pranayama should be performed daily with *sattvika buddhi*."[53] This means the intellect should be predominantly calm and light, with no agitation or dullness.

The third factor in making the breath long and subtle is count. For example in one method one may exhale through *ida* (the left or lunar nostril) first, then inhale three times through *pingala* (the right or solar nostril) followed by retention and exhale, then change back to *ida nadi*, do three internal retentions, and finally exhale through *pingala*. The count for this system, which is one of many, is fifteen. All exhales are on an odd number, which makes them eight altogether. The inhalations are here on even numbers, which makes them seven. Every inhalation is followed by a *khumbaka*, these also totaling seven in number. The term "number" thus relates to the particular techniques we use.

If those three factors — space, time, and number — are observed, the breath becomes long and subtle. Why is this necessary?

Pranayama fulfills the purpose of preparing us for *dharana*, concentration. Concentration, and with it meditation, are not possible if the mind is agitated. With an agitated mind come an erratic breathing pattern and a disturbed flow of *prana*. When the movements of breath and *prana* are made long and subtle through *pranayama*, the mind will flow calmly and move toward single-pointedness. Concentration and meditation will then be possible.

51. *Yoga Sutra of Patanjali*, trans. and comm. J. R. Balantyne, Book Faith India, Delhi, 2000, p. 63.
52. H. Aranya, *Yoga Philosophy of Patanjali with Bhasvati*, p. 233.

53. *Hatha Yoga Pradipika*, II.6.

बाह्याभ्यन्तरविषयाक्षेपी चतुर्थः ॥ ५१ ॥

II.51 When the internal and external spheres are surpassed it is called the fourth [pranayama].

The internal sphere refers to where the origin of the inhalation is observed (*Nabhi chakra, Muladhara chakra*). Alternatively, the inner sphere can also refer to the heart. The external sphere refers to the point of termination of the exhalation, which is twelve finger widths from the nostrils (*dvadashanta*).

The observation of the spheres, together with observation of time and count, has to be practiced during the first three types of *pranayama* until the breath is made long and subtle. When the breath and the retentions have been made long and subtle, the internal and external spheres are said to be surpassed. One then enters into the fourth *pranayama*, which in other texts is called *kevala kumbhaka*, spontaneous suspension. This *pranayama* is not accompanied by supporting aids, just as objectless *samadhi* is not accompanied anymore by supporting objects.

The fourth is rather a qualitative term than a technique. It is the true *pranayama*, which occurs effortlessly, like a true posture. The three previous techniques are ways leading to the fourth. Most people have had experiences where, through intense shock, fear, or bliss, the movement of the breath automatically stops. This phenomenon relates to the fourth *pranayama*, which occurs when *samadhi* is experienced and the breath or *prana* spontaneously suspends, since life itself is experienced and there is no more thirst for an outer manifestation of life. Some commentators take this to mean suspension of breath, whereas others hold that only the *prana* is arrested in *sushumna*, while breath continues its life-sustaining function. There are confirmed reports of yogis who could stop their heartbeat and respiration for extended periods of time, among them Shri T. Krishnamacharya. However, as Krishnamacharya maintained, this was not an essential feature of yoga and in no way required for reaching its goal.

Another natural movement that suspends in deep meditation is the peristaltic movement of the intestine. This is the reason why yoga and many other spiritual disciplines put an emphasis on diet. If heavy foods are eaten, the peristaltic movement cannot stop spontaneously and, if peristalsis cannot stop, spontaneous suspension of the movements of the mind becomes unlikely — not impossible, but less likely.

It is interesting that, when peristalsis stops, movement of the mind and any sexual desire also stop. The sexual urge and charge are produced through a constant massage of the sex center by the peristaltic movement of the intestine. Thus, extended fasting is an easy way to eliminate constant sexual thoughts, which may be preventing higher states of meditation and *pranayama*. After four days of fasting, peristaltic movement will stop, and with it sexual desire. Exalted experiences of meditation are easily accessible then: every breath will become a revelation and *pranayama* will happen by itself. Again, the method of fasting must be learned from a qualified instructor; otherwise it can become a health risk. During the fast, the intestine must be completely emptied and washed daily with an enema. Fasting cannot be combined with *vinyasa* practice, as the body will not have enough energy reserves. Gentle stretches, however, are very beneficial.

Fasting is not a prerequisite for *pranayama*. The *vinyasa* practiced is considered to be strong enough to purify the body without resorting to fasting and the *shatkriya*s (the six actions, described in medieval Hatha texts, that are designed to correct humoral imbalance). For most practitioners a light diet consisting of fruit, milk, and vegetables will keep the peristaltic movement light.

Sticking to a light diet, and having practiced external and internal retention, we become ready for effortless suspension, which may accompany *samadhi*. Some texts go as far as defining *samadhi* as breath retention in excess of 1.5 hours. Patanjali does not say anything about this matter; in fact he does not say retention has to accompany *samadhi*, but it may.

How is it, then, that the breath stops effortlessly and spontaneously? True *pranayama*, like true posture, has the qualities of effortlessness and spontaneity. To understand the mechanism we have to go back to the introductory idea of *pranayama*, which is that breath (*prana*) and mind waves (*vrtti*) move together. If one of the two alters its movement, it automatically influences the movement of the other. The importance of *pranayama* lies in the fact that it is much easier to influence the movement of the breath than to influence the movement of the mind.

If a person in a moment of grace arrests *vrtti*, then *prana* will follow spontaneously. If *vrtti* is arrested for a long period of time, *prana* will perform only that movement that is necessary to sustain life. If the highest form of *samadhi* (*asamprajnata*) is sustained over a long period, no pranic movement whatsoever has any influence on absorption, since true reality is uncreated and indestructible.

ततः क्षीयते प्रकाशावरणम् ॥ ५२ ॥
II.52 Thus the covering of brightness is removed.

"Thus" means when the practice of *asana* and *pranayama* is done in the correct way. The covering refers to the impurities — past *karma*, affliction-based action, conditioning (*vasana*), and subconscious imprints (*samskaras*) — which all collaborate to produce ignorance (*avidya*).

Ignorance, let us recall, is the inability to tell the permanent from the transitory and the real from the unreal. Once this covering of ignorance is removed, brightness and clarity are revealed, which is a prerequisite for going further in yoga. "Brightness" and "clarity," which are qualities of the mind, are here used to translate the Sanskrit term *prakasha*. It can be translated as "light," but that has led modern authors into the trap of taking it to mean the light of the self. But the light of the self (*jnanadiptih*) is the goal of yoga, and it is seen only after practicing the higher limbs. Here what is being talked about is clarity of the mind, which is a prerequisite for concentration (*dharana*).

The proof for this understanding will come in the next sutra.

धारणासु च योग्यता मनसः ॥ ५३ ॥
II.53 Then the mind is fit for concentration.

Patanjali is talking about *manas*, the mind or thinking principle. *Prakasha* (brightness) is used to describe the quality of mind that is fit for concentration (*dharana*). If the last sutra was declaring that the light of the self could be reached through *pranayama*, then no more concentration of the mind would be necessary.

But Patanjali lets us take one step at a time. This sutra really repeats what sutra I.34 has said already: clarification of mind is possible through exhalation and retention of breath. And this is exactly what *pranayama* works on — purification of the mind, not gaining mystical knowledge.

Once the mind has achieved brightness and clarity we are ready for concentration, which is the prerequisite for meditation. In yoga there is great respect for meditation. Most students are considered unfit for spontaneous meditation unless they are prepared. If meditation is done incorrectly it is not beneficial, but in fact detrimental. There are Tibetan Buddhist lamas who say meditation by the uninitiated ends only in one's backside getting flat and flatter, while some of them go as far as to say that whoever meditates wrongly gets reborn as a fish.

If one sits and becomes dull — which, as we have seen, is sometimes called the "white-wall effect" — one should stop meditation immediately and engage in chanting or *japa* (repetition of mantra), because sitting in dullness lets *tamas* (stupidity) rise. If, on the other hand, one sits with an agitated mind, *rajas* (activity) will rise, leading to renewed attachment (*raga*). K. Pattabhi Jois also taught that meditation was not a practice for beginners. He observed further that, once one was established in wrong meditation practice, correction was not possible. This is due to the fact that one's state of meditation cannot be assessed from the outside. In other words the teacher has no way of determining whether the student is doing the right practice. Proper meditation is done in a *sattvika* state, which is possible with the right preparation. If one is not naturally in that state, *asana* and *pranayama* are done as preparation.

स्वविषयासंप्रयोगे चित्तस्य स्वरूपानुकार
इवेन्द्रियाणां प्रत्याहारः ॥ ५४ ॥

11.54 When the mind is withdrawn from the outside then the senses follow and disengage from the sense objects. This is *pratyahara*.

Pratyahara (sense withdrawal) is described next. In some yogic schools it takes center stage, with many different exercises being practiced and much time allocated to it. Patanjali treats it briefly — two stanzas only. As with *asana*, *pranayama*, and *mudra*, the respective exercises were to be learned from a qualified teacher and not from a book.

When we focus on the *Ujjayi* sound in the *vinyasa* practice we do not attend to other environmental sounds, and so the sense of hearing is withdrawn. By gazing toward the prescribed focal points (*drishti*), the sense of seeing is withdrawn. The tactile sense is withdrawn by engaging the entire surface of the body in *asana*. In a similar fashion, the olfactory and gustatory senses are also withdrawn. For example, if the smell of cooking wafts into our practice room we actively disengage from the sensation rather than walk into the kitchen and help ourselves to a meal.

Vyasa uses the metaphor of a swarm of bees. As it flies up when the queen bee flies up and settles down when the queen bee settles down, so also when the mind is agitated and unfocused the senses reach out and attach to sense objects. If two partners have had a hard day at work they are more likely to experience a conflict when they come home. This is due to the mind being in a state of conflict and the senses then attaching to a suitable object. If we are in a state of sexual desire it is more likely that we notice somebody attractive.

If the mind is just plainly unfocused, the senses will attach to anything that is presented and the mind will follow the impulse. This mechanism is used in supermarkets. Close to the exit are positioned so-called impulse articles, like sweets. We did not plan to buy them, they were not on the shopping list, but because they are suddenly presented we follow the sudden impulse "Ah yes, let's have that too." In such ways we fall into many traps

all day long. We might remember there was a moment when there was still choice, and then suddenly we got sucked into the situation and wonder how we ended up there.

If the mind is prepared through the first four limbs, we retain freedom of choice. We are free to be independent of external stimulation.

There are two aspects to *pratyahara*. The withdrawal from the outer world occurs when we realize that external objects cannot make us happy but rather get us into mire. The second aspect is going inside, when we realize that all we yearned for is within us. In this way *pratyahara* is the gatekeeper between inner and outer yoga.

Many of us have experienced *pratyahara*. Whenever we manage to detach ourselves from a strong desire or addiction, that is *pratyahara*. If, years later, we are again confronted with the same object, we realize that something in us does not reach out anymore and attach itself. This mechanism is consciously used in yogic *pratyahara*.

ततः परमा वश्यतेन्द्रियाणाम् ॥ ५५ ॥

11.55 From that comes supreme command over the senses.

Supreme command over the senses is reached when we have become completely independent of external gratification and stimulation. It comes peacefully by itself when we have seen the freedom within. Compared to that freedom, all sensory gratification tastes stale.

There is another way of mastery over the senses. This is where the practitioner, through an act of sheer will, shuts out the entire world and so becomes dead to it. This is a form of cataleptic trance that is necessary on the way to developing superpowers and is similar to the concentration of the magician before he casts a spell. As a state of decreased awareness, cataleptic trance is opposed to the yogic path, since it leads to stupor and a rise of ego, with the powers that come with it. It is the opposite of objectless *samadhi*, which is supercognitive ecstasy or ecstatic trance. In objectless *samadhi* one may fall into trance because the view of millions of universes arising simultaneously out of Brahman is so powerful that one might not be able to react if approached. In the same way, a candle cannot be seen if held against the blazing sun.

This highest *samadhi* is the greatest possible increase in awareness, exactly the opposite of cataleptic or catatonic trance.

It is a tragic error, suggested by some commentators, that freedom might be attained through the childish exercise of completely shutting out the world through willpower. Will is nothing but ego. The world exists, according to sutra II.21, only for the purpose of self-realization, and therefore no shutting out is required. Any act of willpower will only deter us from realizing that the world exists just for us to experience ourselves as infinite consciousness. The world is no trap, but a road to freedom. The body is not filthy, but the vehicle to freedom on that road.

Chapter III: On Powers

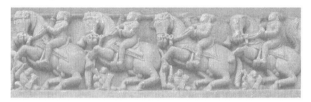

देशबन्धश्चित्तस्य धारणा ॥ १ ॥
III.1 Concentration is fixing the mind to a place.

The five outer limbs (*bahirangas*) have been explained. Now we go on to the inner limbs (*antarangas*). The sixth limb, concentration (*dharana*), is defined as confining the mind to a point in space. Patanjali uses the term *chitta* again here for mind, which encompasses intellect (*buddhi*), ego (*ahamkara*), and mind (*manas*). Vyasa explains that concentration is exercised by fixing the mind on an external or internal object. Internal objects are the lotuses (*chakras*), chiefly the navel center, the heart center, the third eye, and the crown of the head. The tip of the nose and tip of the tongue are also mentioned.

Concentration is focused as well on the inner sound or heart sound (*anahata nada*), which features strongly in the *Hatha Yoga Pradipika*. Binding the mind to the light in the heart lotus (*jyoti*) has been mentioned already in sutra I.36, and a clarifying effect is ascribed to it.

External objects that are suitable for concentration are those that belong to the category of sacred objects. Typically this would be the image of one's chosen deity or something similar. The object must be sattvic in quality, as rajasic objects would agitate the mind and tamasic objects stupefy it. Only sattvic objects fill the mind with effulgent wisdom.

Western observers have often misunderstood India due to its many deities. But the deities are only expressions of the one infinite consciousness (Brahman). They are meditation and concentration devices, and in that context are called *saguna brahman* or Brahman with form. If Brahman is worshiped directly without image, then it is called *nirguna brahman*, the formless. There is no conflict between the two, only a lack of understanding. Kabir has said that *saguna* and *nirguna* are one.

Concentration now means that the modifications or fluctuations of the mind are kept in that chosen place. For instance, if a thought having as its object the light in the heart is brought to an end, it is then replaced by another thought of the same kind. If one thinks continuously of the light in the heart, that practice is called concentration.

If the original thought is replaced involuntarily by thoughts concerning completely different objects, this is not concentration. Some sources say that concentration is achieved only once it can be held for one and a half hours. If in our *vinyasa* practice we keep the mind bound to the breath, which is a sacred object (the *Brahma Sutra* says breath is the Brahman), then this is concentration practice.

तत्र प्रत्ययैकतानता ध्यानम् ॥ २ ॥
III.2 If in that place of *dharana* there is an uninterrupted flow of awareness toward the object, then this is meditation (*dhyana*).

There are many concepts about meditation. The word is often used in the sense of thinking about something. If I am thinking about something, I might be approaching an object from different angles or I might be thinking about aspects that do not represent the object as a whole anymore. This all still comes under the yogic heading of *dharana*, which includes deliberating or reflecting on an object, and it usually creates a beta brain-wave pattern. If, through focusing, I prevent any other object than the one chosen from entering my mind, this creates the brain-wave pattern of concentration, the beta pattern.

In meditation the mind relaxes and switches to an alpha pattern, which brings a deeper communion with the object, but it is only called *dhyana* if there is an uninterrupted flow of awareness toward the chosen object. In yogic meditation we are in *asana* and *pranayama*, with the senses withdrawn and the mind concentrated. If we then add the continuous awareness of an object that is not present in *dharana* (concentration), then it is called *dhyana*. In *dharana* there is a stop-and-go process that we constantly have to kick-start by dodging the distractions. In meditation there is uninterrupted flow toward the object, which means that the connection with the object is not interrupted anymore.

The use of the term "object" is another source of misunderstanding, as it is often taken to mean a thing. But the object is only what we are focusing on — for example the breath in *asana*. One of the ultimate objects of meditation is *shunyata* — emptiness, the great void — which is an aspect of Brahman. In yoga, void is regarded as one of the most difficult "objects" to focus on. The mind has the tendency always to attach itself to the next thought arising, and if it has a choice between void and thought it usually chooses thought. Therefore emptiness is not a good meditation object for beginners. Otherwise we'll be sitting and thinking, then remembering void, thinking then remembering void — which is something in between *pratyahara* and *dharana*, but not *dhyana*.

Shankara describes the difference between *dharana* and *dhyana* thus: "Whereas *dharana* is touched by other ideas imagined about the object, even though the mind has been settled on that object alone — if made on the sun, its orbit and extreme brilliance are also the object of the concentration, for the mind is functioning on the location as a pure mental process — not so with *dhyana*, for there it is only the stream of a single idea, untouched by any other idea of different kind."[1]

1. T. Leggett, *Shankara on the Yoga Sutras*, p. 283.

तद् एवार्थमात्रनिर्भासं स्वरूपशून्यम् इव समाधिः ॥ ३ ॥

III.3 If in that meditation the object only shines forth without being modified by the mind at all, that is *samadhi*.

This is a simple working definition, which defines only objectless (*samprajnata*) *samadhi*. The sutra in fact is almost identical with I.41, which defines *samapatti*, the state of mind during objectless *samadhi*. There the purified mind is likened to a clear crystal that is capable of faithfully reflecting whatever it is placed on. The three inner limbs are as follows:

6 *dharana*: The mind thinks about one object and avoids other thoughts; awareness of the object is still interrupted.

7 *dhyana*: There is a continuous flow of awareness toward the same object.

8 *samadhi*: There is utter stillness and no more movement in the mind. Only the object shines. The mind as we know it has seemingly ceased to exist. Therefore the object can be exactly replicated and we can gain complete knowledge of it.

The usual activity of the mind is to download sensory input relating to an object and then to compare it with all the data it has stored in the past. It then produces the most likely interpretation of what it believes the object to be. For example, the senses report a loud roar to the mind and mind says, "Train approaching fast — step back." This is typical of how the mind works. It always analyzes the impact an object has on us — Does it threaten our survival? Can we gain from it? and so on. The mind is never interested in the object-as-such. Since the mind is analyzing superficial fast-changing appearances, it cannot perceive the underlying deep reality of an object — pure unmodified object-ness or such-ness.

When, now in *samadhi*, the mind waves have subsided, consciousness/self can directly experience the object on which our meditation (*dhyana*) is based. In fact only then, when we do not look anymore through the distorting glasses of our mind, can an object be directly experienced. This is the true meaning of direct experience. If we see an object through our senses and then the information passes through the various filters of our mentation, we can hardly call this direct, but rather relayed experience. Direct experience of the deep reality of an object, its suchness, can only be had in the mystical experience, when the modifying mentation ceases.

The activity of the mind is beautifully shown in the Buddhist story of an elephant being presented to four blind men for identification. The first grasps the trunk and believes the elephant to be a tube; the second takes hold of the ear and believes it to be a sheet of paper; the third gets hold of the leg and believes the animal to be a tree trunk; and the last apprehends the tail and takes the elephant to be a brush. In a similar way our mind sees only part of an object due to our inner blindness, whereas the intrinsic nature of the object is hidden from our view. This process is called misapprehension. By placing layers on layers of misapprehension, it believes it comes closer to the truth. While this might be a great method for acquiring day-to-day skills, if we want to find out about the true nature of things we need to use comprehension instead of apprehension. Comprehension occurs where the ripples of the surface of the mind have subsided and it is so still that consciousness can get an undistorted view of the object.

Vijnanabhikshu affirms in his commentary *Yogavarttika* that the definition of *samadhi* given here is only pertaining to *samadhi* "connected with some place" and "will not cover *samadhi* which is not limited (by some place)."[2] The latter is of course seedless or supercognitive *samadhi*, in which all objects are removed and "*Mahamudra* (consciousness) rests on nought," as Tilopa says.[3] Then we recognize ourselves as consciousness.

त्रयम् एकत्र संयमः ॥ ४ ॥
III.4 If the three are practiced together it is called *samyama*.

If *dharana*, *dhyana*, and objective *samadhi* are practiced simultaneously on the very same object, this process is called *samyama*. Whereas objectless *samadhi* is a technique that eventually culminates in reaching permanent self-knowledge, *samyama* is a method for obtaining complete knowledge of something external. This does not happen in objectless *samadhi*, because in that state the mind is at rest.

Samyama is based on objective (*samprajnata*) *samadhi*. Objectless *samadhi* cannot be combined with *dharana* and *dhyana*, as they rely on objects. Objectless *samadhi* relies on the subject, which can arise only once the objects vanish. The mere definition of *samyama* means that the *samadhi* involved can only be *samprajnata samadhi* — *samadhi* with consciousness of an object.

To get to objective *samadhi* we apply *dharana*, *dhyana*, and *samadhi* sequentially; in *samyama* they need to be applied simultaneously. This is much more difficult than sequential application. Usually the trace of egoity left in *dharana* prevents *samadhi*.

तज्जयात् प्रज्ञाऽऽलोकः ॥ ५ ॥
III.5 From mastery of *samyama* shines the light of knowledge (*prajna*).

Vyasa adds that the more one becomes established in it, the stronger the light of knowledge shines. There is a gradual mastery in this difficult technique, which is the very technique by which the *rishi*s gained all their knowledge. They did not study for a lifetime like scientists, nor did they perfect a particular art, but they first attained self-knowledge and then downloaded all that was to be known about their subject of interest, whether it was medicine, astrology, astronomy, yoga, grammar, law, or whatever.

Thus, at the dawn of time, humanity started out on the highest possible level. Then, because we lost ourselves, knowledge of the world became more and more broken up and scattered until we reached our present state in Kali Yuga (the age of darkness). *Prajna*, which we can translate as knowledge or

2. *Yogavarttika of Vijnanabhikshu*, vol. 3, trans. T.S. Rukmani, Munshiram Manoharlal, New Delhi, 1998, p. 6.
3. G.C.C. Chang, trans., *Teachings and Practice of Tibetan Tantra*, p. 25.

insight, is the property of the intellect (buddhi) after it has been made sattvic. It is a state prior to discriminative knowledge (viveka khyateh) and features prominently in the Yoga Sutra. The seven stages in which prajna arises are set out in sutra II.27.

The reason why samyama is practiced is that it makes the intellect sattvic and therefore fitted for discriminative knowledge. This knowledge arises in the intellect, not in consciousness, the intellect being the seat of intelligence.

The difference between intellect and consciousness is as follows. Consciousness is forever free and aware. Everything exists in it already. Nothing can arise in it; otherwise it would be mutable. The intellect, however, can be aware or unaware of an object. If we suddenly attain discriminative knowledge, whereas we were ignorant before, by definition this means that this knowledge arose in the fluctuating intellect. The intellect, having gained discriminative knowledge, disconnects from consciousness. That state then is called independence (kaivalya), in which the erroneously superimposed identity of intellect and consciousness is erased and the correct knowledge of freedom of consciousness is cognized.

तस्य भूमिषु विनियोगः ॥ ६ ॥
III.6 Samyama is applied in stages.

Samyama is a difficult technique. For this reason the practitioner needs to start with a simple gross object such as a lotus flower. Later, only complex gross objects such as the universe are chosen. Only if gross objects are completely mastered does one switch to subtle objects, which are the subtle essence of the elements — the chakras, the mind, the senses, and so on.

Vyasa points out that, if the higher application is already mastered through the grace of the Supreme Being, one should not go back and engage in the lower form, for example by reading people's minds. There is great responsibility in such powers, but all too often people degrade themselves by using them to manipulate others. Vyasa refers here to sutra II.45, according to which the perfection of samadhi is obtained by devotion to the Supreme Being. Such a person, says Vyasa, should not go back to techniqueing, but rather stay in their high view.

Shankara calls telepathy a petty stage compared to atman realization.[4] Ishvara pranidhana, devotion to the Supreme Being, is here taken as a short cut, a view strongly emphasized in the Bhagavad Gita. If that short cut has been taken, then one should not retrogress by going back to methods whose aims have already been achieved.

Vijnanabhikshu uses the analogy of an archer who first trains to pierce big (gross) and then tiny (subtle) objects.[5] It is in a similar way that the yogi has to proceed with samyama.

त्रयम् अन्तरङ्गं पूर्वेभ्यः ॥ ७ ॥
III.7 These three limbs are the inner ones compared to the prior ones [those covered in chapter II].

Yama, niyama, asana, pranayama, and pratyahara are the outer limbs because they involve us from the mind outward. Called preparatory yoga by some commentators, the outer limbs are not an end in themselves.

Vyasa says the last three limbs are the direct means to samadhi, and Vijnanabhikshu elaborates by commenting that the first five limbs are therefore the indirect means to samadhi. According to him, any outward action must be given up at some point, because it is an obstacle to samadhi.[6] He then quotes a passage from the Yoga Vashishta, according to which, just as the flight of a bird in the sky requires the use of both wings, similarly the highest place is obtained by both knowledge and action. Equating knowledge with the inner limbs and action with the outer limbs, he says the quotation "only suggests, in a general way, the combined practice of both as means and the end. They are not intended as accomplishing liberation together."[7]

Shankara is even clearer. Commenting on Vyasa's reference to the inner limbs as the direct means, he says, "He wishes to show that even though the previous ones [outer limbs] may not have been perfected, effort should be made at these three."[8] This

4. T. Leggett, Shankara on the Yoga Sutra, p. 285.
5. Yogavarttika of Vijnanabhikshu, vol. 3, trans. T. S. Rukmani, p. 9.
6. Ibid., p. 12.
7. Ibid.
8. T. Leggett, Shankara on the Yoga Sutras, p. 286.

means that, even if we have not perfected *asana*, we should make an attempt at the last three limbs, because only these limbs can lead to liberation. From the evidence of *shastra* (scripture), it appears that the ancient masters and authorities accepted *asana* only as a preparation for true yoga. A life confined to *asana* practice appears wasted in the light of *shastra*.

There is a modern, predominantly Western, concept that reduces yoga to *asana* practice. *Asana* is an integral part of yoga, especially for beginners. To reduce yoga to this one limb, however, does it an injustice.

तद् अपि बहिरङ्गं निर्बीजस्य ॥ ८ ॥
III.8 Yet *dharana, dhyana,* and *samadhi* are outer limbs compared to seedless *samadhi.*

This sutra affirms what Patanjali previously said about *samprajnata samadhi*, which is *samadhi* with seed (of new embodiment). *Samadhi* with seed rests on an external object (such as the intellect) and therefore the individual retains its boundaries and conscious identity. It can be used to gain knowledge about the world (in *samyama*) but it still leaves seeds of new *karma* and future lives because we do not leave our boundaries and become one with the ocean of existence.

This happens only in seedless (*nirbija*) *samadhi*, where no trace or seed of egoity is left. It is also referred to as *asamprajnata samadhi*, or superconscious *samadhi*, because we leave our conscious identity and become one with superconsciousness (Brahman).

Seedless *samadhi* is an utterly useless experience. It cannot be used in *samyama* to become more knowledgeable and powerful. And the chances are that, after you experience it, you'll be even less interested in your advantages over others. After you have seen the *atman* in you as the *atman* in everyone, it becomes somewhat less interesting to be better, greater, or more intelligent than fellow human beings.

Samyama and *samprajnata samadhi*, in which we still participate in the game of gain and loss, are nothing but preparations for seedless *samadhi*.

Why are they called preparations or external actions compared to seedless *samadhi*? "On account of its appearance on the cessation of the trio."[9]

This means that seedless or objectless *samadhi* cannot be achieved or produced; it happens from the cessation or letting go of the others (*dharana, dhyana,* and objective *samadhi*). We cannot achieve or practice objectless *samadhi*; we can only abide in it. Shankara states, in his *Brahma Sutra Commentary*, "Liberation is the state of identity with Brahman, and hence it is not to be achieved through purification. Besides, nobody can show any mode whereby liberation can be associated with action. Accordingly, apart from knowledge alone, there cannot be the slightest touch of action here."[10]

No human or superhuman effort can reveal the splendor of infinite consciousness. It is only the cessation of that very effort that makes us recognize that the very presence we are looking for is eternally there in our heart. It cannot be grasped or confined; it will come when we utterly cease to run after it, by grace. We then realize, as the *Samkhya Karika* states, "No one therefore, is bound; no one released, likewise no one transmigrates [incarnates]."[11]

It is consciousness — us — that is never bound, never released and never incarnates. It is only due to ignorance that we believe ourselves to be bound. Objectless *samadhi* is nothing but coming home, coming home to ourselves. This can happen only if we surrender and cease action. It happens through cessation of the inner limbs, which cease after the outer limbs cease.

Why then do we practice in the first place? Vedanta, like Zen Buddhism, suggests surrendering right on the spot. This is the absolute approach, in which the entire distance toward truth is covered in one step. Any technique here is seen as a lie veiling the truth that we are the truth already. For someone who cannot understand this high view, who cannot take this one step, systems like Yoga, Tibetan Buddhism, and Tantra operate within relative truth and approach absolute truth in several small steps.

It is not a logical approach, since you cannot

9. *Yogasutra of Patanjali*, trans. and comm. B. Baba, Motilal Banarsidass, Delhi, 1976, p. 68.

10. *Brahma Sutra Bhasya of Sri Sankaracarya*, trans. Sw. Gambhirananda, Advaita Ashrama, Kolkata, 1965, p. 34.

11. G.J. Larson, *Classical Samkhya*, 2nd rev. ed., Motilal Banarsidass, Delhi, 1979, p. 274.

manifest Brahman. It is always here. But yoga does not deal with Brahman. Brahman is not Patanjali's concern. His concern is our ignorance. If we can reduce ignorance we will eventually see Brahman.

But yoga is not necessary to realize the absolute truth. One who has no ignorance can realize truth in one step simply by ceasing to identify with what is impermanent, such as the mind. Vijnanabhikshu affirms this when he says, "As they [dharana, dhyana, samadhi] are indirect causes [they] are not necessary [directly] to achieve asamprajnata."[12] Shankara goes even further by saying, "Yoga can be effected even without going through the five-fold means [outer limbs], from the mere accomplishment of the triad of concentration, meditation and samadhi."[13]

He also suggests that "mastery of posture [is] not, in the case of distracted people, productive of yoga. Getting rid of the defects, and samadhi — these two will certainly produce it, and nothing else will."[14]

व्युत्थाननिरोधसंस्कारयोरभिभवप्रादुर्भावौ निरोधक्षणचित्तान्वयो निरोधपरिणामः ॥ ९ ॥

III.9 When the subconscious imprint (samskara) of mental fluctuation is replaced with an imprint of cessation [of mental activity], then there is a moment of cessation of mental activity, which is known as transformation (parinama) toward cessation (nirodha).

We know now that consciousness is forever free and unchangeable. So why should we practice if we can't change anyway? And why should we practice, since we are free already?

The fact is that the majority of people can get nothing out of the information that they are free already. Most of us hear that and then just keep suffering. Another reason the information is unhelpful is that, though we are immutable consciousness, we experience constant change and identify with it. For those who cannot spontaneously abide in consciousness, Patanjali presents the psychology of change (parinama). Every negative subconscious

imprint (samskara) is here replaced by a positive subconscious imprint. In this way — slowly, step-by-step — we can transform our personality. Even if we started as a vicious, homicidal thug, we can transform ourselves into a sage, as the yogi Milarepa has demonstrated.[15]

There are some modern forms of therapy in which the content of the subconscious is replaced in a similar fashion to the processes of Patanjali's yoga. The difference between those approaches and yoga is that, in the latter, the question of which imprints are wanted is clearly defined. The choice is not left to the client. The discouraged subconscious imprints are those of mental noise; the encouraged ones are those of mental stillness.

Patanjali gives hope to those who have listened to and understood the lofty discourses of nondualistic teachers but have experienced no positive changes as a result. To those downtrodden ones Patanjali extends his helping hand: "If we slowly change our personality (vasana) from ignorant (avidya) to wise (prajna) we will eventually see the light of knowledge (jnana) even if we weren't able to do so initially."

In this way, yoga is a very forgiving, down-to-earth approach that takes into account the human condition and allows us to progress at our own rate. However big our failures and however deep our despondency initially, we just keep going, knowing that no effort we make is ever lost.[16] Even if we cannot see the light of knowledge now because our mind is clogged up, change (parinama) is possible. The change or transformation toward stillness happens by replacing the subconscious impressions of mental clutter by those of stillness.

There is no mental fluctuation without its subconscious impression. This needs to be deeply understood. It means that our mind will eternally just keep going as long as we let it run wild. If that impression of mental noise is, however, overpowered by a stronger impression of cessation of mental activity, there is a moment of silence in the mind. In that moment we get a glimpse of our true nature as consciousness.

12. *Yogavarttika of Vijnanabhikshu*, vol. 3, trans. T. S. Rukmani, p. 14.
13. T. Leggett, *Shankara on the Yoga Sutra*, p. 287.
14. Ibid.

15. W. Y. Evans-Wentz, ed., *Tibet's Great Yogi Milarepa*, 2nd ed., Munshiram Manoharlal, Delhi, 2000.
16. *Bhagavad Gita* VI.41–42.

The same happens if we have a near-death experience. The mind is overpowered by a much stronger *samskara* and is arrested for a moment. For many people who have had this experience, it has triggered a spiritual quest. In the short time that the mind is arrested, one can experience *jnana*, the knowledge of the self. Even if the experience comes to an end, the memory remains, and that is often enough to start the search for what is real, what does not change in the face of death.

तस्य प्रशान्तवाहिता संस्कारात् ॥ १० ॥

III.10 The mind stays calm through repeatedly applying imprints (*samskara*) of cessation of its activity.

As an imprint of stillness can give us a moment of calm, so can continued calm be achieved by repeated input of the same or similar subconscious imprints. One such method is the use of mantra. To repeat a mantra is to repeat the same subconscious imprint of peace. Again, to meditate on the breath is nothing but placing repeated imprints of calmness. Even to meditate at a certain time of the day or special place means to instill a certain habit that assists the mind to calm down.

Every state of mind has the tendency to call for its repetition. If we are in a state of calmness for one hour, this in itself will set a tendency for the future. If we then get agitated, aggressive, or depressed, this also will call for repetition due to the imprints it leaves. If we constantly put in place imprints of calmness, the mind will slowly let go of its agitation and dullness and become calm.

In placing *samskara*s, one needs to be careful not to wrestle with one's own mind, since that is nothing but agitation, which will make the mind angry. Rather we have to invite it gently into stillness. If an attempt is made to subdue a raging bull, it will get even angrier; if, however, it is led onto a green pasture, with no red rags around, it will calm down.

In order to keep the mind calm, one has to supply a steady stream of imprints of stillness. That is what many meditation techniques do.

सर्वार्थतैकाग्रतयोः क्षयोदयौ चित्तस्य समाधि-परिणामः ॥ ११ ॥

III.11 If the scattering of the mind is replaced by one-pointedness, then this is called the *samadhi* transformation (*parinama*) of the mind.

Patanjali again uses the term *parinama*, this time in the context of *samadhi*. *Samadhi parinama* or *samadhi* transformation of the mind denotes the condition that makes the mind fit for *samadhi*. The *samadhi* referred to here is objective *samadhi*. Transformation toward objectless *samadhi* is referred to as *nirodha parinama*.

Vyasa explains that scatteredness is typical of the mind. After all, it has the tendency to attach itself to the next arising object. But, he continues, one-pointedness is another characteristic of the very same mind. Patanjali will affirm this later in sutra IV.23, where he says that the mind is colored by whatever it is directed to, whether this be the seer or the seen.

Due to the manifoldness of the seen, directing the mind toward the seen results in scattering. If it is directed toward the seer it will become one-pointed, due to the uniformity of the seer. This change of quality is a capacity of the mind and not of the seer, which is immutable.

If, then, the mind turns away from the seen and toward the seer, it thus becomes fit for *samadhi*. This process is called *samadhi* transformation. It is achieved unconsciously through the mere passing of time or consciously through negation or turning away from the seen. If, in our quest to become free, we become disappointed over and over again by the inability of external stimuli to provide lasting happiness, we will eventually turn away from them to find the kingdom within. This process of unconscious *samadhi* transformation is considered to take approximately thirty trillion incarnations per being.

Alternatively, we may consciously negate all objects we are drawn to, which will shorten this time to as little as one life span, as some sources claim. In some cases it may happen in an instant, but traditional authorities hasten to explain that those rare individuals have put in their work in previous incarnations.

The technique of negation works like this. When we sit and meditate and the mind turns, for example, to the accumulation of wealth, we say to ourselves that wealth is transitory and can be lost in an instant. Even if we are prudent, the world could plunge into a global economic crisis, or the country in which we live could be destroyed by war. Therefore it would be unwise to rely for happiness on the accumulation of wealth.

The mind may then suggest making the pursuit of sensual pleasure our quest. To this we say that the body will age and become diseased, and then others may not be interested in experiencing sensual pleasure with us. It is therefore not wise to rely for happiness on the availability of sensual pleasure.

The mind may then turn to friendship and relationships with others as a possible goal. We reject this by pointing out that all those others are transitory and will die, which will leave us alone and disappointed unless we die first. Relationships are transitory. We therefore should not rely on them for happiness. We also need to consider that this attitude would destroy our relationships because we are coming from need. Interest in another just because of their capacity to fulfill one's needs is usage and not relationship.

The mind may then suggest making the body healthy and fit so that it will resist the effects of time. We reject this by pointing out that, however much we care for this body, it is subject to death. It is transitory. If we rely on transitory objects for happiness we will be disappointed.

In this way we negate and reject all suggestions of the mind one by one, since they are all transitory. Eventually, the mind will turn to the only permanent support, which is the seer. This is *samadhi* transformation of the mind.

When working with this process, one shouldn't be discouraged by frequent setbacks. According to Vijnanabhikshu, "There cannot be a total eradication of distraction all at once, nor can there be the achievement of one-pointedness all at once, but only gradually, moment by moment."[17]

ततः पुनः शान्तोदितौ तुल्यप्रत्ययौ चित्तस्यैकाग्रतापरिणामः ॥ १२ ॥

III.12 If there is similarity of that idea that arises to the one that subsides, this is called one-pointedness (eka-grata) transformation of the mind.

If we have come to the point that, during meditation, an arising thought wave has a similarity to the previous one, the mind is transforming to one-pointedness. The word used by Patanjali to describe the relationship between the two thought waves is *tulya*, which can be translated as "similar," "of the same kind," or "equal." If we are meditating on, let us say, the light in the heart, and every newly arising thought wave is roughly equal to the previous one, this is one-pointed mind.

The state of transformation described here is a more modest achievement than the two previous ones, *samadhi parinama* and *nirodha parinama*. It is quite common for yoga masters to start their description with the more advanced states. Since they live from a position of knowledge (*jnana*), they describe first what is close to them, the truth. Only then do they describe the states applying to beginners.

The process described here is called converting mind into intellect. Let us recall that mind (*manas*) is that form of thinking that jumps from one subject to another like a monkey from branch to branch. Mind deals with future or past, which is why it never stops. There are endless possibilities of what the future could bring, and all of them supply fuel to the mind.

Intellect, on the contrary, tends to think about the present. It thinks about one theme until complete comprehension is achieved. To make the mind a yogic tool, we need to convert it into intellect. *Dharana* exercises are used until the thought process can stay with the chosen object. The mind is then called one-pointed (*ekagra*). The transformation toward this state is called one-pointedness transformation (*ekagrata parinama*) of the mind.

17. *Yogavarttika of Vijnanabhikshu*, vol. 3, trans. T. S. Rukmani, p. 19.

एतेन भूतेन्द्रियेषु धर्मलक्षणावस्थापरिणामा
व्याख्याताः ॥ १३ ॥

III.13 By this have also been described the transformations of characteristic (*dharma*), manifestation, and condition pertaining to elements and sense organs.

So far Patanjali has applied his model of three transformations to the mind (*chitta*) only. Now he says the same is valid for the gross (elements) and the subtle (senses). In other words, the transformation of the qualities (*gunas*) of one's mind follows the same laws as the transformation of the gross and subtle world. This explains why yogis who are in control of their minds can control their surroundings as well. By applying the laws of transformation of mind one can transform the world also. This is how the powers (*siddhis*) are produced.

Patanjali talks of transformation pertaining to three aspects: those of characteristic, of manifestation, and of condition. If we look at the mind, transformation of characteristic would be, for example, if the mind changes from single-pointed to suspended (*nirodha*). In *nirodha* the characteristic of the mind has changed so much that we could refer to it now as no-mind.

Change of manifestation would be whether the mind rests in the present on the one hand or in the past and future on the other. If the mind rests in the present moment, *samadhi* transformation of the mind has taken place.

The third category, transformation of condition, relates to what types of fluctuations arise and what types of imprints (*samskaras*) and conditioning (*vasana*) exist in the mind. A case of change of condition would be, for example, when the *samskaras* of focus become strong while the *samskaras* of scattering become weak. Here the mind does not change its fundamental characteristic, nor does it change its time mode (manifestation), but within those parameters it changes its ability to focus on one meditation object. In the previous sutra this was called converting mind into intellect.

Not only the mind but also all objects undergo these three types of transformation. Since the mind is an object too, it undergoes the same transformation. Only consciousness (*purusha*), which is the sole non-object, does not undergo transformation, since it is eternal and immutable.

Gross objects are made up of the gross elements ether, air, fire, water, and earth. The most fundamental type of transformation they undergo is change of characteristic, meaning that after the change has taken place the object is still there, but it has changed its characteristic so much that we cannot recognize it anymore as the object.

Let us choose the human body as an example. When a person dies we usually either bury the body or cremate it. If buried, the body will break down through the process of decay. The main part will transform into ammonia and will be processed through the nitrogen cycle into nitrates and phosphates, which are plant fertilizers. Most of the body will reappear above ground as plant matter. Similarly, if we cremate the body, apart from the minerals, which are left behind in the form of ash, the rest of the body is transformed into a gaseous state. Most of these gases will be returned to earth via rain or filtered out of the air by plants via photosynthesis. In both cases we have a change of characteristic of the object. All the atoms, molecules, and energy that made up the object are retained, but they take on a completely new form. We would say today one object is transformed into others.

The second type of transformation, change of manifestation, is also sometimes called change of temporal character. It is important here to understand that yoga says objects are real. Nothing that is real can ever become unreal and nothing unreal can ever become real. If for example we build a house, and after a hundred years it is destroyed by an earthquake, then yoga says the house was real all the time; otherwise we could never have built it. It changes only its manifestation. Before we built it, the house was unmanifest — in its seed state or potential state. In this state we can receive a vision of it, a vision that can be manifested. The potential state is also called future state. It means this object can manifest in the future. When we build the house it becomes manifest or it moves into the present state. Once it is destroyed it has changed to the residue or past state. Every object that was once manifested leaves a residue in the world. We might remember the house; photos or plans of it might remain.

We can easily understand this pattern when we look at the discovery of America by Christopher Columbus. He had no idea that it was there, but if it hadn't been real he could never have discovered it. Similarly, discoveries of physical laws by physicists can only be made if something real is there.

It is not that we create the laws — we only discover them; they are revealed to us. We have not, for example, created electricity or magnetism. If they hadn't been real all the time we could not have discovered them. Or let us say their discovery would have been a mere concept. As a mere concept, however, it would not have allowed us to use electricity for lighting.

There are indigenous cultures where children are not unconsciously conceived but where one of the parents will go off and dream the child from the seed state into the manifest state. We can recognize here the humble realization that it is not the parents that produce a human: they merely provide the body. The purpose of the dreaming is to find a human being that agrees to be born at this particular time into this particular family. This way we achieved a much more harmonious family life in the past. Interesting here is the ignorance of Western culture, which holds the belief that a human being has its beginning at conception.

There are objects in yoga that are called unreal. They cannot become manifest because they do not exist in the seed state either. They are either conceptualizations, meaning mere words with no objects attached, like the rabbit's horn, the sky flower, or the castle in the sky, or they are illusions like the snake that actually is a rope. These objects are unreal or nonobjects, and therefore cannot become real.

The third type of transformation, change of condition, occurs while an object retains its characteristic and state of manifestation. If we look at the human body we would say it is first young, then mature, and then old. Most structures in the manifest world, like empires, governments, churches, religions, societies, and companies, go through a cycle of three phases — the establishment phase, the consolidation phase, and the dissolution phase.

Through all of these phases the object is still recognizable as the same object, but its appearance may change significantly.

शान्तोदिताव्यपदेश्यधर्मानुपाती धर्मी ॥ १४ ॥

III.14 That essence, which is always there in the past, future, and present, is called the object-as-such.

If we practice deep meditation or *samyama* on an object, we will look through its state of manifestation and observe its essence. Since the essence is unchanged whether the object is in the past, present, or future state, or in other words whether it is in the potential, manifest, or residue state, it is called the object-as-such. This object-as-such also does not change when the object changes from young to old. The object-as-such can be likened to the blueprint of an object. Without it no object can manifest.

There is an important difference here between Yoga and Samkhya on the one hand and Vedanta and Buddhism on the other. In Vedanta, the world of objects is seen as a mirage superimposed on consciousness. In Buddhism objects exist only as momentary notions in the mind. In both systems of thought there are no objects independent of mind: they are created entirely through the misapprehensions of the observer.

Yoga is radically different. The world and objects are seen as real. There is a clear distinction between real objects and conceptualizations such as the sky flower that are based only on words. Not only that, but yoga assigns an eternal aspect to objects, called their essence, which is completely independent of the observer. It is important for the yogi to perceive the object-as-such, or the such-ness of an object, because from perceiving real objects outside ourselves comes discriminative knowledge, the knowledge according to which we are different from the objects. From that eventually comes *kaivalya*, complete independence from the world of objects.

That yoga attests to the reality of the world is very interesting for a Western audience. Everyone who has been to India realizes that a certain "The world does not matter" attitude abounds. When I was traveling there in the mid-1980s I often had to line up for several hours at a train ticket counter. People brought foldable chairs and wrapped lunches, and everyone was fairly content in the queue. The idea was that, if we have thirty trillion incarnations to live through, why not spend a hundred of them in front of the ticket counter. If all objects are only mirages superimposed on consciousness, then the ticket counter is really only consciousness and this place is as good as any other to be.

On another occasion I was swimming in a large lake in India a few hundred yards out when a crowd gathered at the shore and watched quietly. When I returned to the shore, I asked the spectators what was so interesting about a swimming Westerner. A young man told me they were just watching to see whether Mandjula would come and get me. It turned out that Mandjula was a very large crocodile that, according to him, had already eaten twelve people. When I asked why nobody had called out to get me back to the shore, his reply was that whether I was eaten or not was my fate, and interception couldn't change it. Or, if they had intervened, I would only walk into the fangs of a hungry tiger behind the next tree.

I do not want to belittle this view. It is very powerful and definitely has its advantages. However it leads to a certain apathy in Indian society, a belief that it is not really worth changing things. It has its origin in the doctrine of Advaita Vedanta that the world does not matter because it is not real. Shankara himself suggests in *Vivekachudamani* that one should look at the world with the same indifference with which one looks at the droppings of a crow.

It is probably not completely fair to say the world does not matter in the Indian view, but there is a huge difference between the Indian way of happily enduring malfunctions of society that make absolutely no sense and the Western way of frantically changing everything that doesn't work (and often things that do work). Western society made a decision a long time ago that the world was to be looked at as real. On the other hand, however, we denied the existence of consciousness as being completely independent from matter.

Every young Westerner who studies Eastern mysticism should think clearly whether we want to go all the way and adopt a philosophy that denies the reality of the world. And then, if we have made up our minds, we should do that consciously, knowing what it means with all its cultural repercussions and not just unconsciously as a package deal.

Yoga beautifully combines both views, as both world and consciousness are seen as real. It seems to be far easier to reconcile it with our society's values than is the extreme idealistic view of Vedanta.

क्रमान्यत्वं परिणामान्यत्वे हेतुः ॥ १५ ॥
III.15 The differentiation of transformation is caused by differentiation in sequence.

Why is it that Patanjali does not, like most teachers, just talk uniformly of change but subdivides change into three categories?

The answer is that in deep meditation different sequences of change can be recognized. From these sequences three different forms of change can be inferred. Vyasa explains that when dust gets turned into a lump of clay, then into an earthen pot, the pot will eventually break and the piece will disintegrate to dust again. The essence in this sequence is clay, which changes its characteristic in each step.

If we look at the pot as the essence, then, as the pot gets formed from clay, it moves from its potential state into the manifest state. When it breaks, it moves from the manifest into the residue state, which also means it moves from the present into the past, which is the second type of change.

The third type of change is when characteristic and manifestation do not change. Nevertheless after years of use we see that the past changes. It might look worn or cracks might appear.

According to Vyasa the observation of these sequences leads to the conclusion that objects are different from their characteristics, manifestations, and states. In other words if objects were only appearances superimposed on consciousness or momentary notions in the mind, such sequences could not be observed. Understanding the three changes in objects will lead to understanding of the changes of mind. This will help us to change the mind in the direction we want.

परिणामत्रयसंयमाद् अतीतानागतज्ञानम् ॥ १६ ॥

III.16 From *samyama* on the three types of transformation comes knowledge of past and future.

Patanjali starts a series of aphorisms that list the different types of supernormal powers. Having described the term *parinama* (transformation) and its three mental types (suspension, *samadhi,* and one-pointedness) and material types (characteristic, manifestation, and condition), he has defined that their differences are inferred from sequence. Sequence is nothing but succession in time. By practicing the combined form of *dharana, dhyana,* and *samadhi* on the governing aspect of trans-formation, which is succession in time, we get knowledge of time itself and what it seems to hide: past and future.

May I point out here that we are dealing the whole time with the relative world of mind and matter, which occur in time as do transformation and sequence. All of them occur in the absolute world of consciousness, which is timeless. If *samyama* is done now on the characteristic, time aspect, and condition of a particular object, the past and future of that object can be known. *Samyama* reveals not only the essence of the object — the object-as-such — but also when and how it changes.

Samyama on the change of characteristic of an object reveals what kind of object it was before and into what it will transform after it ceases to exist in this form.

Samyama on the change of manifestation of an object will reveal when it becomes manifest and when it will change into the residue state, which means when it becomes past.

Samyama on the change of condition of an object reveals its aging process, which also means how long it has existed in its present form and how long it will continue to exist in this form.

We have to remember, though, that no such knowledge leads to freedom. From the point of view of true yoga, exercizing such powers is a petty achievement. Vijnanabhikshu points out in his sub-commentary to the *Yoga Sutra* that the "respective *samyama* are to be practised only by those yogis who desire those respective powers, whereas those

who desire strongly only liberation should practise *samyama* only on the difference between the intellect and *purusha* (consciousness)."[18]

शब्दार्थप्रत्यानाम् इतरेतराध्यासात् संकरः ।
तत्प्रविभागसंयमात् सर्वभूतरुतज्ञानम् ॥ १७ ॥

III.17 There is always a mix-up between a word, the object referred to, and the concept behind the word. If *samyama* is done on all three consecutively, one can understand the communication of all beings.

In daily use we forget that there is a difference between a word and the object it describes. We be-come aware of it when we meet somebody, usually from a different culture, who uses the same word to describe a different object, or uses a different word to describe the same object.

Vyasa explains that words are made up of letters of the alphabet. Individual letters, or letters that are spoken without being connected, do not refer to an object as a word does. A word is a combination of letters placed in a certain sequence. The meaning of a word grows out of convention. If the letters are uttered in a certain sequence, the intellect recognizes them as a word that is different from the individual letters, which have no meaning.

If the intellect recognizes a certain sequence of letters and connects them to a certain object, which is arrived at by convention, then the word appears as real. In reality, it is only a sequence of letters connected to an object, nothing else. The word "chair" will never become the chair; it is only ever a sequence of five letters. It has meaning only as long as we agree to which object it refers. A sequence of letters might change the object that it refers to when our convention and custom change. For example, nowadays one cannot anymore use the term "wicked" to scold a child, since the word now con-notes something admirable.

Another fact that we have to take into consider-ation is that we may use the same word to describe

18. *Yogavarttika of Vijnanabhikshu*, vol. 3, trans. T. S. Rukmani, p. 73.

roughly the same object, but we have a very different idea of the object. Let us take, for example, two people talking about the jealousy of their partners. One of them may be flattered, taking jealousy as a proof of the true love of the partner; the other may take it as a lack of trust, and in the end a lack of love, since the partner seems to be acting from fear of loss. The two people will find it difficult to communicate about jealousy. Although they use the term to refer to the same phenomenon, they have a completely different concept of it.

We connect ideas to words due to subconscious imprints (*samskaras*) that have been formed in the past and left a trace in our memory. Since we each have a different past, and therefore have collected a nonidentical cocktail of *samskaras*, our ideas related to words are different.

If one does *samyama* on a word, the object behind the word, and the idea behind the word of a particular living being consecutively, then one understands or knows the way of utterance or the mode of communication of that being. If one looks closely at it, there is no great mystery. The reason why we do not always understand each other is that we often use different codes in our expression.

If our codes overlap, some communication is possible.

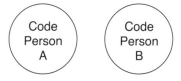

If our codes do not overlap, communication is not possible.

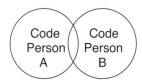

Perfect understanding would be possible only if the codes were identical.

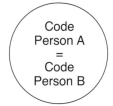

The reason why our codes are not identical is that we are conditioned by the past and communicate on the basis of this conditioning. Since we have a different past and hence a different conditioning, our communication code will also be different.

In *samyama* the yogi suspends his or her past conditioning, as was explained in sutra I.41. Like a crystal, the mind in *samapatti* reflects faithfully everything that it is directed toward. In other words, it duplicates what it perceives rather than produces a simulation of it.

Code
Person A
Duplicated by
Yogi

This is possible because the yogi is in charge of his or her mentation, and not the other way around. By faithfully replicating the code of the examined being and comparing it with the object it refers to, the yogi will understand the communication modes and patterns of that being. Let us remember that only the mind in *samapatti*, which is the state of mind in *samadhi* relying on an object (*samprajnata samadhi*), is capable of truthfully reflecting an object. The mind of the average person is not capable of doing so, since it is likely to be clouded by the past.

In *samyama*, the yogi now compares the truthfully and directly experienced object with the code that the person uses. In this way the erratic nature of the communication pattern of that particular person can be experienced and therefore understood. In other words, the yogi can, in *samyama*, experience the difference between the object-in-itself and the way it is communicated by that being. With that knowledge, the language of that being can be understood. This makes this *samyama* nothing but a code-breaking device.

Vachaspati Mishra says that "the cries of all living beings, tame and wild animals, creeping things, birds and the rest, even the un-phenomenalised speech amongst them and the intended objects (denoted by those cries) and the presented ideas of them"[19] can be understood. The ability to speak in tongues (the Apostles of Jesus) and the ability to

19. J. H. Woods, trans., *The Yoga System of Patanjali*, p. 246.

247

communicate with animals (St. Francis of Assisi) have been reported from many cultures. Here is a scientific approach to it.

संस्कारसाक्षात्करणात् पूर्वजातिज्ञानम् ॥ १८ ॥

III.18 Through direct perception of subconscious imprints (samskaras) knowledge of previous births is obtained.

Vijnanabhikshu suggests the addition of "through samyama" to this sutra, since a direct perception of samskaras by the senses is not possible. From the viewpoint of higher yoga the power mentioned here is very unimportant. It does not matter what got us up to here. Important is what will get us from here to freedom.

This leads us to the question of why, if the siddhis are so unimportant, they are given so much space in the Yoga Sutra. Patanjali describes the siddhis because their manifestation instills trust and conviction that the yogic method works. There is also an important historical and mythological reason for their inclusion. If we look in the epics (Itihasa) and Puranas, yoga was popular as a method to gain powers. If Patanjali had ignored the powers, he would have placed his philosophy in a vacuum that would have isolated it from what yoga was, according to public perception. We can see the third chapter of the Yoga Sutra as an attempt by Patanjali to harness India's magician subculture and turn it toward higher yoga by showing that these powers, if used properly, can lead to freedom.

But if we really understand yogic philosophy we know that the powers are a trap, because they can lead to egoic attachment. To get his point across, Patanjali first proves that he is a master of those powers and only then does he reject them.

To understand the present sutra we must first remember that there are three types of karma, which are all recorded or stored in the form of subconscious imprints.

The three types are:

• Karma that we accumulate now, which will determine who we will be in the future (future karma).

• Karma that we have accumulated in the past, which is awaiting its fruition in the karmic storehouse (residue karma).

• Karma that we have accumulated in the past, which is fructifying right now and has produced this embodiment (fruition karma).

The present sutra is concerned only with knowledge of previous lives. The first type of karma (future) is accumulated now and therefore has not contributed to this embodiment. The second type of karma (residue) is the storehouse. Since it has not contributed subconscious imprints to our present embodiment, we cannot know about it. The last type of karma is called fruition. It is the karma that has been accumulated in the past and has created our present body.

Since the subconscious imprints related to this karma have formed our present body and mind, they are located in our present subconscious right now. If we practice samyama on these imprints, we can know the situations that produced them. By deep meditation on any object, its cause and origin can be cognized. A yogi with a pure (sattvika) intellect, and capable of samyama for extended periods, can uncover anything hidden in her or his subconscious or in somebody else's subconscious for that reason. We know for example that Gautama Buddha had knowledge of future births. Also Krishna says to Arjuna, "Both of us had many lives in this world. The difference is that I know all of them. You do not know."

All these imprints may spontaneously surface in deep insight, as in case of the Buddha.

We have to ask ourselves, however, why we would produce such a memory consciously. The significance of our past lives is on a par with that of the 6 o'clock soap opera on television. Their only value consists in entertainment. Our past lives are gone; we can't change them anymore. What we can change is now. If we exercise what the Rishi Vasishta calls "true self-effort," we can change and create our destiny. Our future is to become real, and to break free into the natural state. Right now we are slaves to our minds, which linger in the past. Entertaining ourselves with the past will increase that tendency.

प्रत्ययस्य परचित्तज्ञानम् ॥ १९ ॥

III.19 By doing *samyama* on somebody's ideas or thoughts, his or her whole mentation can be known.

If we do *samyama* on someone's thought or idea, the entire mentation that produced that thought can be comprehended. The concept used here is that the microcosm is reflected in the macrocosm and vice versa. A thought or idea is always colored by the personality or conditioning (*vasana*) that produced it. By practicing *samyama* on a thought, the thought-producing matrix — the conditioning that produced the thought — is comprehended. Using that understanding, we can then know how this particular personality is going to modify any other sensory input that is presented to it. In other words we can anticipate the person's thoughts, an act referred to in colloquial language as "reading" somebody's thoughts.

The Rishi Vyasa practiced this technique himself on many occasions. In the *Mahabharata* we read that one of Vyasa's grandsons, the virtuous Yudishthira, lived with his brothers in exile in the forest. Still not satisfied with what he had achieved in confining Yudishthira to the woods, Vyasa's other grandson, the evil Duryodhana, went after Yudishthira and the brothers with his army to kill them. The Rishi Vyasa read his thoughts and suddenly appeared before Duryodhana to talk him out of his wretched undertaking. It is important here to note that Vyasa did not use his power for his own benefit, but rather he interfered because somebody else was threatened. Reading somebody's mind to gain personal advantage is not permitted for the yogi, since it comes under the heading of "greed."

न च तत् सालम्बनं तस्याविषयीभूतत्वात् ॥ २० ॥

III.20 The object on which the thought was based is not revealed by this *samyama.*

Let us go back to our example in the previous sutra. Vyasa practiced *samyama* on a thought of Duryodhana. From this *samyama* he understood the matrix that produced the thought, Duryodhana's mind. From

this he came to know all of Duryodhana's thoughts. In our example, Duryodhana's mind-set consisted mainly of hatred for Yudishthira, and from that Vyasa knew that Duryodhana was preoccupied with how to kill him.

In the present sutra Patanjali says that, when we practice *samyama* and read somebody's mind, we will find out everything about him or her, but nothing about the object they thought about. By Vyasa's *samyama* he came to know Duryodhana's thoughts. But the object around which the thoughts circled, in our case Yudishthira, couldn't be known by such *samyama*.

This is important to understand. The purpose of *samyama* is to gain objective knowledge. The mind (*chitta*) of another person distorts an object through its own modifications (*vrtti*). By *samyama* on this distorted image, we can learn about the potency of that particular mind to distort the truth. But a true representation of the underlying object cannot be gained by looking at it through someone else's eyes.

This applies also in daily life. We cannot know a person by what others say about him or her. We cannot comprehend the taste of salt or sugar by hearing about it. If we have never seen the ocean, we cannot understand it through the descriptions of others. We cannot have the mystical experience merely by listening to the words of a great master (unless we have had the experience ourselves but did not understand its significance). The experience itself is not contained in another's words. We need to have the experience ourselves to be free.

कायरूपसंयमात् तद्ग्राह्यशक्तिस्तम्भे चक्षुःप्रकाशासंप्रयोगेऽन्तर्धानम् ॥ २१ ॥

III.21 By practicing *samyama* on the form of the body, its capacity to be seen is suspended. This happens by intercepting the light that travels from the body to the eye of the observer.

To understand this mechanism we need to look into the Samkhya system, which is the philosophy underlying the *Yoga Sutra*. All of our past thoughts and emotions (*samskaras*) densify into conditioning (*vasana*). All of our past *vasana*s (or a dominant

249

combination thereof) densify into the subtle body (*linga*). At death the *linga* then manifests a new gross body (*sthula sharira*), which supplies us with experiences of pleasure and pain until eventually self-knowledge is produced. This manifestation happens through the subtle elements (*tanmatras*), which have the capacity to project themselves out into gross elements (*mahabhutas*). Each subtle element has associated with it a subtle sense. Thus, the element of form is related to the sense of seeing, the element of sound is connected to the sense of hearing.

The subtle elements (*tanmatras*) and the senses (*indriyas*), which are advanced meditation objects, are well known to the yogi from the practice of *samapatti*. In *samapatti* one chooses first gross and then increasingly subtle objects. When the yogi now practices *samyama* on the subtle elements of form (*rupa*), he can intercept its projection into the gross element of fire. (Remember that the *linga* or subtle body manifested the gross body.) The gross body is still there, but it can't reflect any light that could be perceived by the eye of the observer. The visual perception of an object depends on its ability to reflect the rays of light that hit its surface. In our case the surface is removed and the light will travel straight through the body.

In a similar way, says Vyasa, the perception of the other senses is avoided. For example, by practicing *samyama* on the subtle element of sound, we can avoid being heard. Needless to say, to execute this power we first need to be able to perceive the subtle elements (*tanmatras*) in super-reflective *samapatti* (sutra I.44). After that we need to gain the ability to add *dharana* and *dhyana* without falling out of our deep objective *samadhi*.

सोपक्रमं निरुपक्रमं च कर्म
तत्संयमाद् अपरान्तज्ञानम अरिष्टेभ्यो
वा ॥ २२ ॥

III.22 The fruition of *karma* is either imminent or postponed. By practicing *samyama* on *karma* or from observing omens, the time of death can be known.

When death is experienced without prior liberation, a new body needs to be manifested to provide more experience of pleasure and pain. This will happen eternally until the purpose of life, called freedom (*kaivalya*) or liberation (*moksha*), is achieved.

The new incarnation is determined by the strongest impression prevalent in the karmic storehouse (*karmashaya*). All related *samskaras* will collaborate with that particular dominant impression to manifest a new life. All *karma* in the storehouse is postponed or slow fructifying. From the moment it becomes active by participating in producing a body, it becomes immanent or fast fructifying. For example, from our perspective today the *karma* that has manifested our present body is in fruition whereas what is dormant in the storehouse is in residue (slow fructifying).

Similarly, in our life now we constantly produce new *karma*, unless we are in spontaneous suspension of breath (*kevala kumbhaka*) or *samadhi*, have gained *jnana*, are experiencing intense devotion to the Supreme Being (*bhakti*), or are in some similar state. In all of those states no new *karma* is created, because we are in truth or abide in consciousness. The new *karma* that we constantly produce can again be imminent or postponed, depending on the intensity of the act that has produced it. We know from the example of great masters such as Vishvamitra and Vasishta that by practicing with fervor one can break free in one lifetime. But it is true also that acts performed with great viciousness may manifest immediate results. So we are told that when the proud King Nahusha humiliated the Rishi Agastya he was turned into a snake on the spot. Acts performed with a mellower attitude will produce *karma* that accumulates in the karmic storehouse and comes to fruition slowly, in a future life.

By practicing *samyama* on *karma*, one can identify which elements of one's *karma* are imminent or fast and which postponed or slow. By isolating all of one's immanent *karma*, one can identify which part contributes to one's death, and thus the time of death can be known. In this context we need to understand that fast-fructifying *karma* provides the fuel for the body. When this fuel runs out the end of the body is nigh.

The other way by which death can be foreseen is by observing omens. The *Mahabharata* says for example that, in his thirty-sixth year of rule, Emperor Yudishthira saw bad omens. He enthroned his crown prince, Parikshit, stepped down, and awaited the death of Krishna, which marked the beginning of Kali Yuga, and afterward his own death.

Vyasa says in his commentary that omens are of three kinds: personal, impersonal, and divine. Personal omens are when one closes with one's fingers the apertures of the body, such as the eyes and ears, and does not perceive signs of life such as light and sound. Impersonal omens are visitations by other beings that function as messengers of death. A divine omen is the sudden appearance of a heavenly being or deity. From these various omens the time of approaching death can be ascertained.

मैत्र्यादिषु बलानि ॥ २३ ॥

III.23 By doing *samyama* on friendliness, compassion, and joy, one acquires their powers.

This sutra is connected to sutra I.33. There Patanjali suggested that we should be friendly to the happy and compassionate to the downtrodden, experience joy on meeting the virtuous and be indifferent on encountering the vicious. By practicing *samyama* on the first three sentiments, so Vyasa says, unfailing energy results. Indifference, according to him, is not fit to be the object of *samyama*. It is not a sentiment itself, but, as Vijnanabhikshu explains, the absence of a sentiment, like friendliness for example. Since it is only a negation of other feelings, no *samyama* on it is possible and no powers can arise out of it.

The powers that arise from *samyama* on the other three sentiments are to be permanently established in them whatever the circumstance. Vachaspati Mishra says that "the yogi gets the power to make everybody happy and he delivers living beings from pain."[20]

Why is unfailing energy a result of this *samyama*? Yoga considers that we have an endless energy reservoir at the base of the spine in the form of the serpent power *kundalini*. The extent to which this energy is blocked depends on our conditioning, which in turn determines which *chakra*s are open and which are blocked. The *samyama* under discussion makes us free from our conditioning, which is

20. J. H. Woods, trans., *The Yoga System of Patanjali*, p. 253.

nothing but the degree to which we are limited by past hurt. The *samyama* makes us independent because we do not react, in the three cases Patanjali outlined, according to previous conditioning. This enables us to access all our energy resources.

बलेषु हस्तिबलादीनि ॥ २४ ॥

III.24 By *samyama* on any form of strength, such as the strength of an elephant, this strength can be gained.

Vyasa elaborates that by practicing *samyama* on Vainateya we will gain his strength. He believes this strength to be more desirable than an elephant's, which is understandable since Vainateya ate an entire elephant when he was hungry. Who is Vainateya?

"Vainateya" means son of Vinata. It is said in the *Garuda Purana* that, a long time before man appeared on earth, gods and demons fought for supremacy. The gods eventually won by getting hold of *soma*, the nectar of immortality.

The leader of the gods was the powerful Indra, who at times could be very egotistical, proud, and cruel. One day he humiliated a group of tiny, ancient spirits called the Valakhilyas. They approached the Rishi Kashyappa for help in teaching the god a lesson and let all of their power (*tapas*) enter into him. Kashyappa then went and procreated with his wife Vinata.

After five hundred years Vinata gave birth to a son who was invincible. His name was Garuda, the king of the eagles. Garuda was so big that when he spread his wings they would cover the sky and shake the fourteen worlds. He could not be killed because he did not have a mortal body, it being a manifestation of the vibratory pattern of the Gayatri mantra, the most sacred of all mantras. Garuda, against the resistance of all the gods, forced his way into heaven, fought and defeated Indra, and took from him the *soma*, the nectar of immortality. This power of Garuda, explains Vyasa, we can get from doing *samyama* on it.

A similar method is employed today in NLP (neurolinguistic programming). NLP suggests that, if you want to excel in a particular subject, you choose a particular individual who has mastered it and duplicate their experience. If for example you desire to be a composer, you might go and duplicate J. S. Bach's experience. Duplication addresses such aspects as how he felt, how he worked, what his ideas of himself were. In other words you do a meditation on Bach-ness. The concept of duplication is the closest that somebody with a fluctuating mind can get to *samyama*. Duplication means attempting to create in your mind an exact duplicate of your chosen object. Somewhere within that object is the power you are looking for, in this case the genius of J. S. Bach. The success of duplication is limited to exactly the amount by which your thought waves are fluctuating when you perform the duplication. These in turn are, of course, dependent on the extent to which you are a slave to your past conditioning.

Samyama works in a similar way, with the difference that the yogi, having made the mind single-pointed (*ekagra*) in objective (*samprajnata*) samadhi, can download J. S. Bach–ness without being limited by existing conditioning.

Any method for accumulating power, be it *samyama*, NLP, or hypnotherapy, must be questioned from the aspect of liberation (*kaivalya*). In *kaivalya* we go beyond gain and loss, since we become one with the matrix (consciousness) that supports all phenomena. The powers are phenomena, albeit very fancy ones. Phenomena are transitory and therefore cannot lead us to freedom. Why desire transitory phenomena when we can attain to that mystery — consciousness — that alone is eternal?

प्रवृत्त्यालोकन्यासात्
सूक्ष्मव्यवहितविप्रकृष्टज्ञानम् ॥ २५ ॥

III.25 Through directing the luminous light of higher perception onto objects, whether they are subtle, hidden, or distant, one knows them.

This sutra describes the *siddhi* (power) that can arise from the practice mentioned in sutra I.36. There it was suggested that we focus on the effulgent or luminous light in the heart to clear the mind.

The master Vijnanabhikshu explains in his *Yoga*

varttika that this is an indirect *siddhi*, which does not happen by doing *samyama* on an object that is subtle, hidden, or distant. Rather, the *samyama* is done on the intellect (*buddhi*) itself, which has been made sattvic through the prescribed meditation technique. Through the *samyama* there is revealed the effulgent light of the intellect, which is now a manifestation of the pure *sattva guna*. Directed at any object, this shining light reveals it.

This explanation might sound somewhat complicated, but it is exactly what happens. The mechanism can be seen at work in the discourses of many great masters such as J. Krishnamurti. Whatever was placed before him, his intellect appeared to dissect it in a millisecond. The audience can come to the erroneous belief that such masters are all knowing. It is not that they are all knowing; it is the laserlike quality of their sattvic intellect, revealing subtle, hidden, and distant objects, that makes them appear that way.

भुवनज्ञानं सूर्ये संयमात् ॥ २६ ॥

III.26 From *samyama* on the sun comes knowledge of the whole cosmos.

The Rishi Vyasa gives a beautiful description over several pages of the view of the subtle world region, seen through *samyama*. They are primarily spaces inhabited by beings according to their level of awareness resulting from previous actions. The description can be taken from any direct translation of the *Yoga Bhasya* (commentary), and it must not concern us here. Suffice it to say that the subcommentators Shankara, Vachaspati Mishra, and Vijnanabhikshu confirm the order of the world spaces as seen by Vyasa.

Most commentators of the twentieth century have erroneously taken this sutra to refer to the sun in the sky. If we were to do *samyama* on the star "sun" then we would learn all about its orbit, its luminosity, its history, its chemistry, and the like, but not about the world.

Many sutras are expressed in a cryptic way to fool the uninitiated. They were designed as a guide for teachers, along which they could develop their teaching. On reciting a sutra, a vast amount of previously studied material would come to the teacher's mind. In this way no major theme was forgotten. Today students and scholars alike speculate about the meaning of those sutras without undergoing the necessary traditional yogic training beforehand. "Yogic training" in this context means to learn from somebody who has studied the scriptures, has practiced the methods, has had the experiences, and can communicate the content. The many misunderstandings of the *Yoga Sutra* published today come about because such training has not been undertaken.

The key to understanding the present sutra is to know what it is that we have to practice *samyama* on to gain knowledge of all world spaces. Vyasa says, "on the door of the sun," which does not get us much further, but we know it cannot be the sun in the sky — that would give us knowledge only of gross world spaces and not subtle ones.

Vachaspati Mishra gives a more precise description in his *Tattva-Vaisharadi*: "Upon the door of the sun means upon the tube of *Sushumna*."[21] The *sushumna* is the axis and center of the subtle universe, the microcosm. It fulfills the same function as Mount Meru (Kailash) in the macrocosm. As one of the tenets of mysticism says, "As above so below; as within so without." By practicing *samyama* on the center of this subtle universe, we get to know its entire expanse. Hariharananda Aranya agrees that the solar entrance is identical with the *sushumna* entrance. In particular he says that an effulgent ray of light going up from the heart is to be used for this *samyama*.

Vijnanabhikshu, too, says that the solar gate refers to the entrance to the region of Brahman,[22] Brahmarandhra, the gate of Brahman, being another word for the upper end of *sushumna*. If the life force exits the *shushumna* here at the point of death, one does not return into this world to manifest a new body but becomes one with infinite consciousness or "enters the regions of Brahman."

चन्द्रे ताराव्यूहज्ञानम् ॥ २७ ॥

III.27 Through *samyama* on the moon, knowledge of the arrangements of the stars is known.

Neither Vyasa nor any of the historical subcommentators explains this sutra any further. H. Aranya takes "moon" here as meaning lunar entrance, just as "sun" meant solar entrance. When self-knowledge has been obtained, the *prana* will leave through the sun-gate or gate of Brahman at the conclusion of one's life. Having failed to obtain self-knowledge, the life force will exit through the lunar passage, which Aranya equates with the sense openings such as the eyes. The sense organs are apertures through which we apprehend the world, or gross world spaces. As the sun sheds its light on the moon, and it is only through this light that the moon is known, so is the light of consciousness, which shines through the solar passage, reflected onto the lunar passage, the senses. Only through the light of consciousness can our senses perceive.

By *samyama* on the moon gate (the senses), everything that is known through the senses — even the most remote objects such as the stars — can be known. This *samyama* makes the senses more proficient in collecting sensory input from faraway objects such as distant solar systems.

ध्रुवे तद्गतिज्ञानम् ॥ २८ ॥

III.28 Through *samyama* on the pole star the movements of the stars are known.

This *samyama* should be practiced straight after the previous one, Vyasa says. He adds that if *samyama* were made on the celestial vehicles, sometimes translated as "astral chariots," everything would be known about them. Shankara understands this to refer to astrological knowledge, which is knowledge of how conjunctions and oppositions of planetary objects influence the good and bad fortune of living beings.

H. Aranya understands this as the actual movements of the stars in the sky, which can be perceived if one looks steadfastly at the pole star for a long time. Vyasa takes the sutra to refer to both astronomical and astrological knowledge.

21. J. H. Woods, trans., *The Yoga System of Patanjali*, p. 259.
22. *Yogavarttika of Vijnanabhikshu*, vol. 3, trans. T. S. Rukmani, p. 123.

नाभिचक्रे कायव्यूहज्ञानम् ॥ २९ ॥

III.29 From *samyama* on the navel *chakra*, medical knowledge is derived.

Vyasa adds that such things as the three *doshas* (*vata*, *kapha*, and *pitta*) and the seven *dhatus* (skin, blood, flesh, fat, bone, marrow, and semen) are cognized. Those are ayurvedic terms, *Ayurveda* being the ancient Indian system of medicine.

In the traditional chant dedicated to Patanjali, he is credited with being the author of yoga, grammar, and medicine. The *Charaka Samhita*, one of the main treatises on medicine, is ascribed to him.

In this sutra Patanjali describes how he obtained his understanding of medicine — not by decades of research but simply by practicing *samyama* on the center of the body. In this way all systems of the body are comprehended. Vijnanabhikshu explains that the navel is chosen for this *samyama*, since the limbs and organs of a fetus grow out of the bulb of the navel (where it is connected to the mother) as a banana plant grows out of the bulb of its root.

The bulb (*kanda*) is an intricate detail of subtle anatomy. It is said to be the point of termination of all 72,000 *nadi*s. The Rishi Vasishta points out that the navel constitutes the middle part of the *kanda*, from which the *chakra*s originate.[23] An *asana* called *Kandasana* is designed to stimulate *kanda* by pressing both heels into the abdomen.

कण्ठकूपे क्षुत्पिपासानिवृत्तिः ॥ ३० ॥

III.30 *Samyama* on the cavity of the throat brings cessation of hunger and thirst.

According to Western medicine, metabolic activity, and with it decreases and increases in hunger, is directed by the thyroid gland, which is situated in the throat. When thyroid activity is high, one will be hungry and metabolize fast. People with an active thyroid gland often eat a lot and yet do not put on weight. Those with low thyroid activity experience minimal hunger but, since the body metabolizes

slowly, they put on weight even if they eat little. The *samyama* on the right location will switch off any experience of hunger and thirst.

This *samyama* would have incredible commercial applications, since it is the ultimate slimness "pill." Unfortunately Patanjali is not specific, and Vijnanabhikshu says the exact method can only be learned from "special yoga *shastra*" or from a guru who teaches it.

कूर्मनाड्यां स्थैर्यम् ॥ ३१ ॥

III.31 *Samyama* on the *kurma nadi* leads to complete steadiness.

The *kurma nadi* is a particular energy channel. Vyasa says this *samyama* leads to the motionlessness of a snake or lizard, in other words motionlessness of the body. Vijnanabhikshu and H. Aranya, however, take this sutra to be referring to the motionless mind, and Aranya takes *kurma nadi* to mean bronchial tube. The calming of the breathing mechanism will, according to his exposition, make the body motionless. This will lead to the mind becoming motionless.

Vijnanabhikshu says this *samyama* will lead to a steady state of mind. He interprets *kurma nadi* (tortoise channel) to mean the heart lotus, since it is formed by a collection of nerves "in the shape of a tortoise."[24] This could be right. His interpretation would lead to the reading of the sutra as "*Samyama* on the external form of the heart lotus leads to steadiness of the mind." In linking the heart and the mind, this would anticipate sutra III.34, in which Patanjali says understanding of the mind is gained from *samyama* on the heart.

मूर्धज्योतिषि सिद्धदर्शनम् ॥ ३२ ॥

III.32 By practicing *samyama* on the effulgence in the head, the *siddhas* can be seen.

Some beings, in their quest for freedom and their consequent effort to map possible paths for others, did not just merge into infinite consciousness upon

---

23. Sw. Digambarji, ed. and comm., *Vasishta Samhita*, Kaivalyadhama, Lonavla, 1984, p. 20.

24. *Yogavarttika of Vijnanabhikshu*, vol. 3, trans. T. S. Rukmani, p. 127.

liberation, but consciously manifested again and created a large body of teachings over several manifestations. The Rishi Vyasa's ability to "appear" or "disappear" is often mentioned in the *Mahabharata*. In a similar way Patanjali reappeared in the form of Charaka to give teachings on medicine, while Patanjali himself is seen as a manifestation of the serpent of infinity. The masters of the Advaita lineage — Gaudapada, Govinda, Shankara — are seen as a reappearance of the masters of the yoga lineage.

Accomplished masters who can project appearances at will are called *siddha*s in India. Here Patanjali suggests getting the *darshana* or view of such beings. In the *Purana*s (a category of scriptures) many stories are related where the practice of a yogi was greatly accelerated by getting the *darshana* and the instruction of a *siddha*. The method for getting such an audience, according to Patanjali, is to do *samyama* on the light in the head.

Vachaspati Mishra explains that the light in the head here means *sushumna* but doesn't elaborate. This light arises when *kundalini* rises through *sushumna* and then creates effulgence at its upper end, which is the gate of Brahman inside the head. The *samyama* on this light will lead to the view of celestials. Stories are told, for example, that at the enlightenment of Gautama Buddha, at the death of Milarepa, and during the discourses of Yajnavalkya to Gargi and of Vasishta to Rama, the sky was full of *siddha*s and celestial beings.

प्रातिभाद् वा सर्वम् ॥ ३३ ॥
III.33 Otherwise everything will be known from the rising glow of illumination.

Vyasa explains that this rising glow is the anticipation of discriminative knowledge, which will make us free or deliver us. Vijnanabhikshu declared earlier that all the previously described *samyama*s are to be done only by those who desire the powers they make available. To all of those who desire only liberation, the *samyama* on the difference between intellect and consciousness is sufficient. In this present sutra Patanjali states that all those powers will automatically come at the dawn of self-knowledge. We cannot help but be reminded of the attempted

seduction of Jesus Christ by the Prince of Darkness in the desert. Gautama Buddha had the same experience under the bodhi tree when Mara tried to seduce him.

The powers are traps that might seduce an immature practitioner. They are attempts of the ego to attach itself yet again to appearance and claim it as its own. Just before self-knowledge is attained, pure intelligence is cognized and then rejected as not being the true self. In this cognition of pure intelligence, all powers of this world are contained. If we hold on to pure intelligence and use it for our own satisfaction, we can have all the power of this world. This moment is represented in the stories of Jesus and Buddha by the devil and Mara appearing and offering them all the world's empires.

The devil and Mara are metaphors for the ego. The ego knows that when one step further is taken and the self is seen, the ego will be rendered powerless forever. In mysticism this is called the destruction of the ego, which again is only a metaphor. The ego now plays the last drawcard that it has, which is its identification with the last object that appears before the sun of self-knowledge rises. This last object is pure intelligence (*buddhi*).

The ego promises us that, if we sustain identification and declare this intelligence as ours, we can own the entire world. That is true. Pure intelligence, once freed from the shackles of *tamas* and *rajas*, will be able to penetrate any object. But it comes at a price. If we sustain identification, self-knowledge and therefore freedom are obstructed. It is only through the surrendering of all identification that what is intangible (consciousness) can be realized.

The following footnote is offered to those who want to understand the fine differences in Indian schools of thought. Shankara says, in his subcommentary *Vivarana*, "When the yogi makes *samyama* on the self (*atman*)…"[25] This quote identifies the author as a Vedantin, which is indeed what Shankara is. Patanjali, who follows Kapila's school of Samkhya, defines *samyama* as a combined effort of *dharana dhyana*, and *samprajnata samadhi* (sutra III.4). *Samprajnata samadhi* is *samadhi* that relies for its arising on an object (such as the intellect) and is therefore called "*samadhi* with object." *Samprajnata samadhi*

25. T. Leggett, *Shankara on the Yoga Sutras*, p. 336.

excludes the *atman*, which is not an object but the subject. If we sustain *samadhi* on *atman* (consciousness) then this is "*samadhi* beyond object" (*asamprajnata* or *nirbija samadhi*). According to Patanjali, *nirbija samadhi* cannot be combined with *dharana* and *dhyana*, since both these methods imply the sustenance of ego. For a Vedantin like Shankara this poses no problem, since all appearances, including the ego, are seen only as mirages superimposed on the one true reality, consciousness.

हृदये चित्तसंवित् ॥ ३४ ॥

III.34 Through *samyama* on the heart, understanding of the mind (*chitta*) is gained.

In this sutra Patanjali explains how he himself gained knowledge of yoga. According to him, yoga is the discipline of stilling the fluctuations of the mind (sutra I.2). In this definition, yoga is declared a discipline that deals mainly with the mind, it being the main obstacle that prevents us from abiding in consciousness. Students who do not experience the mind as an obstacle can go on to study the science of consciousness (Vedanta) directly. The Vedanta is explained in the *Brahma Sutra*, which starts with "athato brahmajijnasa," meaning "Now then inquiry into consciousness."

The term *athato* implies that in order to undertake this inquiry certain requirements need to be fulfilled beforehand. The principal requirements are that cognition needs to be free from error and the fluctuations of the mind (*chitta*) need to be predominantly sattvic. If this is not the case, we are not ready for the science of consciousness and should study the science of the mind first, which is yoga. For students who cannot meditate on consciousness directly, yoga provides the opportunity to become free.

Patanjali displays in his *Yoga Sutra* such complete understanding of mind that all subsequent masters accepted him as the authority for yoga. How did he get such a complete understanding, such comprehension of the matter? He did so through mastery of *samyama*.

Before Patanjali there were masters such as Hiranyagarbha who wrote treatises on yoga, but Patanjali's replaced theirs. The method of *samyama* was possibly not as refined before Patanjali.

The understanding of the mind (*chitta*), and with it the understanding of yoga, is gained by *samyama* on the heart. The *Maitri Upanishad* states that, when the fuel of the senses is withheld, the mind is reabsorbed into the heart. It is reabsorbed into the heart because it was projected out of the heart in the first place. The heart is the source of the mind. That is why *samyama* on the heart is required if we want to understand mind.

The *Chandogya Upanishad* says, "Inside of the city of Brahman there is a house with nine doors. Inside this house there is a small shrine in the shape of a lotus flower [the heart]." On this lotus the *samyama* is to be made. Vijnanabhikshu confirms that, by the practice of *samyama* on that abode called the heart, there is direct perception (knowledge) of the mind.[26] The location that is understood here is obviously not the gross structure but the heart lotus in the form of the *anahata*, which is also called the center or the central channel.

सत्त्वपुरुषयोरत्यन्तासंकीर्णयोः प्रत्ययाविशेषो भोगः परार्थत्वात् स्वार्थसंयमात् पुरुषज्ञानम् ॥ ३५ ॥

III.35 Experience that serves the purpose of another is defined as the erroneous commingling of intellect and consciousness, which are really completely distinct. Through *samyama* on that which exists for its own purpose some knowledge concerning *purusha* can be obtained.

This is a difficult but highly rewarding sutra, once it is properly understood. The Sanskrit term used here for intellect is *sattva*. Through practice, study, and detachment, the common intellect has to be freed from all stupor (*tamas*) and frenzy (*rajas*). Only the intellect that has been made sattvic is a fitting tool for liberation. According to Samkhya, intellect in the form of pure *sattva* is the first evolute to arise out of

26. *Yogavarttika of Vijnanabhikshu*, vol. 3, trans. T. S. Rukmani, p. 130.

nature (*prakrti*). This makes the *sattvika* form the natural form of the intellect. However, due to evolution, which in yoga is viewed as degeneration from the pristine, original, and natural state, it has been soiled and stained. Once the intellect has been returned to its original state, we can meditate on the difference between intellect and consciousness. This meditation eventually will lead to liberation.

The term "experience" now needs to be defined. The Sanskrit word used is *bhoga*, which can also be translated as "enjoyment" or "consumption." The *Mundaka Upanishad* relates the story of two birds that sit on the same tree of life. One is enjoying or "eating" the fruits of the tree, the fruits of pleasure and pain. This bird is the conceptual, phenomenal, or egoic self, sometimes called *jiva* in Indian thought. The other bird just silently looks on and witnesses. This is the true self or consciousness, usually called *atman* or *purusha*. The first bird, through eating the fruit of pleasure and pain, falls into despair and ignorance. On turning around, however, and recognizing the glory of its friend, the true self, the first bird becomes free.

The conceptual or phenomenal self believes that it can own, accumulate, and consume phenomena, a process that is called *bhoga* or experience. The true self or consciousness is only silent awareness or witnessing. This state is true yoga or freedom. *Bhoga* and yoga are opposed. Either we believe in the game of gain and loss, the illusion that we can accumulate or lose phenomena, which is called experience, or we are forever free. The student of yoga who has experienced the whole breadth of human emotion now, in her or his thirst, asks for an experience (*bhoga*) of yoga and consciousness. But consciousness is beyond experience, since experience by definition is impermanent and fluctuating. Consciousness, however, is eternal and immutable; it is beyond experience and must be realized. Realization leads to freedom from thirst for experience. No experience can quench this thirst. On the contrary, experience always creates new thirst for new experience.

The sutra explains that experience exists for the purpose of the seer, as Patanjali states. This is why the seer is called "deep reality," the reality that cannot be reduced to a deeper layer. That which exists only for its own purpose is, according to the *Samkhya Karika*, the *purusha* (consciousness). If consciousness did not exist for itself but for another, we would have to propose a yet deeper layer of reality underneath consciousness. This is not possible, since consciousness is already the formless absolute.

What is it exactly, then, that we have to do *samyama* on in order to get an idea of the self? Let us recall that *samyama* includes objective *samadhi*, which according to Patanjali's definition cannot be directed at *purusha*. This is affirmed by H. Aranya, who says, "*Purusha* by himself cannot be the object of *samyama*."[27] The *samyama* here is done on the image or concept of *purusha* that the intellect has developed. "By *samyama* on the form of knowledge of *purusha*, a knowledge regarding the real *purusha* is acquired."[28] Now we understand why only the *sattvika* intellect is suitable for such inquiry. The intellect distorted by *tamas* and *rajas* could never come to right knowledge. Vyasa says in his commentary that practicing *samyama* on the idea or conception of consciousness leads to insight (*prajna*), which has *purusha* as its object.

Why is that important? Is not insight (*prajna*) still only a property of the intellect?

As we know from sutra II.27, insight is sevenfold and is the pre-stage and prerequisite for discriminative knowledge (*viveka khyateh*). Discriminative knowledge is the medicine that cures the disease-conditioned existence, which has been caused by ignorance (*avidya*), and returns us to the healthy state, which is freedom (*kaivalya*).

Discriminative knowledge now does arise in the intellect. How is that possible? Does not liberation mean to abide in consciousness? One either does have or does not have discriminative knowledge, which makes it changeable. When something previously unknown comes to our awareness, it arises in the intellect. Consciousness, however, is forever aware and unchangeable.

Discriminative knowledge is nothing but the final stage of the awakening of intelligence. Once it is obtained, the illusion that the intellect forms a functional unity with consciousness is destroyed. The conceptual bond with consciousness is severed and consciousness then shines in its own glory. This happens without consciousness going through any

27. H. Aranya, *Yoga Philosophy of Patanjali with Bhasvati*, p. 312.
28. Ibid., p. 311.

mutation whatsoever. Only through isolation from the staining intellect are the independence and aloneness of the consciousness realized. The insight (*prajna*) obtained through the *samyama* described in this sutra is a pre-stage to it.

ततः प्रातिभश्रावणवेदनादशार्स्वादवार्ता जायन्ते ॥ ३६ ॥

III.36 From that arise illumination, supernormal hearing, supernormal touch, supernormal sight, supernormal smell, and supernormal taste.

"From that" means from the *samyama* previously described. This is another clear indicator that the previous sutra was not talking about self-knowledge. Such powers do not arise out of self-knowledge. They are in fact an obstacle to self-knowledge, because the ego or I-am-ness attaches itself to the powers and claims them as its own. Any such form of identification will, however, stop one from becoming one with the ocean of infinite consciousness.

How do these powers (*siddhi*s) arise? The first one, illumination (*pratibha*), has been described already in sutra III.33. It is a quality of the intellect that arises prior to discriminative knowledge (*viveka khyateh*). The other five are supernormal developments of the five senses. Let us recall that in Samkhya the senses and the five gross elements are projected out from the five subtle elements (*tanmatras*). The *tanmatras* can be looked on as subtle essences of the senses and gross elements. In a similar fashion the *ahamkara* or ego can be looked on as the subtle essence of the world as we know it, and cosmic intellect can be understood as the subtle essence of ego.

When the yogi has attained the stage of sattvic intellect and practiced the *samyama*s mentioned in the previous sutras, one perceives the subtle essence directly. For example, instead of seeing, one sees divine light — which is seeing-as-such — and with it all that is to be seen. Instead of hearing, one hears divine sound and with it all that is to be heard.

Vyasa explains that all things subtle, hidden, remote, past, and future are perceived, and many mythological stories are related of people obtaining those powers. When the blind king Drtharashtra looked over the battlefield Kurukshetra, on which all his sons and relatives had assembled to kill each other, his charioteer Sanjaya was given the celestial ear so that he could report all occurrences to the blind king. With his newfound ability he was able to hear all that was said on the battlefield and relay it to Drtharashtra.

Another example is the celestial eye that Arjuna obtains when he asks Krishna to reveal his cosmic form (*Vishvarupa*), to behold the Lord containing all universes in him. The next sutra will explain further.

ते समाधाव् उपसर्गा । व्युत्थाने सिद्धयः ॥ ३७ ॥

III.37 All these are powers for the fluctuating mind, but they are obstacles for samadhi.

Vyasa explains that the superpowers hinder one from realizing the highest truth, which is the self-in-itself. All the powers are still just fluctuations of the mind, which prevent us from realizing the glory of the self.

To be able to see into the past and future might look very powerful to the fluctuating mind, offering a great opportunity to obtain advantage over others, but seen from consciousness it is absolutely insignificant. Time is a phenomenon that occurs in *chitta* (mind), which is *achit*, unconscious. *Chit* (consciousness) witnesses all time modes simultaneously and knows everything presented to it.

All phenomena, whether past, present, or future, are identical in their purpose. They are supplied only for us to realize ourselves as infinite, pure consciousness. The powers, however, because they are seen as extraordinary by the fluctuating mind, invite us to cling to them, and so prevent us from entering into seedless *samadhi*.

Vachaspati Mishra says, "Occasionally a man acquires those perfections, and thinks because of the power of these, that he has effected his purpose, and so might cease the *samyama*."[29] There are in fact many stories related of practitioners who acquired such powers and then fell from grace by pursuing them instead of the realization of consciousness. One might, for example, be a beggar in the waking state

29. J. H. Woods, trans., *The Yoga System of Patanjali*, p. 266.

and a billionaire in dreams, and on acquiring powers one might set one's sights on becoming a billionaire in the waking state as well. All these states, however, beggar and billionaire, waking and dreaming, are only transitory appearances arising to the eternal awareness of consciousness. If we "own" them, whatever they are, seedless *samadhi* cannot arise. For this reason all these states are an obstacle to *samadhi*.

बन्धकारणशैथिल्यात् प्रचारसंवेदनाच् च चित्तस्य परशरीरावेशः ॥ ३८ ॥

III.38 Through loosening the cause of bondage and by knowing how the mind moves, one's mind can enter another body.

The cause of bondage is ignorance. From ignorance are produced afflictions (*klesha*s), affliction-based actions, new *karma,* and more negative subconscious imprints (*samskara*s). Altogether they produce more ignorance (*avidya*). *Avidya* and all the related impurities are gradually removed, first by Kriya Yoga (yoga of action) and then by Ashtanga Yoga (eight-limbed yoga). This process is also referred to as loosening the cause of bondage.

Knowing how the mind moves is achieved by *samyama* on the heart. Vyasa explains that the bonds brought into being by previous actions become weak when yogic power increases. The bond between body and mind exists only because of subconscious imprints. Once those are removed, which is accomplished by objective *samadhi*, the yogi can withdraw his mind from one body and project it into another.

An interesting story relates how the great Shankara did exactly that. Some Western scholars and Vedantins have put significant effort into portraying Shankara exclusively as either a philosopher or a Vedantin, but from his treatises and his biography we can see that he was a great yoga master as well. He traveled the entire length and width of India by foot twice in an attempt to restore the correct understanding of the *Upanishads*, and in the course of his travels he defeated, in learned dispute, many scholars of rival schools.

One of his prominent victims was the famed ritualist Mandana Mishra. Shankara did battle with Mishra for a whole month until Mishra conceded defeat, which meant he had to become Shankara's disciple. At this point Mandana Mishra's wife Bharati stepped in, she being a great scholar in her own right, and persuaded Shankara that his defeat of Mandana was not complete until he had defeated her as well. Upon accepting the challenge, however, the surprised Shankara found that the subject of the renewed debate was to be *kama shastra*, treatises teaching sexual pleasure. He realized that, having been a monk from boyhood, he was ill-equipped to face the challenge, and asked for the debate to be adjourned for a month.

Shankara had heard that in a nearby kingdom the king had just died and was to be cremated that day. He instructed his disciples to take care of his unconscious body while he was gone; then, through the method described in our sutra, he withdrew his mind from his body and projected it into the body of the dead king. The body became animated by Shankara's *prana shakti*, just as his own body became lifeless. For a whole month Shankara "studied," in the body of the king and with the king's wives, all that a monk usually does not get to study. The theory behind it, as you might have guessed, is that since he did not use his own body, he did not suffer any "pollution." After fulfilling his mission, he returned to his body and defeated Mandana's wife in debate using his newly acquired knowledge.

The story is omitted from some but not all accounts of Shankaracharya's life. Some orthodox hardcore Vedantins feared it could put some confusing ideas into the minds of devotees. Its interest to us is that there is historical evidence the great Shankara successfully practiced Patanjali's technique.

उदानजयाज्जलपङ्ककण्टकादिष्वसङ्ग उत्क्रान्तिश्च ॥ ३९ ॥

III.39 Through mastering the *udana* current, one stays untouched by water, mud, and thorns, and at death one rises up.

There are five principal vital airs. Vyasa describes them thus: *Prana* extends from the nose to the heart.

Samana distributes food and goes up to the navel. *Apana* is a downward current that goes from the navel to the feet. *Vyana* pervades the entire body. *Udana* is an upward current that extends from the feet up to the head. Altogether they are known as *prana*.

By mastering the upward current, *udana*, lightness is achieved. This lightness expresses itself in two ways. One is that the yogi, when traveling over mud, water, or thorns, which would normally lead to immersion or entanglement, now remains in non-contact. In other words the yogi hovers above the terrain. The second manifestation is related to the endpoint of the *udana* current, which is *brahma-randhra*,[30] the upper end of *sushumna*. Through mastery of the *udana*, at death one exits the body through *brahmarandhra*. The exit point is related to the type of embodiment one will encounter in one's next life. Vyasa states that the method enables one to die at will.[31] This claim reconciles with accounts of masters who consciously left their bodies once their work was completed.

This rising at death is also exercised through the Phowa meditation, which is one of the *Six Yogas of Naropa*. The Tibetan Karma Kagyu School, which used to center around Mount Kailash, practices Naropa's yogas. Ramamohan Brahmacharya, who was living at Mount Kailash, taught some of these techniques, such as *Tummo* (yoga of inner fire), to Shri T. Krishnamacharya.

समानजयात् प्रज्वलनम् ॥ ४० ॥

III.40 By mastering the *samana* current, effulgence is acquired.

As described in the previous sutra by Vyasa, the *samana* current is responsible for distributing food and is located at the navel. In other words, *samana* fans and supports *agni*, the digestive fire. *Agni* cannot be controlled directly, but through *samana* it can be directed.

The sutra says this can be taken to such an extreme that the yogi's body shines. There are reports of yogis using their bodies as torches in the dark

forest. This is again related to Naropa's six yogas, in this instance to *Tummo*, the yoga of inner fire. In one case the fire is used to create light, in the other to create heat. In *Tummo*, which is taught in Tibet, the yogi learns to melt ice to a diameter of several yards around the body.

श्रोत्राकाशयोः संबन्धसंयमाद् दिव्यं श्रोत्रम् ॥ ४१ ॥

III.41 Through *samyama* on the relationship between space and the sense of hearing one gains the divine ear.

The divine or celestial ear was considered under sutra III.36. There it is said to derive from *samyama* on the image of consciousness (*purusha*) arising in a sattvic intellect. Here we have a similar but slightly different method for arriving at the same goal.

According to yoga, space is the medium in which sound waves travel. In Samkhya, space (*akasha*) is the gross element (*mahabhuta*) that develops, together with the hearing sense, out of the subtle element (*tanmatra*) of sound. In other words, space and hearing depend on the subtle element of sound that is its origin. If we do *samyama* on the relationship of two objects (in this case space and hearing), we will recognize their common source. In our case the *samyama* on hearing and space will lead to the revelation of the subtle element of sound. Once the subtle element is cognized, the divine ear can be developed.

कायाकाशयोः संबन्धसंयमाल् लघुतूलसमापत्तेश्चाकाशगमनम् ॥ ४२ ॥

III.42 Through *samyama* on the relationship between space and the body or by *samapatti* on objects that have a quality of lightness, such as a cotton fiber, traveling through space is possible.

What is the relationship between space and the body? The body consists of four elements, but these four elements depend for their manifestation on space. No manifestation is possible without space. Vyasa writes that the relationship between the two

---

30. *Yogavarttika of Vijnanabhikshu*, vol. 3, trans. T.S. Rukmani, p. 151.

31. H. Aranya, *Yoga Philosophy of Patanjali with Bhasvati*, p. 315.

is that space pervades the body. Through *samyama* on this relationship, the ability to place the body in space at will is gained.

All objects are made up of vibratory patterns. In yoga we call those patterns "sound," even if the vibrations are not audible to the human ear. According to H. Aranya, the *samyama* is done on the unstruck sound (*anahata nada*) that pervades the body.[32] The unstruck sound means of course an inaudible sound. *Akasha* being the medium through which sound travels, the unraveling of the sound or vibration pattern of the body leads to the ability to place the body in space wherever one wishes.

A similar effect can be gained by meditating on objects that have the property of lightness. This effect is used today in NLP (neurolinguistic programming). If one wants to attain the performance of, let us say, a certain athlete, one focuses completely on that athlete, and in that way duplicates his or her entire experience. The main reason somebody is able to perform a certain action is that they have associated this ability with their sense-of-I (*ahamkara*). It is a well-known fact that a belief that one will succeed in whatever one undertakes has the tendency to manifest that very result. This tendency is greatly enhanced by hypnosis, which can change unconscious beliefs about oneself. *Samyama* is even more effective, as one consciously replaces undesirable subconscious imprints (*samskaras*) with desirable ones.

बहिरकल्पिता वृत्तिर्महाविदेहा ततः प्रकाशावरणक्षयः ॥ ४३ ॥

III.43 The "Great Bodiless" is a method that functions outside of the gross body and beyond imagination. Through its application the veil over brightness is destroyed.

This is an advanced meditation technique. Westerners have a concept of meditation that is often strongly influenced by Buddhist Vipassana meditation and Japanese Zazen. The main technique in those forms of meditation is to be alert and to simply watch

what happens, whether it is the breath, mental activity, or physical sensation. We have to let go of this concept if we want to understand meditation according to the *Yoga Sutra*.

Like Tibetan Buddhism and Tantra, Ashtanga Yoga proposes a much more elaborate system of meditation that is claimed to show results much faster, depending on our starting point. The *Vijnana Bhairava*, a collection of 112 meditation techniques, suggests looking at one's daily life as if it were a dream and to act in one's dreams as if one were awake. The purpose of the method is to realize that both states are not reality in itself but can be reduced to a third state, which is deep reality or consciousness.

Then we find in the *Six Yogas of Naropa* a technique called Illusory Body Yoga. In the instructions we read the following: "Within the crude and karmic human body lies the pure essence of the Buddha body concealed by men's clingings and confusions. Through the practice of the Illusory Body Yoga *samadhi*, these clingings and confusions will gradually be cleared away.…As a result the samsaric *pranas*, *nadis* and *bindus* are purified."[33] It is in this context that our sutra has to be understood. The three systems of Tantrism, Ashtanga Yoga, and Tibetan Buddhism all employ methods that are occult, magical, alchemistic, shamanic, and transformatory. In this regard they are similar to each other and differ from the more rational and intellectual systems — Vedanta, Samkhya, Theravada Buddhism, and Zen Buddhism. We will understand now that a Tibetan Buddhist or an Indian tantric will be able to relate to the following description, whereas a Vedanta swami or a Sri Lanka Buddhist will discard it as abracadabra.

The sutra describes a method called *mahavideha* — "the Great Bodiless" — according to which we project our mind out of the body and imagine ourselves to be somewhere else. If this is achieved but we still perceive our gross body, then it is called imagined (*kalpita*). If we are completely established in our projected body and have become independent of the gross body, then it is called unimagined (*akalpita*) or actual. The *kalpita* is practiced first and leads then to the *akalpita*. Once it is perfected it is called the Great Bodiless.

---

32. H. Aranya, *Yoga Philosophy of Patanjali*, p. 318.

33. G. C. C. Chang, trans., *Teachings and Practice of Tibetan Tantra*, p. 87.

As with Illusory Body Yoga, we project a body created by our imagination. And as with the *Vijnana Bhairava*, we hypothetically accept something as real that we know to be unreal (our dreams). This is done to reduce attachment to and identification with our gross body and the waking state. The attachment consists of ego (*ahamkara*). It is the belief that "I am the body" that prevents us from realizing ourselves as consciousness.

Vyasa explains that the practice reduces the afflictions, *karma*, and their threefold fruition. It is also said to eliminate *tamas* (stupor) and *rajas* (frenzy), which cover the *sattva* (intelligence) in the mind. In this way, as the Buddhist text explained, the "clingings and confusions" are reduced and the "*pranas*, *nadis*, and *bindus* are purified."

स्थूलस्वरूपसूक्ष्मान्वयार्थवत्त्वसंयमाद्भूतजयः ॥ ४४ ॥

III.44 The elements can be described in terms of five attributes, which are grossness, essential nature, subtleness, inherence, and purpose. If *samyama* is done on the five attributes successively, then mastery of the elements is obtained.

The literature of the subcommentaries on this sutra is quite extensive. It is surprising to see such precise and in-depth analysis of nature and experience developed by the ancient sages of India. It is especially interesting then to look at contemporary man's beliefs that he has invented science and thinking and that our ancestors were barbarians.

The five attributes that describe the elements are:

• Grossness: What we can perceive with the senses, such as the shape of an object or whether it is sound, light, or water.

• Essential nature: For example, liquidity of water, obstruction of earth, gaseousness of air, and so on.

• Subtleness: An element's subtle essence (*tanmatra*). The *tanmatra* of a particular element is the subtlest form in which that element can still be perceived. It is perceived in *samadhi* and can be reduced

only to ego (*ahamkara*) and intellect (*buddhi*). In that form, however, it is not related anymore to a particular element, which is why it is said that the *tanmatra* is the essence of the element.

• Inherence: The combination of the qualities (*gunas*) *sattva*, *rajas*, and *tamas* present in an element. Every element has a particular makeup of *gunas*, which can be known in deep meditation.

• Purpose: What an element is here for — namely, to provide first the opportunity for experience and second, when there has been sufficient experience of pleasure and pain, liberation.

The meditation technique suggested here consists of a successive penetration of deeper and deeper levels of elements until we reach their core. If we take water, for example, *samyama* is done first on its external form, which is water. Then *samyama* is done on its essential nature, which is liquidity. The next *samyama* is practiced on the *ap-tanmatra*, which is the subtle essence of water, perceivable only in *samadhi*. The fourth *samadhi* is done on the combination of *gunas* that constitute water, which is in this case a much higher level of *rajas* than *tamas* since water is very mobile and can engulf other objects. The last *samyama* is the most important. One perceives that the object does not exist for itself, but its purpose is to bring forth consciousness and quality of awareness (which is experience), and then its ability to know itself (which is liberation).

The sutra finally says that mastery of the elements can be gained from that *samyama*. To master the elements means to fulfill their purpose, which is to realize what they are here for.

ततोऽणिमादिप्रादुर्भावः कायसंपत् तद्धर्मानभिघातश्च ॥ ४५ ॥

III.45 From that *samyama* come the eight *siddhis*, which are not obstructed by the characteristics of the element.

The eight *siddhis* are:
• to become minute
• to become light
• to become large
• to reach far into the distance

- to be able to penetrate substances
- to make manifest whatever one chooses
- to be able to control appearances
- to be able to fulfill all one's desires (omnipotence).

These eight *siddhi*s are said not to be obstructed by the elements. Indeed, the last three embrace manipulation of the elements at will. But, says Vyasa, the yogi will not or cannot use this power to change anything in this world. This is because the order of the elements in this world is willed so by the one who has been perfected right from the beginning. That perfected being is, of course, the Supreme Being. In other words, although the powers are not obstructed through the elements, they are obstructed by the order established by the Supreme Being.

रूपलावण्यबलवज्रसंहननत्वानि कायसंपत्
॥ ४६ ॥

III.46 Perfection of the body is beauty, strength, grace, and adamantine solidity.

Instead of commenting, Vyasa repeats the sutra by saying that perfection of the body consists of loveliness, radiance, unsurpassed strength, and adamantine hardness. Shankara and H. Aranya refuse altogether to comment on Vyasa, while Vachaspati Mishra and Vijnanabhikshu merely repeat Vyasa's words — which are virtually a repetition of Patanjali's! We are looking here at the only one of 195 sutras on which none of the authoritative commentators wishes to comment.

The reason for their silence is that the body is seen as crystallized ego. When we make the body perfect, we make nothing but the ego perfect. The cause of freedom is to let go the identification with ego and body. They are silent because they want to avoid leading the student onto the wrong track — the search for perfection of the body.

ग्रहणस्वरूपास्मितान्वयार्थवत्त्वसंयमाद्
इन्द्रियजयः ॥ ४७ ॥

III.47 From *samyama* on the process of knowing, the essential attribute, the ego, inherence, and purpose comes mastery of the senses.

The sutra is related to sutra III.44, but this time with the process of knowing or process of perception as the object.

- The first *samyama* is done on the process of knowing, which we may exemplify by consideration of the visual sense. Rays of light are reflected by an object, then collected by the eye, passed on to the mind, and compared to previous data collected about such objects. The process of knowing involves the presentation of an object, a sense organ such as an eye or ear, and the mind to recognize the object.

- The essential attribute is the intellect/intelligence. According to Vyasa, it is the nature of intelligence to illuminate whatever is presented. Miraculously, we could add. It is called the essential attribute because, without this essence of shedding light on objects, no knowing is possible. Intelligence is like light, like a torch in the darkness. Once it is switched off, even if objects, eyes, and mind are still present, seeing is not possible.

- The ego is the agent that owns the perception. Whereas the intelligence is pure knowing, the ego says it is I who knows; I perceive this object. Without this owner, perception is there, but there is nobody who perceives.

- The inherence is that which is inherent in all aspects covered so far. The process of knowing, the intellect, and the ego are all formed by the three *guna*s of *prakrti*: *rajas, tamas,* and *sattva*. The inherence therefore is the *guna*s.

- As in sutra III.44, the last *samyama* is done on the purpose. Here it is the purpose of perception, but it is identical with the purpose in III.44 nevertheless. The purpose of the world is to be seen. The purpose of perception is seeing. Both are there for the intellect to deduce the existence of the subject, the consciousness. From that, eventually the seer abides or rests in the true self, which is consciousness. This state, then, is freedom (*kaivalya*).

Mastery of the senses is a reversal of the process of projecting oneself outward. The normal process is to project oneself out through intelligence, ego, and the process of knowing, and eventually to identify oneself with objects such as house, car, social status, or one's ability to conquer yoga postures. This process is also called evolution.

Opposed to this is involution, which leads from normalcy to the natural state. The natural state is not projecting ourselves out through the process of knowing but knowing ourselves as consciousness. Mastery of the senses in this context means accepting that permanent freedom and bliss are found only within, and therefore not letting the senses reach out and grasp the objects of desire.

ततो मनोजवित्वं विकरणभावः प्रधानजयश्च ॥ ४८ ॥

III.48 From that [mastery of the senses] comes the ability to move the body with the speed of the mind, independence from the body, and mastery over the cause of manifestation.

To move the body with the speed of the mind means to be wherever one projects oneself. Ancient masters such as Vyasa have demonstrated the method.

Independence from the body is the ability to perform actions that would normally require a body but not resort to one. This means to project a mind and from that projected mind a body is manifested. This will be discussed further in sutra IV.4.

The cause of manifestation is nature (*prakrti*). But identification with that manifestation starts only because we observe it without self-knowledge, without self-remembrance. By giving up the erroneous belief (through *samyama*) that we are the world, *prakrti* ceases to manifest (at least as far as we are concerned: she will still manifest for others). This is mastery over the cause of manifestation. Mastery is not the manipulation of creation at one's whim, because that would imply one has an agenda in this world. Any need to manipulate this world reflects an erroneous owning of phenomena, which stems from lack of self-knowledge.

सत्त्वपुरुषान्यताख्यातिमात्रस्य सर्वभावाधिष्ठातृत्वं सर्वज्ञातृत्वं च ॥ ४९ ॥

III.49 From knowing the difference between intellect and consciousness comes sovereignty over all states of being and omniscience.

This is one of the key sutras of the third chapter. Everything heard so far aims at purifying and empowering the intellect. Finally, the intellect has been made purely sattvic or a pure manifestation of *sattva guna*, which is wisdom and intelligence. In such an intellect eventually arises the knowledge that the quality of awareness, the observer, is not located within it, but is a separate and deeper layer (or entity). The main difference between the two is that the intellect is fluctuating: it may be or may not be aware of an object. The consciousness, however, is eternally and unchangingly pure, quality-less awareness.

From knowing the difference between intellect and consciousness come supremacy and omniscience.

Omniscience is knowing everything that is to be known. Once one lets go of identification with the intellect, one can rest in true nature as consciousness. Once one rests in consciousness, the world is known. This is due to the fact that the world arises only through the onlooking of consciousness and for the purpose of consciousness realizing itself. In other words the intrinsic nature of all phenomena is only to provide knowledge for consciousness. Once this knowledge is gained, the intrinsic nature of all phenomena is understood.

The same fact accounts for the sovereignty of all states of being. All states of being, from suffering the greatest torment to being the most powerful ruler in the world, are identical in the regard that the experiencer identifies with the content of the experiences, the phenomena. This makes the experiencer impermanent, since all phenomena fluctuate. It is also said that all such beings go from death to death. Since they do not attain self-knowledge with this death, but still identify with the body, future deaths (and lives) have to be provided until the truth is seen.

Superior to all these states of being is that state in which one knows oneself as the eternal indestructible consciousness. In this state one separates at death from the body as a ripe fruit from the vine. Since consciousness is permanent, such a person is said to be immortal. Immortality in yoga is a bodiless state. All that is born must die, since birth carries the seed of death. To be immortal therefore means not to be born again.

तद्वैराग्यादपि दोषबीजक्षये कैवल्यम् ॥ ५० ॥

III.50 Through supreme detachment toward even sovereignty and omniscience, the seeds of future *karma* are destroyed, which results in freedom (*kaivalya*).

The state of sovereignty described in the previous sutra has to be surrendered in order to become free. If we hold on to the powers, the ego will arise and say it is I who is powerful. This union with the transitory will plunge us back into conditioned existence. All powers and all knowledge are transitory because the intellect itself is impermanent.

Vyasa explains how this supreme detachment (*vairagya*) comes about. The yogi realizes that discriminative knowledge did arise in the intellect and is a property of it. Since the intellect is therefore fluctuating and mutable, it is nothing but a manifestation of the *guna*s. Patanjali expresses this by calling the intellect *sattva*, which is nothing but the name of one of the three *guna*s. The yogi knows that the *guna*s started to manifest the world only due to our ignorance. In this way discriminative knowledge can be seen as the final link in a long chain that started with ignorance (*avidya*).

Once this is understood, the yogi realizes that consciousness is eternal, immutable, and forever free, it being completely untouched by the presence or absence of discriminative knowledge or intellect. From this realization comes complete detachment from the intellect, which severs the illusory link between consciousness and conditioned existence.

Along with detachment from the intellect comes the dissolution of any sense of agency, the illusion that we are the doer. There follows the destruction of the seeds of future *karma* and rebirth. From this destruction of all shackles and bonds arises the state of cosmic consciousness or *kaivalya*.

स्थान्युपनिमन्त्रणे सङ्गस्मयाकरणं पुनः अनिष्टप्रसङ्गात् ॥ ५१ ॥

III.51 The invitations of celestial beings should cause neither pride nor attachment, since that would again cause undesirable consequences.

According to Vyasa there are four types of yogis. The first type is practicing, and for them the light is just dawning (sutra I.36). The second type has achieved super-reflective (*nirvichara*) *samapatti*, and therefore receives truth-bearing knowledge (sutra I.48). The third type has mastered the elements and senses but is still practicing (sutras III.44 and III.47), while the fourth has gone beyond practice and is approaching liberation.

Of these four types, the first is of no interest to celestial beings and the third and fourth are out of their reach. According to Vyasa the second type will, however, arouse their attention. They will try to seduce him by offering physical immortality, the services of compliant nymphs, satyrs, spacecraft, and wish-fulfilling trees as well as clairvoyance and clairaudience. Furthermore, one will be promised meetings with the great masters, be given an adamantine body and so on. All those, so the celestials will say, one has rightfully earned through one's practice. The problem is that, on accepting such invitations, pride and attachment to the newfound acquisitions will develop. These will quickly consume the merit of one's practice and plunge one again into ignorance and darkness.

One needs to realize that those celestials are in the claws of death due to their own attachment to pleasure. The yogi needs to detach from these invitations to gain freedom.

क्षणतत्क्रमयोः संयमादविवेकजं ज्ञानम् ॥ ५२ ॥

III.52 From *samyama* on the moment and its sequence comes knowledge born of discrimination.

A moment (*kshana*) is defined as the ultimate particle of time, as the atom is the ultimate particle of matter, according to Vyasa. He offers a second definition, which is the time taken by an atom to travel from one point in space to the adjacent point.

If we observe a continuous flow of such moments, this is called *krama*, sequence or succession of moment. Such a sequence is not, however, an accumulation of moments. In truth, one moment turns into the next moment and again into the next. We only ever observe one moment. Concepts such as an hour or a day give us the idea of time, but in fact there is no time. Time is only a construct of the mind, which is incapable of understanding momentariness. Nobody has ever seen future or past, as there is only ever the present. The mind develops concepts of future and past to understand why it cannot perceive certain objects.

It claims they have disappeared into an elusive past or will appear from an even more elusive future. Everything exists in all directions simultaneously. Phenomena become manifest and return to their potential state in this very moment. Nothing has ever happened in the past or future. Because our mentation cannot understand that everything is happening in the present, it develops the concept of time. But time exists only in the mind. It is its technique to organize phenomena one after the other because it does not comprehend the world.

People who have had near-death experiences have reported that they saw their life flashing past in one instant. This happens because the mind suspends at death. Then we rest in consciousness until it transforms again. From the viewpoint of consciousness our entire life happens simultaneously in a moment.

When we take a moment and look back we find there is something in us that was always there and has never changed. It appeared ancient when we were young, somewhat unabated by our youth. In old age this same aspect of ourselves suddenly feels young, timeless, and completely untouched by what is called the course of time. This aspect of ours is the true self, the consciousness. It has no past and no future. It is there simultaneously at our birth, in our youth, during our mature years, and at death. In the same way, a river is simultaneously at its source, in the mountains, in the plains, and at its mouth. It's not that the river spends time to get from source to mouth: it is there in all places simultaneously. In the same way the consciousness spends no time

to get from birth to death. Everything happens in a moment.

When we pass from one moment into the next this is called sequence. A sequence of moments, according to Vyasa, does not amount to time, as there is only ever the present moment. Individual moments differ from each other, though, since all aggregates of *prakrti* are in constant flux.

If *samyama* is done on the moment and its succession, knowledge born of discrimination arises. This is due to the fact that this *samyama* will highlight anything that fluctuates. Whatever fluctuates is a product of *prakrti* and therefore not us — not *purusha* (consciousness), our true nature. In this *samyama* whatever is permanent will stand out from anything that is transitory. Discrimination comes about in this way.

जातिलक्षणदेशैरन्यताऽनवच्छेदात् तुल्ययोस्ततः प्रतिपत्तिः ॥ ५३ ॥

III.53 From that, two objects that are identical in type, characteristic, and position in space can be distinguished.

In the sequence of moments it has passed through, every object has undergone a different history of mutation from any other object, even if that other object has the same function and even is in the same place. From the *samyama* on succession of moments such difference can be cognized.

The sutra says that a yogi can distinguish even two objects that are absolutely identical. If we place two identical objects — let us say two coins of the same denomination — before a blindfolded yogi and then exchange the position of the objects, the yogi can distinguish which of the objects has been in which position beforehand.

This is possible because, although the objects appear superficially identical, they have undergone a different history of change — for example object A was first in location 1 and then in location 2, whereas object B was first in location 2 and then in location 1.

तारकं सर्वविषयं सर्वथाविषयम् अक्रमं चेति विवेकजं ज्ञानम् ॥ ५४ ॥

III.54 Discriminative knowledge enables one to cross over. It is all-comprehensive and it is beyond time.

That which enables one to cross over (the ocean of conditioned existence) has to arise in every single practitioner. It cannot be gathered from a teacher's instruction. For this reason the three stages of contemplation are always mentioned.

• *Shravanna* — listening to a teacher who is expounding the truth according to scripture. (It is important that a teacher does not make up his or her own truth, but that it reconciles with the teachings of literally hundreds of generations of masters.)

• *Manana* — reflecting and contemplating on the truth. Doubt is encouraged. Ask the teacher if you are not convinced. Don't be satisfied with belief. Only when you have absolute conviction can the next step happen.

• *Nidhidhyasana* — realizing and permanently abiding in the truth.

Only with this last step has the truth become ours; mere listening or reading is not enough.

"All-comprehensive" means that nothing is hidden from this knowledge. "Discriminative knowledge" means to be aware of that which is different, the consciousness. Once this awareness is there, one knows everything that arises to consciousness. Since there is no other entity to which phenomena arise but consciousness, everything that arises is known — all-comprehensiveness.

"It is beyond time" means that this knowledge does not arise in time. It is a knowledge that discriminates between the phenomena and the container in which they arise. Time is only another phenomenon arising in this container. All phenomena arise simultaneously with this awareness. Discriminative knowledge is beyond *manas* (mind) and can only be gained by *buddhi* (intellect).

सत्त्वपुरुषयोः शुद्धिसाम्ये कैवल्यम् इति ॥ ५५ ॥

III.55 When the intellect has been made as pure as consciousness is already, liberation results.

This sutra points out the importance of the intellect. The consciousness plays no part in liberation since it is forever free and inactive. This is also stated in the *Samkhya Karika*. The consciousness (*purusha*) can never be bound, because it is forever free and therefore it cannot be liberated. Similarly the *Karika* says that the consciousness sits back like a spectator and only sees. It is *prakrti* that in a selfless way provides liberation (and bondage). This selfless role of *prakrti* led to the concept of the mother goddess Shakti in the later tantric philosophy, where the consciousness is identified with Shiva.

The purity of the consciousness consists in its unstainability through the phenomena that are projected onto it. The mind is impure because it is stainable by phenomena like afflictions (*kleshas*), ignorance (*avidya*), and actions (*karmas*). These phenomena leave imprints (*samskaras*), which force us to act according to previously acquired conditioning. The mind is therefore unfree and the consciousness free.

Patanjali here again uses the term *sattva* for intellect. It means that through the practice of yoga all traces of *tamas* (stupor) and *rajas* (agitation) have been removed, and we have reached a state of pure intelligence. In this state all misapprehensions are replaced by correct knowledge or truth (*rta*).

Because we now perceive things as they really are, no more afflictions can develop and no future *karma* can accumulate. It is only in this state that the intellect can comprehend the nature of consciousness, and all attachment and identification with the aspects of *prakrti* are given up. The self now rests in itself.

Chapter IV: On Liberation

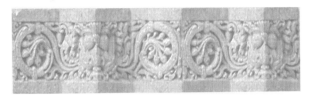

जन्मौषधिमन्त्रतपःसमाधिजाः सिद्धयः ॥ १ ॥

IV.1 Supernatural powers (*siddhis*) can arise from previous births, drugs, mantras, austerities, and *samadhi*.

How those powers arise from *samadhi* was covered in the third chapter. The same powers can also be acquired through other means, in which case they are not yogic. Four different ways to accumulate such powers are cited by Patanjali apart from *samadhi*. He lists them in hierarchical order, beginning with the lowest form.

The first way is acquisition of powers through birth. Some children display special gifts at birth. These can only be understood as being acquired in a previous life. Mozart's extreme musicality at four years of age must be seen in this light.

Another way to acquire powers is through the use of herbs, chemicals, and drugs. Vyasa hastens to state that this method is used in the abode of the demons. H. Aranya mentions the potions of the witches, which enabled them to leave the body.[1] Shankara writes of the soma,[2] the drug mentioned in the *Veda*s by which the *deva*s (gods) achieved immortality. Some interesting research published by R.G. Wasson points to the likelihood that the vedic soma can be identified with the mushroom *Amanita muscaria*, which was also used by Siberian shamans.[3]

Another Indian tradition is that of the Rasa Siddhas who, like the European alchemists, used herbs and drugs to gain powers and achieve longevity. James Gordon White tells of historical testimonies of yogis in India who extended their life span to more than 275 years through the combined application of purified mercury and *pranayama*.[4] Vijnanabhiksu mentions the turning into gold of lesser materials through medicinal herbs. Again, both the Rasa Siddhas and the alchemists sought to achieve this.

The next method mentioned by Patanjali is *mantra*. This technique is used in yoga mainly under the headings *pratyahara* and *dharana*. For example the *pranava* (the mantra OM) is described as being uttered by the Supreme Being (Ishvara). The *Upanishad*s assure us in many passages that, by repeating this mantra and eventually hearing it, the Supreme Being can be known. The second limb of Kriya Yoga as taught by Patanjali is *svadhyaya*, which includes the repetition of mantra.

The use of mantra mentioned in this sutra is, however, different from the yogic approach. Here mantra is used as a spell that is cast to get some type of advantage. In the *Atharva Veda* many spells are mentioned that can bring all type of results, but not knowledge of one's true nature. The only object of desire here is the acquisition of powers.

The final nonsamadhic method for achieving power mentioned in this sutra is austerity (*tapas*). This is the most popular method in Indian history. Arjuna went to the Himalayas to increase his martial capacities by performing *tapas*; the might of the demon king Ravanna was produced through austerity; the demon king Bali accumulated his power by the same means. Again, this use of austerity is not part of yoga, as the yogi does not seek power but freedom. Austerity in Patanjali Yoga is the first limb of Kriya Yoga, the aim of the approach being only to become independent of external stimuli. Self-torture to

1. H. Aranya, *Yoga Philosophy of Patanjali with Bhasvati*, p. 347.
2. T. Leggett, trans., *Shankara on the Yoga Sutras*, p. 366.
3. R.G. Wasson, *Soma: Divine Mushroom of Immortality*, Harcourt Brace Jovanovich, 1970.

4. J.G. White, *The Alchemical Body*, The University of Chicago Press, Chicago, 1996.

accumulate powers is rejected by Lord Krishna, who says in the *Bhagavad Gita*, "Those who torture the body outrage me, who is the indweller [in the body]."

These four ways to come to power are therefore seen as inferior by the yogi. They are inferior because accumulation of power here will always lead to accumulation of new *karma*.

जात्यन्तरपरिणामः प्रकृत्यापूरात् ॥ २ ॥
IV.2 The transformation into a new birth comes through nature (*prakrti*).

All of our actions, words, and thoughts, according to whether they are virtuous or vicious, produce subconscious imprints (*samskaras*). All those subconscious imprints provide a frame or mold. Once a new body is needed, the elements of nature (*prakrti*) rush into this mold and fill it out, as water fills the shape of a receptacle. According to those *samskaras*, nature will produce a new body. How exactly does it happen that a new body manifests?

The answer is that it is a mechanism inherent in *prakrti*. In other words *prakrti* is designed to perform this action. According to Yoga and Samkhya, the body, also called the outer instrument, consists of ten organ systems. They are the five sense functions (seeing, hearing, feeling, tasting, smelling) and the five functions of action (speaking, walking, grasping, excreting, and procreating).

These ten organ systems are manifested by the five gross elements (ether, air, fire, water, earth). The five gross elements are manifested in turn through the five elementary potentials (*tanmatras*), which are called sound, touch, taste, form, and smell.

The elementary potentials or infra-atomic potentials consist of various combinations of the three *gunas*: *rajas*, *tamas*, and *sattva*. The three *gunas* are *prakrti* made manifest.

Prakrti is the creative cause of all manifestations and particularly of the body. Although the body is produced by *prakrti* and not by us, it is we who, through our past actions, manifested the conditions in which *prakrti* creates.

निमित्तम् अप्रयोजकं प्रकृतीनां । वरणभेदस्तु ततः क्षेत्रिकवत् ॥ ३ ॥
IV.3 Our actions are not the creative cause of the new body; they only remove the obstruction, like a farmer.

We cannot claim to be the creative cause of our bodies. They are created by nature (*prakrti*). However, through our actions we create subconscious imprints (*samskaras*), which form the blueprint according to which nature then manifests a body in an instant. While nature is the creative or quantitative cause of the body, our actions perform the role of the qualitative cause. The kind of body, life span, and related experience we get depends on our actions and not on *prakrti*.

The simile used in the sutra is that of a farmer irrigating a rice field. On opening a floodgate the farmer removes the obstruction and the water can flood the field. The creative cause here is still nature, which manifests water and gravity, both necessary for the flooding of the field. The farmer is not pumping the water through physical force but only directing the forces of nature. Similarly, with our actions we only open a floodgate, and in an instant *prakrti* manifests a body according to conditions determined by us.

The particular way in which the body is manifested is determined by actions, thoughts, and speech that leave *samskaras*. The act of manifesting, however, is performed by *prakrti*.

निर्माणचित्तान्यस्मितामात्रात् ॥ ४ ॥
IV.4 Created minds arise from one I-am-ness (asmita) only.

To understand this sutra we first have to understand what Patanjali means by "created mind" (*nirmana chitta*); we also have to remember that the fourth chapter of the *Yoga Sutra* deals with liberation (*kaivalya*) and all related themes. To a yoga novice some of those themes will seem remote, but they were reasonable considerations to the ancient masters.

The present sutra discusses the situation of a master whose mind has gone beyond the habitual state of suspension (*nirodha*). When my mind is in

269

the state of suspension, that means I will use it like a muscle. Using the mind like a muscle means using it only when there is work for it. At other times the mind is suspended and I will abide in the heart.

To go beyond that stage means to enter the final stages of the sevenfold insight described in sutra II.27, called freedom from the mind. Although mind itself is regarded as eternal in yoga, for the yogi who is approaching liberation it loses its grip. It is said that the constituents of the mind (the *gunas*) then return to their source (*prakrti*). This stage is reached when the yogi realizes there is absolutely no more work for the mind, which means that he or she has achieved completion. However, although all the yogi's work might be completed, there could be work to do for others or for the greater good.

In this case the yogi will go on to become a *siddha*. One cannot train for this. The decision whether one becomes a *siddha* is not made by the individual but, depending on our favored philosophical viewpoint, by *prakrti*, by cosmic intelligence (which is a product of *prakrti*), by the Supreme Being (which, if we follow Vedanta, is the cause of *prakrti*), or by Shakti, the Mother Goddess (a personification of *prakrti*).

A *siddha* is a liberated master who can manifest bodies and appearances at will, often for the purpose of teaching. According to popular Indian belief, the masters Patanjali, Vyasa, and Shankara were such *siddha*s. It is said about Shankara, for example, that he did not die but transformed his body into a rainbow. Vyasa and Patanjali are said to be either immortal or manifested in consecutive embodiments in order to serve.

According to Vyasa the present sutra answers the question whether the different bodies manifested by a *siddha* are directed by individual minds or share one common mind. If it were proposed that the *siddha* manifested bodies from one mind, that would contradict the very definition of *siddha*. The *siddha* is a being who has attained freedom from the mind; in other words no mind is present in between the different manifestations.

Patanjali says now that many minds are created by the same I-am-ness (*asmita*). This means that the only aspect that *prakrti* retains of a *siddha* in between manifestations is his or her I-am-ness. This answer is the only philosophically correct one. If the mind were

retained, the *siddha* would not be a *siddha* after all. If the *siddha* were reduced to pure intelligence (*buddhi*), we could not argue that we are still looking at one and the same *siddha* through subsequent embodiments.

I-am-ness (*asmita*) is a function of egoity (*ahamkara*). Patanjali uses *asmita* also to mean egoism when he talks about the afflictions, but in a more general sense he uses it instead of *ahamkara*, and then it means cosmic egoity.

According to Samkhya, from *prakrti* rises cosmic intellect, which does not include a feeling of identity. From cosmic intellect now rises cosmic egoity (*ahamkara*), which says "I am" and "all this is perceived by me," whereas intellect is just pure intelligence without that notion.

From *ahamkara* arise the body (the five functions of sense and the five functions of action) and the mind. We have to realize from this scenario that egoity (*ahamkara*) is necessary for the process of manifestation. Without egoity there is no separation from consciousness, without that there is no manifestation, without that no bondage, without that no experience, without that no liberation. Egoity is therefore one of the constituent aspects of manifestation and creation.

Egoity or I-am-ness is also one of the objects fit for meditation. Precisely speaking, it is one of the highest objects to be meditated upon, second only to intellect (*buddhi*). Consciousness is not counted as an object for meditation, since it is the subject.

To meditate on egoity / *ahamkara* in yoga does not mean to think "I have such a wonderful big ego" or the opposite of such a thought, such as "I hate my ego and want to destroy it." Meditating on egoity / *ahamkara* means, whenever a thought arises, becoming aware of the faculty that says "I am thinking that thought." If we claim identity with that faculty, that is called evolution, manifestation, bondage, and eventually suffering and "going from death to death." If we stay detached from egoity, which according to Samkhya and Yoga is not ours but, like mind and intellect, owned by *prakrti*, then we are on the road to involution, dissolution, liberation, and finally bliss and freedom.

This egoity, this owner, is the prerequisite for the arising of mind, which makes sense after the previous explanation. Mind is a simulator of reality for the purpose of sustaining (survival) a separate identity (egoity) from the underlying cause of existence (consciousness). Without there being an owner (egoity) of perception, there can be no use for a faculty of organizing perception (mind) for the purpose of being owned.

Patanjali now says that from one owner (*asmita*) a multitude of minds can spring forth or can be projected out. In this way the question is answered whether several bodies manifested from one being have several minds or one mind. Each has an individual mind, created from one I-am-ness.

प्रवृत्तिभेदे प्रयोजकं चित्तम् एकम् अनेकेषाम् ॥ ५ ॥

IV.5 One mind directs the different activities of the created minds.

The question that this sutra answers is, "If the original mind of the *siddha* is dissolved when the *siddha* becomes unmanifest, how can a *siddha* appear to be in several places at the same time in the next embodiment?"

Patanjali answers this by saying that the *siddha* creates one central mind from which the activities of the individual projected minds are created. Although the many minds are not created from the one mind but from pure I-am-ness, nevertheless the central mind of the *siddha* directs the individual ones.

H. Aranya discriminates in his explanation between pure I-am-ness and what he calls mutative ego.[5] The pure I-am-ness from which different minds are projected would be free from what we normally call egoism, which is a later-arising mutation.

तत्र ध्यानजम् अनाशयम् ॥ ६ ॥
IV.6 Of the five ways of accumulating *siddhis*, the one born from meditation is without karmic residue.

In the first sutra of the chapter Patanjali talks of five ways to accumulate supernatural powers (*siddhis*). Of those, the accumulations through birth, drugs,

mantra, and austerity come with karmic deposit, residue, and subconscious imprint. In other words they do not make the practitioner free.

In those four cases the *siddhis* develop prior to achieving discriminative knowledge. This means the yogi will now claim or own the powers, which leads to an erroneous commingling of consciousness on the one hand and the powers on the other. But exactly that commingling constitutes ignorance, as sutra II.24 states.

If the powers develop after discriminative knowledge, the yogi will reject them as something nonessential, impure, transitory, and not pertaining to the self. They are now seen as produced by nature (*prakrti*) and not as belonging to our true self. In the first four ways of accumulation, the powers if used will leave new subconscious imprints that will lead to more *karma* and actions based on ignorance. If they are used by one who has gained them in *samadhi*, they will usually be used for the greater good, such as in the case of Patanjali, who, in order to be understood, addressed all his students in their own mother tongue. However, if the powers are associated with objective *samadhi*, egoity can still arise. They are only to be used by the liberated one, who is beyond gain and loss, beyond virtue and vice. These pairs of opposites are explained in the next sutra.

कर्माशुक्लाकृष्णं योगिनः त्रिविधम् इतरेषाम् ॥ ७ ॥

IV.7 The *karma* of the yogi is neither white nor black; of the others it is threefold.

Altogether, four types of *karma* are referred to here.

The *karma* of the villain is black, since he performs actions with the intention of harming others. This type of *karma* will lead to future suffering and ignorance.

The *karma* of the average person is mixed, which means white and black. H. Aranya explains that the mere attempt to preserve one's wealth involves effort to keep others from obtaining it. This means imposing suffering on them. Our whole society is arranged around the idea of competing with others for limited resources. The more competitive a society becomes, as is the case with a highly industrialized society, the more successful it becomes in using up resources that belong to less competitive societies. Being part of such a society, and adhering to its basic ideas, makes us co-responsible for extinguishing endangered species, destroying indigenous cultures, and keeping the majority of the inhabitants of this planet in poor conditions.

Although there are ample opportunities to do good, we will, as the *Mahabharata* shows, not always be able to make the right decisions. Human lives are so complex that we are bound to make wrong choices. The majority of people therefore have a *karma* that is a mixture of white and black, virtue and vice.

For a person to accumulate white *karma* only, it is necessary to tread the path of selfless service for others without pursuing any personal goals whatsoever. We may say, however, that the goal of such a person is the accumulation of exclusively white *karma*. Karmic merit, according to Indian thought, leads to a life in one of the heavens. Life is infinitely more pleasant there than on earth, but because this is so no steps toward liberation are undertaken. Once the karmic merit is exhausted, one falls back to earth.

These three types of *karma* are those of the others, meaning the nonyogis. The *karma* of the yogi is neither white nor black nor mixed: it is of the fourth type. The path of yoga is thus something entirely different from that of the doer of good. In the yogic scriptures and the *Upanishads* there is repeated talk of him who goes beyond virtue and vice and him who goes beyond gain and loss.

The path of the saint deals with accumulating heavenly merit through performing virtuous deeds. Yoga agrees that there is a heaven that can be attained through such action, but then it goes on to say that this heaven is not what the yogi seeks, since it is a state that is created and therefore impermanent. It is impermanent because first it is absent and then it is present. It is created because, through performing certain actions, we can create this state in ourselves.

The state of freedom that yoga describes is eternal and uncreated, and cannot be produced and created by any action. In this regard it agrees with Advaita Vedanta. And Shankara has shown in his commentary on the *Brahma Sutra* that the Brahman cannot

be attained through action. Everything created has a beginning and therefore an end. Everything that is created, achievable, and changeable in yoga is by definition a part of *prakrti*. In other words, it is not our self.

Everything that is created, produced, and achieved will dissolve, crumble, and disappear. The state, however, that was here before everything arose, has been here during the existence of creation, and will still be here after everything created disappears is *purusha*, the eternal consciousness. This state cannot be achieved by virtuous action; therefore one needs to go beyond virtue and vice, beyond gain and loss. In virtuous action it is still the ego that wants to gain, even if the aspiration is toward heaven. Beyond virtue and vice is the awareness that is unchanged during all states, the state that is prior to the mental notions of virtue and vice, the state to which virtue and vice arise.

तततस्तद्द्विपाकानुगुणानाम्
एवाभिव्यक्तिर्वासनानाम् ॥ ८ ॥

IV.8 From the three types of *karma* result conditionings, which will produce, again, corresponding actions.

As explained in sutra II.13, the result of all actions is appropriate conditionings (*vasana*s), which will lead to the performance of corresponding actions. Any experience, whether it be of pleasure, pain, hatred, fear, love, or whatever, will therefore have the inherent tendency to produce similar experiences. Thus, the performance of virtuous deeds may be the mere product of conditioning, and as such it cannot lead to liberation.

Virtuous and vicious deeds alike lead to conditioning (*vasana*), which is a robotlike programming of our subconscious. This conditioning leads to fluctuating of the mind, which is the coloring of reality according to our conditioning. Whether we live in the reality tunnel of the villain or that of the saint, it is still an artificially produced reality that is not truth or such-ness (reality as it is) or deep reality. Virtuous actions must be performed, but without any attachment to the outcome. The yogi does not perform good actions to get recognition or any form of merit, since the merit would lead to attachment and the new rise of egoity. From the point of view of egoity, it is not a matter at all of whether we arrive at it through good or bad actions. Any type of action to which we attach ourselves makes us separate from the ocean of infinite consciousness.

The fourth type of *karma*, which is the yogi's, is neither white nor black nor mixed. The yogi's *karma* produces *samskaras* that obstruct other imprints (sutra I.50). These are imprints of mental stillness. This leads eventually to the cessation of mind.

जातिदेशकालव्यवहितानाम् अप्यानन्तर्यं
स्मृतिसंस्कारयोः एकरूपत्वात् ॥ ९ ॥

IV.9 The connection between memory and subconscious imprint exists even if they are separated by birth, time, and space.

Conditioning arises from karmic deposit (*karmashaya*) and consists of subconscious imprint (*samskara*). The two reinforce each other. Memory, according to H. Aranya, is the "cognitive transformation" or "re-cognition" of subconscious imprints.[6] Memory exists only due to *samskara*. Subconscious imprint encourages the production of related memories, which will lead to more imprints leading in the same direction. A violent upbringing will create a subconscious tendency to accept violence as normal, and it will create memories of violence. Both together encourage violent action later on, such as hitting one's own children, and this in turn will produce more subconscious imprints and memory.

If a conditioning (*vasana*) is stored but not active in our present life, it is called karmic deposit (*karmashaya*). This means it is waiting to come to fruition. Over several lifetimes we might collect impressions related to being a violent person. Even if we are in every individual life peace-loving, righteous people, there will always be a residue of violence present, which is concealed. This residue will slowly build up and gather force in the karmic storehouse. In due time it will come to fruition,

6. H. Aranya, *Yoga Philosophy of Patanjali with Bhasvati*, p. 359.

and then all deposits relating to such an embodiment will come suddenly to the surface and manifest, whether they have been gathered in many lifetimes, in many different places, or even in different historical periods.

To be in a good position now does not mean we will encounter that again in the next life. Possibly we have used all our merit for this life, and lower embodiments could be around the next corner. Similarly, if we see a person who we perceive as wretched, they could just exhaust their last demerit and have an embodiment as a great saint coming up next. There is a popular Indian folktale that illustrates this dynamic. A saint lived opposite a prostitute. The saint observed the prostitute being visited daily by many men and he really loathed her for that. He was so absorbed in his disgust that he often found it difficult to meditate. The prostitute on the other hand observed the saint and took great delight in him. Whenever she could, she watched him, and he became a beacon of light in her otherwise bleak life.

When the saint died, all members of the community came together and provided a great ceremony, for everybody held him in great esteem. When the prostitute died nobody attended, since nobody wanted to have anything to do with her. When it was time for the saint to be reborn he found out to his great horror that he was to be reborn a prostitute. He had not only exhausted all his previously acquired merit in his life as a saint, but he had also created in his mind, through his constant despising of the prostitute, subconscious imprints (*samskaras*) that made him a prostitute in his next life.

The prostitute was to be reborn as a saint. Through her constant meditation on saintliness she had created a conditioning (*vasana*) that made her a saint in her next life. This story shows that, although we are in a good position now, that does not mean it will continue in the future. There is no reason to rest on our laurels. Similarly we need not judge somebody who presently appears to be in a less advantageous position. This can change quickly.

The sutra continues the line of argument that accumulation of good *karma* will never make us free. It just produces enjoyable moments, which might turn sour at any time. Martin Luther King and Mahatma Gandhi were arguably the greatest

visionaries and philanthropists of the twentieth century. Nevertheless they suffered violent deaths. In
the ocean of conditioned existence, one wave might
lift us up and in the next moment another wave
might drag us down again. Since our past *karma*s are
concealed, we will never know what is next in store
for us. It is for those reasons that all attachment to
action must be surrendered. Action is performed in
all cases by *prakrti*, as stated in the *Bhagavad Gita*. If
we realize ourselves as consciousness, we are free of
all future *karma*s, whether white, black, or mixed.

तासाम् अनादित्वं चाशिषो नित्यत्वात्॥ १० ॥

IV.10 These *samskaras* and memories are without beginning, since desire is beginningless.

There is a desire in living beings to perpetuate their
own existence. Since this desire exists in all beings, it
must be due to eternal and uncreated subconscious
tendencies (*vasana*s). We would call that today the
collective subconscious. These uncreated *vasana*s
lead us to the conclusion that the mind (*chitta*) itself
is uncreated and all-pervading. This understanding
is opposed to the Vedantic view, in which *samskara*s
and mind represent only the erroneous superimposition of a mirage onto the real (consciousness).
If we realize that a snake is in truth only a rope, the
wrong idea of the snake ends. In this way the subconscious mind and the world are said to disappear
once their true essence, the consciousness
(Brahman), is realized.

This is the reason why Vedantins find it difficult
to interpret yoga correctly. Some widely published
Vedantins have done much damage by erroneously
interpreting yoga to suggest that practitioners "curb
each thought," "cut off the senses," "kill the senses,"
"kill the mind," "obliterate the ego," or "kill the ras-
cal ego." Those suggestions might work in the context of Vedanta, but if transferred to yoga they create
the impression of an esoteric self-annihilation cult,
which in fact some people believe yoga to be. In
yoga we look at the world as real and the mind and
ego as eternal. There is nothing wrong with these
three, but if we want to become free we need to stop
identifying with them. Only then can we recognize

ourselves as what was forever free: the consciousness. No cutting, killing, or obliterating is necessary;
in fact these are pastimes that increase egoity.

Since the mind, the ego, and the world are accepted
as real, beginningless and uncreated, it is not the
mind itself that we delete, but its makeup, which
consists of fluctuations (*vrtti*). What is unreal in
yoga is the erroneous commingling of consciousness
on the one hand and the evolutes of *prakrti* — the
world, mind, and so on — on the other. This erroneous commingling or false union (*samyoga*) ends
when *vrtti* are subsiding and the mind is still. Then
consciousness rests in itself.

हेतुफलाश्रयालम्बनैः संगृहीतत्वाद् एषाम् अभावे तदभावः ॥ ११ ॥

IV.11 The subconscious impressions are held together by cause, result, base, and supporting object. If these cease the *samskaras* will also cease.

This sutra discusses the makeup of subconscious
imprints. They are said to depend on four facts:
cause, result, base, and supporting object.

• The cause of our subconscious impressions is
ignorance (*avidya*). Through ignorance we project
ourselves out into the phenomenal world, believing
ourselves to be the phenomena. From ignoring our
true nature, which is consciousness, we develop
egoity (*asmita*). Egoity is to take the seer and the seen
as one single entity. From egoity we develop desire
and hatred, which could not arise if we accepted
that the world is completely separate from us.

• The results that come from subconscious impressions are vicious or virtuous actions. If we do
not have imprints of fear and hatred in our subconscious, we will not be able to commit destructive
acts. Any actions performed will of course lead to
new imprints that will strengthen the existing
conditioning.

• A subconscious imprint needs a suitable base.
An impression of ignorance or desire, for example,
cannot be located in a suspended mind (*nirodha chitta*)
and it will have difficulty in getting a hold in a single-
pointed mind (*ekagra chitta*). The confused or oscillating

mind (*vikshipta chitta*) is, however, a suitable breeding-ground or base for all types of *samskaras*. This confused mind is changeable; it is unstable and can tilt in any direction. This makes it a suitable base for imprints.

• The supporting object is the object that, on its presentation, will cause the subconscious imprint to trigger action. For example we might believe ourselves to be peaceful, but in a war situation hatred and fear suddenly surface and we become capable of killing. If the supporting object (war) is absent, the subconscious imprint (hatred) is not capable of producing the result, which is the action of killing. This does not mean that the subconscious imprint is nonexistent. Being subconscious, it can come into the foreground as soon as a suitable situation arises.

The whole chain of cause, result, base, and supporting object forms what is called the wheel of *samsara* (conditioned existence) or wheel of endless rebirth. As has been explained at sutra II.12, an action performed due to a subconscious imprint produces more *karma*, more forms of suffering, and more subconscious imprints based on ignorance and egoism. In this way the wheel of conditioned existence keeps revolving. It is kept in motion by the mechanism that continuously puts in place subconscious imprints. If our actions did not lead to subconscious imprints, if we completely forgot everything as soon as it happened, our actions would not color us.

Patanjali says that the subconscious imprint will cease if the four aspects of cause, result, base, and supporting object cease. He has said in sutra I.50 that the "conditioning" imprints described there can be deleted by superimposing "liberating" imprints of mental stillness. In this sutra he suggests that the conditioning can also be avoided by taking away the constituting elements of the circle or wheel of conditioned existence. We will now examine how these constituting elements can be taken away.

• The first obvious element to take away would be the supporting object. We would avoid if possible any situation that triggers strong negative responses in us. This would also include avoiding people who have a negative influence on us, or support negative sides of our personality.

• To take away the base of the *samskaras* means not supplying anymore the type of mind in which they flourish. Of the five types of mind, the restless mind (*kshipta*), which tends to violence, and the infatuated mind (*mudha*), which tends to materialistic stupor, rarely choose to study yoga. Most students come to yoga with a confused or oscillating mind (*vikshipta*). The two remaining types of mind are *ekagra* (single-pointed) and *nirodha* (suspended). *Ekagra* means to be established in yoga; *nirodha* means to be liberated or close to liberation. To remove the base of *samskara* is to change the mind from confused to single-pointed. It is done, of course, by practicing the eight limbs and particularly by studying the scriptures, chanting of their stanzas, reflecting on the truths contained in them, and finally being established in them. A mind that is capable of the relentless analysis and rigorous reasoning of philosophy becomes *ekagra*.

• To take away the results of the *samskaras* means to strictly adhere to the *yamas* and *niyamas*. If at first we only grudgingly submit to the ethical rules, thinking that they mainly benefit others, we realize later that they benefit us by protecting us from ourselves.

• To take away the cause of the *samskaras* means to overcome ignorance and egoity. In the case of a confused mind (*vikshipta chitta*) they are overcome by a full course of the eight limbs. In the case of a single-pointed mind (*ekagra chitta*), the practice of the last three limbs is recommended.

अतीतानागतं स्वरूपतोऽस्त्यध्वभेदाद् धर्माणाम् ॥ १२ ॥

IV.12 The notion of past and future exists only due to distinction in the path of characteristic (*dharma*).

Yoga subscribes to what is called the *satkaryavada* doctrine. According to *satkaryavada*, everything real is eternal and uncreated. A thing that does not exist cannot come into being, such as a hare's horn or a flower in the sky. Everything that does exist can never disappear. A carved image is said to exist as a seed-state in a rock or in the carver's head. An ornament is said to exist as a seed-state in gold. Multiple universes are said to exist in a potential form in nature (*prakrti*). Subconscious imprints do exist in a potential form in mind (*chitta*), and mind exists in potential form in nature.

This sutra explains or, rather, relativizes the statement of the previous one. As we heard in IV.10, subconscious imprint and mind are beginningless. In IV.11 Patanjali states how the disappearance or deleting of subconscious imprints can be achieved. The discrepancy between the two statements is explained now by saying that deleting subconscious imprints — or in fact anything — is a relative statement, because nothing is ever lost. All things real only ever change from a potential state, which we call future, through a manifest state (present), into a residue state (past). This does not mean that they become nonexistent: they only become unmanifest. The characteristic (*dharma*) of the object does not change in this process, only its temporal aspect (*lakshana*).

This amounts to yoga's rejection of time, which is said to be again only a relative thing existing in the mind. Time is said not to exist to the extent that it can never change the characteristics of things — the objects-as-such.

The process of yoga aims at realizing things or knowledge as things-as-such. A thing-as-such — the information blueprint of a perceived object — does not change whether it moves from the potential to the manifest or the manifest to the residue state. Yogis are said to see future and past because they see objects stripped of their temporal phases, leaving the pure object only. This way of seeing leads to complete knowledge of objects (*prajna*), and it is gained through objective (*samprajnata*) *samadhi*.

If we look now at the world as an object, it means that before the manifestation of the world it was there as a potential state. Even if an omnipotent God had created it, it would have been, according to yoga, in the consciousness of that God as a potential state. A *samskara* that arises in a mind must have been in that mind as a potential state. For this reason yoga says both world and *samskaras* are uncreated. This does not mean that everything is uncreated and eternal. The human mind can develop many ideas that have no reality at all — the scriptures often mention the hare's horn, the flower in the sky, or the castle in the clouds. Those are mere conceptualizations (*vikalpa*). If one contemplates on them

one realizes there is no such thing. It has no potential state (past), no manifested state (present), and no residue state (future). It is just a fancy without corresponding object.

Just as subconscious imprint (*samskara*) is eternal and uncreated, so also is the state of liberation (*kaivalya*). This means it is not something entirely new, but contained as a potential state in every single one of us. While its characteristic (*dharma*) is unchanged, its temporal state (*lakshana*) is moved from potential (future) to manifest (present) when we attain it. This movement or development is called the course or path of the characteristic. Due to distinctions in that course, meaning distinctions between the potential, manifest, and residue states, the notion of past, present, and future arises and with it the notion of time.

Time is a concept mind has to develop to explain our lack of sensitivity. It is only due to lack of sensitivity and ignorance that we cannot perceive things in their such-ness and in their potential and residue states. Because we cannot see them anymore, or not yet, we say they are past or still to come.

ते व्यक्तसूक्ष्मा गुणात्मानः ॥ १३ ॥

IV.13 The three temporal states are manifested or subtle and are formed by the *gunas*.

If an object can be perceived, it is said to be manifested. That means its temporal state is present. It is perceptible then by the senses, since it has a make-up consisting of gross elements (*mahabhutas*). If the object cannot be perceived directly by the senses, it is in a subtle state, which means its temporal state could be either potential (future) or residue (past).

There are examples where we are aware of this fact. In almost all human cultures a grieving person is consoled by the belief that a deceased loved one has not really become nonexistent but only vanished from sight. Various cultures suggest that the dead go to the ancestors, to heaven, to the netherworlds, or back into the elements. These suggestions, for our purpose, all have one thing in common: that the deceased person leaves a residue behind. We acknowledge this in our Western culture by maintaining cemeteries in which crosses or stones are placed to commemorate our dead. Each grave, and particularly the gravestone, is a statement that this person has left a residue in this world; the person is not gone altogether. Again, when we hang up photographs of our ancestors we state that the residue of these people continues to exist. In many cultures the proper disposal of the dead has led to very elaborate ceremonies, this also showing that the residue of the dead is important.

Some indigenous cultures practice the astonishing wisdom of dreaming or calling their progeny into the manifested state from the potential state. Those cultures realize that there is an aspect in us that is unchanged whether we are manifest or not. How could a man and a woman create a new being? It is not possible. We can only create a dead body. The body becomes alive only with the entrance of a being that comes from the potential into the manifest state.

Those objects that change from potential to manifest to residue are all made up of the *guna*s. In our case, the mind (*chitta*), the subconscious (*vasana*), the ego (*ahamkara*), and the intellect (*buddhi*), which can go from potential to manifest to residue, are still made up of the qualities (*guna*s) of nature (*prakrti*). This means they will always be transitory and changeable — they will always be object and never become subject. The only aspect of us that is untouched — unchanged by temporal phases and changes of characteristic — is the eternal consciousness (*purusha*).

The consciousness within us is completely unchanged when we die. It does not even change into residue, because it is unchangeable. This is why Krishna says to Arjuna, "Do not grieve. No being can ever be killed. Nor can you ever kill another being."

परिणामैकत्वाद् वस्तुतत्त्वम् ॥ १४ ॥
IV.14 The such-ness (tattvam) of an object is produced by the unitariness of transformation (parinama).

Patanjali continues to develop the physics of yoga through this important sutra. The keen student needs to contemplate deeply upon and thoroughly understand it. It is vastly complex and difficult to translate into English. This sutra and many others can be understood only by undertaking excursions into the history of Indian thought.

The such-ness or that-ness of an object is an important concept to understand. It is also called the object-as-such or the object-in-itself. All those terms imply that we follow a school of thought that understands the world to be real, as Yoga and Samkhya do. As explained earlier, Yoga looks at both the world and consciousness as real, and since it accepts two separate real identities it is called a dualistic school. A monistic school is one that accepts as real only one category to which all other categories can be reduced.

We can divide the monistic schools into two classes. There are the materialists, who believe that only matter exists and mind can be reduced to matter. For example communism and Western science (excluding new developments in quantum mechanics) are monistic schools of materialism. On the other hand there are the idealists, who claim that matter is a notion that occurs only in mind/consciousness. These schools of thought claim that matter can be reduced to mind. In India the Buddhist idealists (Vijnanavadins) and the Vedantins were popular schools of idealism. In Europe, Hegel and Fichte developed idealism as a philosophical concept.

The Shunyavadins, the school of Buddhist nihilists (Latin *nihil* — absolutely nothing), are neither materialists nor idealists. They hold that neither mind nor matter is real but only a momentary notion of the nature of emptiness.

This sutra starts a sequence of sutras that criticizes idealism with the aim of proving it wrong. India had and still has today a proud tradition of arriving at the truth through relentless logic, fierce reasoning, and learned dispute. Torpid belief and faith were never considered to lead to freedom. The aim has been clarification of the mind until a state of pure intelligence is reached. Discriminative knowledge, as the name says, cannot be gained by a believer but by one who knows. Even this knowledge is, however, only a pre-stage to the mystical experience, which itself is only a pre-stage to liberation.

Western yogis associate India today with belief in a guru or deity that bestows some state of happiness. This view does ancient India an injustice. For never has another culture worked to such an extent, through the effort of hundreds of generations of masters, to arrive at the correct view of what deep reality is. As sincere students of yoga, we have to recapitulate the findings of the ancient masters and not just take them at face value. It is then that the depth of their analysis will profoundly humble us.

The term "such-ness" of an object implies that there is a deeper, real blueprint of an object behind its appearances. This object-in-itself is to be seen by the yogi through higher perception (*samyama*). "Object-in-itself" means the object that really exists outside us. The Buddhist idealists and Vedantins have argued that an object comes into reality only by our perceiving it, and it becomes unreal as soon as we cease to perceive it. In this system of thought, the falling of a tree in some remote forest would be unreal since nobody is there to perceive it. To support that argument, the Buddhists and Vedantins say that in our dreams we produce a sensory experience of objects such as sight, sound, and taste without any object being there; similarly, the objects in the waking state vanish when we fall asleep to give way to dream objects. The idealists derive from that the notion that objects are unreal. Only the mind or consciousness in which they occur, whether waking or dreaming, is real.

In the yoga system all images in the mind are produced from perceiving real objects, albeit usually in a distorted form: the mind can reorganize images in such a way that they do not correspond anymore to any existing object. For example we separately perceive a flower and the sky. Our imagination is now capable of connecting the two to arrive at the sky flower, the flower growing in sky. Similarly we fancy the castle seen on the ground as being up in the clouds. This process is called imagination (*vikalpa*), which is still dependent on impressions gained from real objects.

All impressions form memories in the mind and imprints in the subconscious. These are lived through dreams mixed with imagination. The dream world, according to yoga, is just a reorganization of previously gained impressions of real objects. If those objects had never been perceived they could never appear in our dreams. Thus, the dream experience is no second reality based on itself but only a result of the waking state commingled with conceptualization.

We are rejecting therefore the view of the idealists, according to whom the dream state is a second reality, disproving the existence of the first reality, the waking state.

If we refute the views of other schools, this does not mean that we believe them to be worthless. No school can be completely right, since all schools of thought are products of the human mind. The human mind in itself is incapable of reproducing the universe, since the universe does not fit into our minds. What we arrive at in our minds will always be a reduced copy of the creation. Why then do we still produce philosophical systems?

Philosophical systems derive their value from their ability to lead people to a state of freedom. This ability Yoga, Vedanta, Samkhya, and Buddhism have all proved. All systems are but many modifications of the one truth that has been uttered in the *Upanishad*s. The systems were developed because the majority of the people could no longer understand the highest truth of the *Upanishad*s. Because all systems are an explanation of the one truth, true mystics such as Vyasa, Vachaspati Mishra, Gaudapada, Shankara, and Vijnanabhikshu can comment on all schools of thought. Since they have realized their underlying truth, they can contribute to all of them.

It has been asked how so many highly differentiated objects can be created by the same three *guna*s. Patanjali's reply is, "through the unitariness (*ekatvat*) of transformation (*parinama*)." This means the *guna*s don't act individually but always together, and their various combinations end up in millions of differentiated stable objects.

To explain this mechanism I will liken the three *guna*s to the three elementary particles of nuclear physics — the proton, neutron, and electron. Every atom is formed by the three elementary particles, and in various combinations they form 108 elements. These 108 elements, in their multifarious combinations, form thousands of organic and inorganic compounds. Out of these compounds develop the millions of shapes and appearances that make up the universe. By forming various patterns and orbits, the neutral and positively and negatively charged elementary particles produce the vast structure of trees, rocks, mountains, rivers, continents, planets, galaxies, and universes. To form this multitude is an ability inherent in matter. We can only describe how the different atoms are structured; how exactly the electrons know how to organize themselves in complex layers of orbits to form the elements is difficult to say.

In a way similar to the production of matter from three particles, the *guna*s, according to yoga, produce this world. The main difference at this point between yoga and Western science is that yoga says the three particles are mass (*tamas*), energy (*rajas*), and intelligence (*sattva*). Yoga says it is the process of unitary transformation by which these three particles arrive at millions of stable elements. "Unitary transformation" means that an inherent quality makes the three particles (*guna*s) move in unison to produce the world.

वस्तुसाम्ये चित्तभेदात् तयोर्विभक्तः पन्थाः ॥ १५ ॥

IV.15 One and the same object is represented by different minds in completely different ways. This proves that mind and object are two separate identities.

Here is another proof that refutes the thesis of the idealists that the world is only a mirage occurring in the mind. One and the same object perceived by different people is represented completely differently in their minds. Vijnanabhikshu gives the example of a beautiful woman seen differently depending on whether she is seen through an attitude of virtue or vice. If seen by her husband, she may stimulate happiness; if seen by another man, she may trigger a reaction of desire. If she is seen by another woman she may provoke jealousy, while a liberated one will remain indifferent to her.

We can see from this example that the four minds perceived the same object, because the external representation of the woman, such as color of hair, would be the same in all four perceptions. If it was not the case that they were seeing a real object separate from themselves, we would not be able to ascertain that it was in fact one and the same woman perceived by all four people. If each of the four minds had created its own woman, there would not have been so many correspondences. This assures

us that all have perceived the same woman, the one who is the wife of that particular man.

The different reactions to the object, such as desire and jealousy, let us infer that we are not looking at one mind through which four different people perceive, as the Buddhist idealists suggest, but four completely separate minds. Furthermore, if all four minds were representations of one and the same mind, how could it be that the woman provokes four completely different reactions? The differences in perception of the object arise from the individual histories and different conditionings of the four separate minds.

The Buddhist idealists (Vijnanavadins) say that the object comes into existence only when it is perceived and ceases to exist when perception of it ceases. This would lead us to the conclusion that the very same woman comes into existence four times and ceases to exist four times after she has been perceived by four minds one after the other. Yoga deduces from the same occurrence that, since she has been seen by four separate minds, she cannot be a conceptualization (*vikalpa*) and therefore must be real. Reality in yoga means that an object exists for itself as a completely separate identity whether mind perceives it or not.

न चैकचित्ततन्त्रं वस्तु तद् अप्रमाणकं तदा किं स्यात् ॥ १६ ॥

IV.16 An object cannot be said to depend on one mind. If it were so, what would happen to it if not cognized by that mind?

This sutra develops the train of thought of the previous one. The Buddhist idealist school says that the only support of an object is the mind in which it arises, meaning it has no separate existence apart from that mind. Let us say we walk along a certain street and look at a house with a certain address. We can describe the architecture, the color, the materials, and its age. If we walk away from that house, according to the Vijnanavadins, it will cease to exist, since its only support was our mind.

If we now give the address to others and tell them to describe the house, how is it that they will offer the same description, although it had ceased to exist when it vanished from our perception? The idealist would have to say that through some mystical power a second witness had recognized the content of our mind and managed to describe it.

If we let a second person enter the house and describe it from the inside, it must be conceded that he or she couldn't have derived that information from the first person. The idealist would have to propose now that the external and internal descriptions were of two separate objects, created by two minds, which fortuitously seem to be identical. Rather, it has to be admitted that there is a real object that can be described by different minds and be recognized as such. Therefore this object has a completely separate identity.

Vyasa says that an object has a distinct existence perceptible by all. How could it otherwise be explained that the same object is still in position when seen by the next person? If it were to become nonexistent, another mind would cognize a different object in the same place, because that second mind has a different past and conditioning.

Another criticism leveled by Vyasa is the fact that if we see the front of an object we do not necessarily see the back of it. This would lead us to the conclusion that the back is nonexistent, because there is no supporting perception for it. If the back of a thing is nonexistent we must conclude that the front is nonexistent also, since all visual objects — people, trees, houses, mountains — always have two sides. From this example we can see that we must accept the existence of things even if we cannot perceive them. In other words, just because we can't perceive a certain thing doesn't mean it does not exist.

तदुपरागापेक्षत्वात् चित्तस्य वस्तु
ज्ञाताज्ञातम् ॥ १७ ॥

IV.17 The mind (chitta) either knows an object or does not know it, depending on whether that object colors the mind.

Vyasa says that objects act like magnets that attract the mind, which he likens to a piece of iron. It is interesting that he ascribes magnetism to the objects themselves and not to the mind. This reflects the importance of objects and of the external world, as taught by yoga.

It also reflects the problem of meditation on emptiness or the self/consciousness. In yoga, beginners are advised not to meditate on consciousness or emptiness, as is done in Vipassana meditation. Only after the mind is trained to become single-pointed and the intellect is made sattvic is this last step in meditation taken.

If the mind has a choice between meditation on consciousness, which is the subject, and any object, it will always be drawn to the next object. Due to the magnetic property of objects, the mind gets diverted toward them. In other words one is distracted.

The present sutra defines how knowledge arises in the mind. It involves the process of cognition as well as mere perception. Recognition means that the mind identifies an object seen previously; cognition is the mere identification of an object seen for the first time.

If we merely see an object and the mind does not cognize, then no knowledge is produced. If many objects are produced simultaneously, the mind will be attracted to the one exercising the strongest magnetism. (Since consciousness is formless, it does not exercise magnetism.) Knowledge of that object is then produced.

The advertising industry uses this mechanism by presenting a product together with a second unrelated object that has the function only of attracting attention, which is then diverted to the prime object. This second unrelated object is often the body of a female.

The process of cognition is described in the sutra as the coloring of the mind. Whenever knowledge occurs, a particular object has modified or colored the condition of the mind. We know this from a visit to the cinema. Depending on whether a movie is depressing or uplifting, it will change the condition of our mind. The novice yogi especially needs to exercise a wise choice over which objects to present to his or her mind. Once a yogi is established in suspension (nirodha), no presented object will impinge on his or her state of permanent freedom. A yogi established in single-pointedness (ekagra) will usually sustain focus, although it might take effort. A novice yogi with a distracted (*vikshipta*) mind will lose focus but regain it after an indefinite period. Those with an infatuated (*mudha*) or a restless (*kshipta*) mind are thrown from object to object like a nutshell tossed about on the ocean.

The process of coloring also shows that it is very hard for the mind to gain complete knowledge. The coloring alone is not enough to achieve complete knowledge. Rather the mind has to be made like a clear crystal; only then can it reflect the object truthfully (sutra I.41).

We also have to understand that the mind will be in constant flux unless it is in suspension (*nirodha*). Since different objects are provided constantly, each will change the color of the mind. The coloring of the mind in an average person can be likened to the light show during a rock concert. This, of course, corresponds to the daily roller-coaster ride of our emotions. There is, however, something within us that is different from the fluctuating mind. This will be described in the next sutra.

सदा ज्ञाताश्चित्तवृत्तयस्तत्प्रभोः
पुरुषस्यापरिणामित्वात् ॥ १८ ॥

IV.18 The unchangeable consciousness (*purusha*) always knows its servant, the fluctuating mind.

The mind either knows or does not know about an object, which is why we call it fluctuating. The consciousness, however, is ever aware of the state of the mind. From this very fact, says Vyasa, the immutability or changelessness of consciousness is established. If this were not the case, we would sometimes know our thoughts while at other times they would be unknown. However, we always have to listen to our thoughts, whether we like it or not, and this means that consciousness is ever aware.

If we observe for a whole day all phenomena that we encounter, we realize there is something that is unchanged. This eternal aspect of us is our awareness. The objects that are presented all change, but the awareness to which they are presented is changeless.

This awareness is a property of consciousness. If it were a property of the mind, the mind would have to have permanent knowledge of all objects. This is not the case, however, since the mind variously has or does not have knowledge of an object.

There is another serious reason why the mind cannot have awareness. It is discussed in the next sutra.

न तत् स्वाभासंदृश्यत्वात् ॥ १९ ॥

IV.19 The mind does not possess the light of awareness since it is of the nature of the seen.

The consciousness is also called the seer, *drashta*. It is called so because it is pure contentless, qualityless awareness. This is important to understand. If consciousness contained character, personality, past, and so on, it could not permanently be aware of the contents of the mind. Character, personality, memory, ego equate to blind spots in our mentation. Because we have a certain memory about something, it will color any new experience. We see that in daily life, where things tend to manifest according to previously acquired beliefs. If we change our belief system, the world will suddenly look different. If certain things do not fit into our belief system, we tend to blend them out or prefer not to see them.

For example, a sexist tends to overlook achievements and great performances by women; a white supremacist tends to overlook the great cultural achievements of people of color. In other words, the mere nature of the mind, with all its contents, prevents complete awareness. From the fact that consciousness is ever aware of the mind, we know that it is contentless and pure. If it had contents beyond awareness, these contents would prevent its permanent awareness of the mind.

The fact that consciousness is pure awareness also means that we cannot observe it directly. Consciousness is discovered on an inward journey by rejecting all that we can observe as being nonessential and transitory.

We know that we are not the body, since we can observe it. Being observable, it must be an external object. The same is true for the mind. Since we can comfortably lean back and observe it in all its facets like a TV show, we know that the mind is an object and an external agent. It is observed by an even deeper layer, which is the consciousness or seer. This seer cannot be seen; otherwise it would itself become an object and we would need to look for an even deeper layer.

Although we cannot perceive the seer directly, we can abide in its nature, which is called "truth" or "the natural state." Giving up the artificial act of outward projection leads to objectless (*asamprajnata*) *samadhi*. To give up the false union with the seen means to stop identifying with the egoic body-mind complex. The fact that we can give up this identification, as many masters have shown, is only possible because we are not the body/mind.

The presence of ideas such as "My mind drives me crazy" and "I changed my mind" shows that there is a deeper layer that owns and operates the mind and is not located in it. It is this layer that is awareness. If awareness were located in the mind, then we would be somewhat like an animal: aware only of our outside world and following our urges and impulses all day long without reflecting on our behavior at all. The term "somewhat" has been used here because animals do not completely follow this pattern. However, when we say to another human "You behave like an animal," we imply that he behaves unreflectively, as if awareness were located within his mind, and not deeper, so that he is incapable of observing himself.

एकसमये चोभयानवधारणम् ॥ २० ॥

IV.20 And we cannot ascertain both the mind and the external objects in the same moment.

This sutra is aimed against another Buddhist doctrine, the doctrine of momentariness held by the Buddhist nihilists (Shunyavadins). Not only do they deny the existence of matter, as do the idealists, or the existence of mind, as do the materialists, but they deny the existence of both. The Shunyavadins claim that neither mind nor matter has an existence of its own.

Let us recall that Yoga and Samkhya accept the separate existence of both. According to the nihilists, mind, matter, and the self, which they deny as well,

are only momentarily arising ideas. When the idea of matter and mind ceases, they lose their existence as well. The Shunyavadins say the world is only a concept arising in mind, but the mind is also only a concept, which is contained in an idea or thought. As soon as that thought or idea subsides, both matter and mind are annihilated. In this school of thought, perceiver, perceiving, and object are not separate, but only aspects of the one arising-and-disappearing notion.

The present sutra refutes this teaching by saying that both the mind and the external world cannot be watched at the same moment. Let us say we sit in meditation and watch the world. Then we shift our awareness and watch the mind. In other words we watch ourselves watching the world. This shift takes a split second. If we shift the awareness back to the world, again it will take a split second. We notice this shift especially if we are in a situation that needs intense concentration. In such moments, self-awareness might be greatly reduced. We are always surprised at the atrocities that people can commit in war situations. This is because self-reflectiveness falls away in a combat situation.

Similarly, we can meditate driving a car, or watch ourselves driving. If we get into a demanding situation we have to shift our awareness to the external world in order to react faster. If the focus is on the mind, meaning if we are introspective, then we first have to shift to the outer world and then react. If we are extraverted already, the reaction time will be shorter.

From this momentary shift, from this inability to observe both simultaneously, Patanjali deduces the invalidity of the doctrine of momentariness. Since the two — observing the mind and observing the world — are separated by a moment, they cannot be contained in the same idea or notion. Therefore the doctrine of momentariness, which declares both mind and matter to be nothing but momentary ideas, is seen as refuted.

There is more evidence that mind and phenomena are separate things. Especially when we study descriptions of life-threatening situations and near-death experiences, we recognize that observing the mind and observing the world are two separate things. Years ago I was involved in an accident in which a thirty-ton truck swiped me off my motorbike. I was on a country road overtaking the truck when the driver, without any warning, veered over onto my side of the road. There was absolutely nothing I could do in the split second before the impact. I felt that I was suddenly being sucked inward and things started to move really slowly. I realized I was not watching the world anymore but only myself. The light and perspective of my vision changed and I felt suddenly completely detached. It was more as if I were watching a movie and not my own life. Through shock, the connection with my mind was suddenly severed and there was only consciousness watching mind. The reaction of my body/mind seemed to occur completely without my contribution. I observed how in a slow, robotlike movement my hands pushed against the tank of the bike and I hopped up onto the seat in a squatting position. When the impact came, I leaped off the motorbike toward the safety of the roadside. This movement pushed the bike under the truck, where it was crushed. I felt my body, or rather the body of this stranger, skidding and tumbling until it finally came to rest.

Several observations are interesting here. First, I experienced what the *Gita* calls "all actions [being] performed only by *prakrti*," since my body/mind saved itself without any contribution from me. Second, the consciousness appeared to be, as the ancient texts say, completely inactive — completely separated from that which acts. Third, there is a notable difference between consciousness observing mind directly and observing the world through mind. The difference is stark and dramatic. In extreme situations, when the time simulation of mind is switched off, we can perceive the difference between the two.

From this and similar near-death experiences described by many people, we can infer that mind and the world are not ascertained simultaneously and that awareness is not located in the mind.

चित्तान्तरदृश्ये बुद्धिबुद्धेरतिप्रसङ्गः स्मृतिसंकरश्च ॥ २१ ॥

IV.21 If awareness of mind came from a second mind, then this would lead to an infinite regress and a confusion of memory.

The Shunyavadins say that no mind exists separate from the idea that arises in it and that no permanent self exists to be aware of mind. This leads us to the proposal of a separate mind arising with every idea, which illumines or is aware of the previous idea. This is similar to the modern psychological concept of literally thousands of consecutive selves (the postmodernist view) opposed to only one solid self (the modernist view).

Patanjali rejects this solution by pointing out that it leads to an infinite regress. An argument that entails an infinite regress is unacceptable because it offers no solution. So, for example, Ramana Maharshi has pointed out that mind control is not possible because we need a second mind to control the first one. The problem is now that we have one controlled mind and a second free mind running wild. We need a third mind to control the second mind and then a fourth to control the third. The reason why this infinite regress is rejected is that it always leaves one mind uncontrolled and therefore leads nowhere.

Similarly, the argument presented here is of one arising mind being aware of the previous subsiding mind. Since, according to the Shunyavadins, mind does not exist but is only a notion arising with perception, we have to ask how it is, then, that I remember my previous perceptions. This is answered by proposing that with every memory a new mind arises that remembers the previous one, but in the intervals nothing exists. Patanjali rejects this proposal by pointing out that it always leaves one mind unaware and is therefore not a solution but only postponement of a solution, an infinite regress.

The second problem encountered is the confusion of memory. If we propose that there is not one mind in which notions exist but only consecutive notions that support each other, then the continuity of memory cannot be explained. During life our memory is constantly filled with impressions. These memories cannot be accessed by another mind under normal circumstances, so our memories are distinctly different from anybody else's. If there was not one perpetually existing mind, but only momentary notions, then we could not ascertain whose memories we were looking at. This, however, is not the case. If separate people were to write down their memories we could distinguish which memories belong to which person. From the continuity of memory we can deduce the continuity of one mind. We therefore reject this solution also.

चितेरप्रतिसंक्रमायास्तदाकारापत्तौ
स्वबुद्धिसंवेदनम् ॥ २२ ॥

IV.22 In the process of shedding awareness on the intellect, the consciousness appears to take the form of the intellect.

After having refuted the views of opposing schools, the standpoint of the school of yoga is stated here. This sutra repeats what has been set out in sutra II.20.

Some scholars regard the fourth chapter of the *Yoga Sutra* as a later add-on. This view is supported by the fact that the third chapter ends with the word *iti*, which means end of quote. *Iti* is then found again at the end of the fourth chapter. Furthermore, some of the criticism against Buddhism is addressed against schools that flourished after the date that is usually given for Patanjali. For example some sutras are taken as being aimed against the teaching of Nagarjuna, who is thought to have lived around 400 CE. The counterargument to proposing an early date for the *Yoga Sutra* contends that, even if Nagarjuna did further develop certain concepts, they were common Buddhist ground even in earlier centuries.

The traditional Indian view is that the battle of Kurukshetra, the central theme of the *Mahabharata*, occurred five thousand years ago. Veda Vyasa, the divider of the *Veda*, who authored the *Mahabharata* and is one of the epic's main figures, is therefore placed by tradition at 3000 BCE. Since Vyasa commented on the *Yoga Sutra*, and the eight-limbed

yoga with twenty-six categories (*tattvas*) is mentioned in the *Mahabharata*, tradition places Patanjali at approximately 4000 BCE.

If we propose a second Vyasa who authored the *Yogabhasya*, the *Brahma Sutras,* and the *Gita*, he would have lived around 450 BCE, which is a possible date for the *Gita*. Since he commented on Patanjali's *Yoga Sutra*, we would have to place Patanjali no later than around 500 BCE, shortly after Buddha. This leaves some room for speculation that the fourth chapter of the *Yoga Sutra* actually is a later addition.

Since this sutra is a repetition, its concept will be explained only briefly. Consciousness itself is the seer, and it is formless. Whatever object we direct it to, using the mind as a tool, that object it illuminates. In that process we then perceive the object mixed with awareness. Since awareness can only be deduced and not perceived directly, unless by an advanced meditator, what we perceive is the form of the object. From a superficial point of view, we come then to the conclusion that consciousness is whatever we are conscious of. This view leads to union (*samyoga*) with the seen, which is suffering (*duhkha*).

Through the practice of yoga we slowly isolate body, mind, ego, and eventually intellect from our true essence. The final step is to realize that consciousness is not contained in intelligence/intellect. It is only through the process of observing, which is also called proximity, that the intellect seems to be conscious, and consciousness appears to modify sensory input. In reality they are both completely separate. Thus is briefly stated the view of the dualistic school of yoga.

द्रष्टृदृश्योपरक्तं चित्तं सर्वार्थम् ॥ २३ ॥

IV.23 It is the purpose of the mind to be colored by seer and seen.

The mind is that instrument by which apprehension or cognition of the world is possible. In other words the mind is responsible for the process of grasping or seeing. For seeing to be possible we need two more categories: the seer and the seen.

The seen is the universe and all the objects that comprise it. Each object leaves an imprint in the mind and colors it. This trait is called the stainability of the mind. After having accumulated various stains, we relate more to previously collected data than to the present object, a process called conditioning.

After having existed in a conditioned state for some time (those thirty trillion incarnations) we realize that freedom and bliss cannot be had through objects and we turn inward. We realize then that another factor apart from the seen has colored the mind, and that is awareness. Through correct philosophical inquiry, which is possible after the intellect has been prepared through yoga, we realize that awareness cannot be located in the mind, since mind is mutable and awareness is not.

We come to understand now that the mind has been colored by two entities, one inside, one outside. This is the purpose of the mind. Vyasa in his commentary pities those who believe the mind itself is conscious and those who believe only the mind is real. In *samadhi*, he says, one realizes that an object is completely separate from the mind that reflects it. Similarly there comes the realization that the seen is completely separate from the mind. According to Vyasa, it is those who manage to isolate the three entities of knower (consciousness), knowing (mind), and known (world) that will know consciousness in itself and thus break free — and not those who manage to unite seer, seeing, and seen as one.

तदसंख्येयवासनाभिचित्रम् अपि परार्थं संहत्यकारित्वात् ॥ २४ ॥

IV.24 The mind, being colored by countless subconscious conditionings, exists for the purpose of another, since it acts conjointly.

The idea here is that everything that is one whole exists for its own purpose. The consciousness cannot be subdivided into smaller units and it is not put together from components. For this reason it has as a purpose only itself. Objects like houses and bridges are put together from pieces, and they serve the purpose of external agents — the people that use them.

The world also consists of objects that are made up of elements and atoms. Therefore, according to yogic philosophy, it must exist for the purpose of another. Sutra II.21 tells us that the world exists only for the purpose of consciousness.

When we look at the mind, which is colored by our entire evolutionary past, there arises the impression that it exists for its own purpose. This is reflected in the concept that our purpose is survival, individually and as a species. According to yoga, however, the mind — like everything that has component parts and depends on other elements for its existence — acts only to serve another. The *chitta* (mind) is a construct consisting of *manas* (thinking agent), *buddhi* (intellect), and *ahamkara* (ego). All of these three constituents themselves are made up of the three *guna*s: *sattva*, *rajas*, and *tamas*.

The mind also cannot act or exist independently. It cannot come to any conclusion by itself, but has to act conjointly with others for the process of cognition (seeing) to take place. We need to add sense organs, external objects, and awareness to the mind for experience to happen. Having established that the mind is a construct, we know now that it acts for an outside entity, which is consciousness.

विशेषदर्शिन आत्मभावभावनाविनिवृत्तिः ॥ २५ ॥

IV.25 For one who sees the distinction, there is no more wondering about one's nature.

All seekers start by reflecting on their nature or on their lack of knowledge thereof. We may ask, "Who am I?" "What is my purpose in life?" "What happens when I die?" or "Where did I come from?" A person who wonders about his or her nature in such a way is thought to have the right attitude for yoga. Those who never ask such questions but are happy to continue wallowing in ignorance, are understood to have no previous link with the search for truth. Students who practice only yogic *asana*, and none of the other limbs of yoga, are believed to be associated with yoga for the first time, whereas others who naturally take to all the eight limbs are thought to have practiced in previous embodiments.

All this wondering, this questioning, this searching is, however, only a function of the mind. Although seeking is an essential starting point — an acknowledgment of one's own ignorance — the solutions offered will be only models of the mind and will never truly satisfy. Since the mind is eternally fluctuating, none of its models and metaphors will be permanent. The wondering and searching will stop, however, in one who can distinguish between mind and consciousness.

Consciousness does not look for its true nature because it is true nature. Consciousness does not look for answers: it is the answer. Consciousness does not ask about death: since it is uncreated and without beginning, there is no destruction and no end.

तदा विवेकनिम्नं कैवल्यप्राग्भारं चित्तम् ॥ २६ ॥

IV.26 Then the mind is inclined to discriminative knowledge, and liberation is not far.

"Then" means when the sort of reflection described in the previous sutra has ceased. This does not mean that one suppresses such a reflection. To want to know the truth about life is a sacred thirst, and we should never suppress it. It marks the starting point of yoga, and the journey can be only successful if this thirst is strong. Vyasa says that a sign for a sufficient thirst is that one's face becomes awash in tears and one's hair stands on end when one finally hears about the path to freedom. The thirst will come to a natural end when it is quenched. Only the understanding that our true nature is eternal, immutable consciousness quenches it.

When we begin to discriminate between the eternal and the transitory, the notion of consciousness is established in the mind of the practitioner. This leads eventually to permanent discriminative knowledge, for which the intellect has to become purely sattvic. With that achieved, the final freedom is not far. This final step is beyond achievement, but one automatically gravitates toward it.

Since receptivity and letting go are required on behalf of the yogi, some schools ascribe the attainment of this final state of liberation to the grace of the Supreme Being.

तच्छिद्रेषु प्रत्ययान्तराणि संस्कारेभ्यः ॥ २७ ॥

IV.27 During intervals arise other thoughts, depending on one's subconscious imprints (samskaras).

Permanent discriminative knowledge is exactly what the words say and not more. It means one is capable of distinguishing at any moment between the eternal and the transitory, between the stained and the unstainable, between the mutable and that which never changes. It does not mean that no conflicting thoughts will ever arise in one's mind, and it especially does not mean that one never thinks. This needs to be understood deeply; otherwise one will be disappointed on attaining this coveted state.

A vivekinah (one who has attained discriminative knowledge) will experience thoughts based on egoity from time to time. Being established in discriminative knowledge, however, one knows them as being part of the transitory, stainable, and mutable. In other words they do not pertain to one's nature, and therefore won't result in actions based on afflictions (kleshas). Such thoughts cannot produce suffering in the vivekinah, since she or he has achieved permanent nonidentity with such thoughts.

Why is it, then, that even in this state we still experience conflicting thoughts? Discriminative knowledge is the highest result of samprajnata samadhi, samadhi pertaining to objects. From this samadhi we learn everything about objects, including the mind. We finally learn that there is a something that is not an object that is not perceivable. We also learn the difference between the objects and the only non-object — the subject (the consciousness) — by way of inference.

What we do not get here is direct knowledge of consciousness, which is only gained in objectless (asamprajnata) samadhi. The objective (samprajnata) samadhi, which has taken us thus far, is also called samadhi with seed (sabija). It carries this name because the seeds of karma, the seeds of affliction-based action, the seeds of future rebirth, have not been parched and destroyed. What are those seeds?

They are nothing but our subconscious imprints (samskaras) and afflictions (kleshas). These imprints are finally destroyed only through the state of seedless (objectless) samadhi. Since the vivekinah has not yet experienced this state (otherwise we would call him or her *jnanin* or liberated one), the subconscious imprints are still capable of producing conflicting thoughts.

हानम् एषां क्लेशवदुक्तम्॥ २८॥

IV.28 The subconscious imprints (*samskaras*) are reduced through the same process as the afflictions (*kleshas*).

The second chapter of the *Yoga Sutra* described the process by which the five afflictions are to be reduced. A similar process is used to reduce subconscious imprints (*samskaras*), which produce conflicting thought. Let us recall, however, sutra II.10 stating that the subtle or seed state of the afflictions is only destroyed when their support, which is the mind, is dissolved into its source. The source of the mind, however, is *prakrti* — procreativeness or nature. On liberation, the mind disconnects and is dissolved in *prakrti*. The *Katha Upanishad* calls this more poetically "absorbing of the mind into the heart."

Another important sutra to recall in this context is I.50, in which it is stated that the subconscious imprint of knowledge (*prajna*) is used to delete the subconscious imprint of fluctuation of mind, which produces suffering. In sutra III.9 Patanjali says that subconscious imprints of fluctuation of mind can be overpowered by subconscious imprints of stillness, indicating a slow process of deconditioning.

Whereas the subcommentators agree in their interpretation of the sutra, they are at odds in defining at what point exactly this deconditioning takes place. Vijnanabhiksu says that the fire of insight (*prajna*) will slowly destroy the *samskaras*. For a faster result, however, he suggests objectless *samadhi*. Vachaspati Mishra believes the problem to be only one of maturity of discriminative knowledge. He says, "Whereas in the case of one in whom discriminative thinking is mature, the subliminal impressions (*samskaras*) have dwindled and are not capable of generating other presented ideas…"[7] H. Aranya also believes that subconscious imprints of insight (*prajna*) are sufficient to render sterile the subconscious imprints of fluctuation of mind.

7. J. H. Woods, trans., *The Yoga System of Patanjali*, p. 340.

प्रसंख्यानेऽप्यकुसीदस्य सर्वथाविवेकख्यातेर्धर्ममेघः समाधिः॥ २९॥

IV.29 If in permanent discriminative knowledge (*viveka khyateh*) one detaches oneself from any gain to be had from meditation (*prasamkhyana*), one enters into the cloud-of-characteristics-dispersing *samadhi* (*dharma-megha-samadhi*).

All forms of yoga described so far, including meditation and *samadhi*, have a purpose, a goal — something to be achieved or to be gained. So are all phases of objective (*samprajnata*) *samadhi* designed to gain complete knowledge and understanding pertaining to objects. This knowledge (*prajna*) then enables us to experience the world as such. The *samyama*s described in the third chapter of the *Yoga Sutra* are performed to produce powers (*siddhi*s). The ultimate achievement of objective (*samprajnata*) *samadhi* is discriminative knowledge.

As already hinted at in sutra II.27, there is a point to come when effort, practice, becoming, developing, growing, and succeeding will not carry us any further but will have to be relinquished. At this point we have to completely let go of the idea that yoga will get us anywhere. We have to give up the mere idea of progress and gaining. As long as we want to get somewhere, we are still climbing ladders — whether the corporate ladder or the spiritual ladder does not matter. Climbing ladders involves ego, effort, willpower, and the mind. It requires the effort to become something we are not as yet. The mere wish to become, however, means denying our true nature as consciousness. Consciousness is immutable. It is in an eternal state of freedom. In this final and objectless *samadhi* the great mystical realization appears that we are all that already.

Appearances, objects, and phenomena have in the course of our lives formed a cloud around us that prevents us seeing the sunlight of the self and the open blue sky of consciousness. The light of the self is formless; it does not have a characteristic. Our mind, on the other hand, is drawn to everything that has form and therefore characteristic. This function of the mind — to look away from our true nature toward phenomena for the purpose of gain — is called the cloud of characteristic. This cloud hides the self, and it is this cloud that *dharma-megha-samadhi* disperses, thus enabling us to abide in our true nature, the consciousness. For this reason it is called cloud-of-characteristics-dispersing *samadhi* (*dharma-megha-samadhi*).

There has been considerable confusion around the term *dharma*, which forms part of the Sanskrit name of this *samadhi*. As we know from sutra III.13, Patanjali uses the term *dharma* to mean characteristic or attribute. It is one of the three forms of transformation (*parinama*) that an object can undergo. The essence of an object — the object-as-such — Patanjali calls *dharmin*. It is surprising to find that many translators have taken *dharma* to mean righteousness or virtue. In the *Mahabharata*, dharma is used with this meaning, but not in the *Yoga Sutra*. This misunderstanding is parallel to taking "yoga" as meaning "union" in the context of Patanjali's *Yoga Sutra*, or to take *adhyatma* as pertaining to the true self.

To read "virtue-showering cloud" into *dharma-megha-samadhi*, as some modern authors have done, makes little sense. Vyasa states on several occasions that true yoga goes beyond virtue and vice. According to sutra IV.7, some collect *karma* associated with wicked actions, some collect *karma* associated with virtuous actions, whereas most of us collect mixed *karma*. The yogi, however, collects neither of them. Virtue and vice are part of the pair of opposites that we leave behind in sutra II.48. Virtue and vice are categories used by the mind to judge the world. If we go beyond mind in this highest *samadhi*, how can it be called the virtue-showering cloud? This amounts to nothing less than a return to conditioned existence.

From the bird's-eye view of liberation there are no virtue and vice. The Rishi Ashtavakra puts it this way: "As the sky is not touched by smoke, so is the heart of one who knows consciousness not touched by virtue and vice."[8] All beings perform their action out of a desperate, painful urge to achieve happiness. Most acts of hatred are committed because the perpetrator is incapable of expressing love. According to the *Upanishads*, at the end of each world age (*kalpa*) all universes are inhaled by Brahman, which

amounts to annihilation of the entire world: all beings are terminated. From the point of view of the victims it seems to be a vicious act; from the bird's-eye view it is the swinging of a pendulum between existence and nonexistence, which appears natural — like the heartbeat or the pulse of the cerebro-spinal fluid. It is certainly neither virtuous nor vicious, but neutral. So is consciousness. If consciousness were virtuous it would have quality and content. The definition of consciousness is, however, pure awareness. For awareness to be pure it needs to be content-less and quality-less.

As we have seen in sutras III.13–14, Patanjali uses the term *dharma* to mean not virtue but characteristic. The cloud or mist of characteristics refers to the erroneous commingling of the world and the seer. In the cloud-of-characteristic *samadhi*, that cloud is revealed and for the first time recognized as such. In the mystical experience the sun of consciousness then dispels the mist. The taint of ignorance by which the seer (consciousness) is commingled with the world of characteristics, attributes, objects, and mind is removed and the seer abides in itself. This is the state of true yoga.

This *samadhi* does not depend for its arising on an object but on the subject, which is consciousness. The problem with objective *samadhi* is that objects are transitory and therefore the *samadhi* based on them is also. Since this objectless *samadhi* is based on consciousness, which is eternal and immutable, the *samadhi* is as well. From the moment of dispelling the mist of the phenomena, we have become one with the sun of consciousness. Once we have recognized our true nature as consciousness, we have reached a state of permanence, for consciousness has no beginning and no end.

ततः क्लेशकर्मनिवृत्तिः ॥ ३० ॥

IV.30 From that *samadhi* the modes of suffering (*kleshas*) and *karma* cease.

Vyasa affirms that from this cloud-of-characteristics-dispersing *samadhi* (*dharma-megha-samadhi*) comes the state of liberation while still in the body. In other words the cloud-of-characteristics-dispersing *samadhi* is seedless (*nirbija*) and objectless (*asamprajnata*)

8. *Ashtavakra Gita* IV.3.

samadhi. Only this second and higher type of *samadhi* can bring liberation. Some authors have erringly understood the cloud-of-characteristics-dispersing *samadhi* to be yet another form of objective *samadhi.*

Vyasa states that this liberating *samadhi* finally destroys ignorance (*avidya*) and all the modes of suffering (*kleshas*) that are produced by ignorance. Furthermore the accumulated *karmas* in the store-house (*karmashaya*), whether wicked or virtuous, are destroyed, together with wrong knowledge (*viparyaya*). With the destruction of wrong knowledge, which is the cause of and seed for rebirth, no more future conditioned embodiment is necessary — nay, even possible.

This *samadhi* is called "seedless" because the seed of future rebirth, ignorance, and suffering is destroyed. It is also clearly said here that it is only this mightiest of all *samadhis* that can render such seeds sterile and not the weaker objective (*samprajnata*) *samadhi* — as, again, modern writers claim. This is an important point to remember. If we wrongly project such expectations onto objective *samadhi* we will not realize when objective *samadhi* happens to us and we will also expect too much of those who have experienced it.

Only through extensive objectless *samadhi* will the mind (*chitta*) be habitually suspended (*nirodha*), which means it is reabsorbed into *prakrti*. If the yogi needs a mind after this point he projects it forth on appropriate occasions only (*nirmana chitta*). In the interval when no mind is needed, he returns into the infinity of *nirodha*, which is consciousness. This means that such a yogi resides in the heart, is in the natural state, and permanently abides in his or her true nature.

For this reason, only the teachings and statements of a *nirodhin*, one with suspended mind, are binding. Examples of such teachings are the *Upanishads.* The Upanishadic sages were in the state of *nirodha* and could see to the bottom of their hearts. Their teachings are therefore also called *shruti* — that which is heard. Because their minds were still, they were free to hear the sacred wisdom of their hearts. "Heart" here is a metaphor for consciousness, and the wisdom heard is contained in the sacred sound OM, which is produced by Brahman (consciousness).

Again it is very important to understand the

distinction. Prior to *dharma-megha-samadhi* the mind of the yogi is only single-pointed (*ekagra*). From the viewpoint of the beginner this is an incredible achievement, but as a teacher the *ekagrin* — he or she with single pointed mind — is not yet sacred authority. His or her statements are probably very deep and meaningful, but they come from a human mind and not from the depth of the heart. Teachers with single-pointed minds have given us an incredible canon of teachings, called *smrti. Smrti* means that which is memorized, and it is a term for tradition. All *smrti* are understood to be of human origin whereas the *shruti* are considered to be of divine origin.

तदा सर्वावरणमलापेतस्य
ज्ञानस्याऽनन्त्याज्ज्ञेयम् अल्पम् ॥ ३१ ॥

IV.31 Then, when the covering impurities are removed from the infinity of knowledge, the knowables become insignificant.

"Then" means when the cloud-of-characteristics-dispersing *samadhi* is attained. The covering impurities are ignorance (*avidya*) and wrong cognition (*viparyaya*). When those covering impurities are removed, says Patanjali, the infinity of knowledge becomes visible. What is the infinity of knowledge (*jnanasya ananta*)?

The *Upanishads* describe deep reality (Brahman) in terms of three words: truth (*sat*), consciousness (*chit*), and ecstasy (*ananda*). However, some old passages such as *Taittiriya Upanishad* II.1.1 mention *sat, chit,* and *ananta* (infinity).[9] It was later that *ananta* (infinity) was replaced by *ananda* (ecstasy). The *Upanishads* with the older reading are prior to the *Yoga Sutra.* At the time of Patanjali, *ananta* was still used to describe Brahman.

Patanjali does not use the concept of Brahman, since it implies a single entity deeper than *purusha* and *prakrti*, which reconciles their difference. He uses the term *purusha* to refer to the consciousness of an individual. When Patanjali talks about consciousness that is not bound by the confines of an

9. S. Radhakrishnan, ed., *The Principal Upanishads,* HarperCollins Publishers India, New Delhi, 1994, p. 541.

individual, he uses the term "infinity" (*ananta*). Patanjali himself is considered a manifestation of the serpent of infinity, *Ananta*.

The term "infinity of knowledge" means, then, to abide in or to be one with the ocean of infinite consciousness. In today's language, which is strongly influenced by Vedanta, we would say to be one with Brahman.

In that state, when the infinity of consciousness is known, the knowables become insignificant. The knowables are the world with all objects and phenomena — mind, ego, intellect, *gunas*, and so on. Compared to the infinity of consciousness, these knowables or things to be known become so insignificant that Vyasa compares them to fireflies in the sky. Compared to the vastness of the sky, which is here the knowledge of infinite consciousness, all that we can know about objects is like mere insects.

The yogi is now abiding in his true nature as consciousness, which is the container that holds the world and all beings. Compared to the infinity of that container, its content — the world of objects — is little. The yogi is now in a state where he realizes that, compared to knowledge of the infinity of consciousness, knowledge of the world is like a candle held before the blazing sun — or like fireflies before the vastness of the sky.

ततः कृतार्थानां परिणामक्रमसमाप्तिर्गुणानाम् ॥ ३२ ॥

IV.32 Thus, with the *gunas* having fulfilled their purpose, the sequence of their transformation concludes.

Another result of the cloud-of-characteristics-dispersing *samadhi* (*dharma megha samadhi*) is described here. Initially the proximity of nature (*prakrti*) and consciousness (*purusha*) set in motion the dual function of experience and liberation. Stirred into action through the proximity of consciousness, "mother" *prakrti* provides through the *gunas* a seemingly endless sequence of transformations. The term "transformation" (*parinama*) is used here to affirm that the world, although eternal, is at no time in a stable state but in constant flux. If at any time the *gunas* ceased to act, the world would not freeze like a photograph

but would become unmanifest. "Unmanifest" does not mean "nonexistent" in yoga, as nothing that is existent can ever become nonexistent or unreal, and nothing that is nonexistent can ever become real.

When the yogi becomes liberated through the cloud-of-characteristics-dispersing *samadhi*, the purpose of the *gunas* is fulfilled. As explained in *Samkhya Karika*, *prakrti* ceases to perform her dance once she has been seen. The sequence of transformations of the *gunas* is nothing but the dance of nature (*prakrti*). *Prakrti* ceases to dance, the *gunas* become reabsorbed into their origin (*prakrti*), and the world swings back from manifest to unmanifest, as far as the liberated yogi is concerned. This does not change the reality of the world, which remains existent but unmanifest. It will still be manifest for others.

क्षणप्रतियोगी परिणामापरान्तनिर्ग्राह्यः क्रमः ॥ ३३ ॥

IV.33 Sequence, which consists of instants, ends through the conclusion of transformation.

This sutra states that when the *gunas* have concluded their activity, and therefore the constant transformation (*parinama*) of one phenomenon into the next ceases, time ceases as well. This might be a disturbing concept at first, but it becomes clearer and less threatening when inquired into.

We know time only from changes in nature. We observed that the earth turns around its axis and called it one day. Apart from that movement and its result, the changes in daylight, there is no justification for the idea of the day. Hours, minutes, and so on are only subdivisions of the concept "day." We observe that the earth circles around the sun, and we call it a year. We watch a certain movement in nature and call the sum of instants that passed "time." If for some reason the earth lost contact with the sun, our time units would become meaningless, and we would have to look for other changes in nature. Time is a conceptualization (*vikalpa*). *Vikalpa* is defined as a word that does not have a corresponding object. Time has no corresponding object in nature; it is merely deduced by the human mind, based on observation.

Our universe is said to be billions of years old and is predicted to last for another fifteen billion years. Prior to the Big Bang, all matter was condensed in one spot. Time is dependent on observation of change, an external reference point, and an observer. None of them can be ascertained prior to the Big Bang. This leads us to the conclusion that there was no time either.

Everything that has a beginning must have an end. When the universe ceases in fifteen billion years, time will cease as well. As we know from Einstein's relativity, time is dependent on the observer. With no observer left at the end of the universe, there will be no time. According to Indian logic, however, what is not real in the beginning or at the end is not real in the middle either.

According to Yoga, time is connected to mutability. Since consciousness is immutable, there is no time in consciousness. Time is an intellectual construct of the mind, a conceptualization. Time is born from mind; it is a child of the mind. Once the mind is dissolved into *prakrti*, time is dissolved with it.

What is time, then, if it has no true reality as such? As explained in the previous sutra, the *guna*s manifest the world as being in constant transformation. If we observe an object, let us say our body, we see that it constantly changes. Through the constant flux of the *guna*s our body appears first as young, then as mature, and later as old. The change from young to old is called "change of state" (*avastha parinama*). When the body eventually dies and disappears, it changes from a manifest into a residue state. Similarly, when it is born it changes from a potential to a manifest state. This type of change is called "change of manifestation" (*lakshana parinama*). This means that time is a mental concept that describes change of manifestation.

We can look at it from another point of view as well. The body does not actually disappear, only its form does. All elementary particles that formed the body will continue to exist, albeit forming different compounds. This type of change is called "change of characteristic" (*dharma parinama*). Underlying those three forms of change are "sequences" (*krama*). The change from young to old does not happen all at once; only after a certain *krama* is observed do we call it change. The smallest unit during which any change is still observable is called an instant (*kshana*). An instant is perceivable only if a change has occurred, even if that was only our breath or the ticking of a clock. If no change whatsoever is perceivable, we won't notice that an instant has passed and a sequence is happening. If we were isolated in a situation where we could not observe sequences, we could not say time had passed.

Time therefore is abstracted from change. If we cannot observe any of the three types of change and their sequence, we will not deduce the passing of time. The conceptualization of time will cease when sequence and instant cease. Sequence and instant cease when change (*parinama*) ceases. *Parinama* ceases when the *guna*s cease their work. The *guna*s cease to work when their purpose is fulfilled. Their purpose is fulfilled when *dharma-megha-samadhi* is experienced and the seer abides in his or her own form (consciousness).

पुरुषार्थशून्यानां गुणानां प्रतिप्रसवः कैवल्यं स्वरूपप्रतिष्ठा वा चितिशक्तिरेति ॥ ३४ ॥

IV.34 When the *gunas*, having lost their purpose, return into their source (*prakrti*), then liberation takes place, which is pure consciousness established in its own nature.

The purpose of the *guna*s is to manifest the world, a process that provides experience for *purusha*. From experience comes bondage, which is the illusionary union of the seer and the seen. From bondage, through supply of pleasure and pain, comes eventually the realization of the existence of consciousness (*purusha*) as one's true nature.

At this point we realize that the intellect, which is the highest manifestation of the *guna*s, was never commingled with consciousness, which was always free and untouched. This realization is called *kaivalya*, the independence of consciousness.

The liberated yogi is established now in his or her true nature as consciousness, which is the self-in-itself. It is a permanent state of unlimited freedom and supercognitive ecstasy. Supercognitive here means that we have gone beyond the need for phenomena, manifestation, and world. It is these that limited our ecstasy and freedom before.

We are free now to recognize that we were never reborn, were never bound by ignorance, and never an isolated egoic entity. Since the consciousness in which we abide now is eternal and immutable, it existed all along as a state of unlimited freedom that was not recognized by us in our delusion.

The *gunas*, having fulfilled their purpose, are reabsorbed into their source, which is nature (*prakrti*). This means that, in regard to the liberated yogi, the world has transformed into the residue state. This does not mean that it is nonexistent, since it is still manifest to serve others.

Here ends the path of Yoga. The liberated yogi, permanently abiding in consciousness, stays embodied until the body comes to its natural end. The yogi then becomes one with eternal, bodiless, supercognitive ecstasy.

Is there something left to do?

The school of Yoga is silent in regard to a state even higher than that, which is the state of identity (as Shankara has it) or identity-in-difference (as Ramanuja has it) with the Supreme Being. This does not mean Yoga and the school on which it is based, the Samkhya, are ignorant of that state.

The "founders" of both schools, Bhagavan Patanjali and Rishi Kapila, are seen as manifestations of the very same Supreme Being. Nevertheless their aim was to devise a path to freedom that does not rely on knowing (in the case of Yoga) or surrendering (in the case of Samkhya) to the Supreme Being.

The yogi may, as soon as the mind is free from wrong cognition, go on to study the Vedanta instead of continuing to follow the path of Yoga.

Alternatively the yogi may, after attaining realization of his or her own consciousness, go on to realize the one that was never ignorant.

The one that is the first and foremost of all teachers.

The one that has been known by various names such as the Brahman, the Dao, the Lord, and the Mother, and that, after all names are left behind, is still there as the incomprehensible, luminous, vibrant, silent, vast emptiness in our hearts.

GLOSSARY

ABDUCTOR Muscle that draws a bone away from the midline of the body.

ACHARYA Teacher, one who has studied the texts, practiced the methods, achieved the results, and is capable of communicating them.

ADDUCTOR Muscle that draws a bone toward the midline of the body.

ADVAITA VEDANTA Upanishadic philosophy propounding unqualified monism, founded by Acharya Gaudapada and developed by Acharya Shankara, holding that the individual self (*atman*) and the deep reality (Brahman) are identical.

AFFLICTIONS The five forms of suffering (*klesha*s).

AHAMKARA Egoity, I-maker, the one that owns the perception, not to be mistaken for the Freudian ego.

AKASHA Space, ether.

ALLOPATHY Western medicine.

ANAHATA CHAKRA Heart *chakra*, a subtle energy center.

ANAHATA NADA The unstruck sound, sound of the heart lotus, an object of meditation.

ANANDA Ecstasy, bliss.

ANANTA Infinity, a name of the serpent of infinity.

ANTERIOR Forward, in front.

ASAMPRAJNATA Objectless *samadhi*, supercognitive *samadhi*.

ASANA Posture.

ASHTADYAYI Ancient treatise on Sanskrit grammar, authored by Panini.

ASMITA Literally I-am-ness. 1. Egoism, to take seer and seeing as one, one of the five forms of suffering.
2. A form of objective *samadhi* that arises when pure I-am-ness is witnessed.

ATMAN The true self, consciousness. Term used by Vedanta instead of *purusha*.

AVATARA Divine manifestation.

AVIDYA Ignorance.

AYURVEDA Ancient Indian medicine, one of the four subsidiary *Veda*s (*Upveda*s).

BANDHA Bond, energetic lock.

BHAGAVAD GITA Song of the Lord, most influential of all *shastra*s. The Supreme Being in the form of Lord Krishna amalgamates the teachings of Samkhya, Yoga, and Vedanta.

BHAGAVATA PURANA Also called *Shrimad Bhagavatam*, a *Purana* that deals with devotion to the Supreme Being

in the form of Lord Vishnu. All *avatara*s of Vishnu are described, including Krishna.

BHAKTI Yoga of love, the practice of devotion to the Supreme Being.

BHOGA Consummation, experience, bondage.

BONDAGE Erroneous identification with the transitory, being bound up with the phenomena.

BRAHMA SUTRA Principal treatise of the Vedanta, authored by Rishi Vyasa.

BRAHMACHARYA Recognition of Brahman in everything, later to mean celibacy.

BRAHMAN Infinite consciousness, deep reality, the reality that cannot be reduced to a deeper layer.

BRAHMARANDHRA Gate of Brahman, upper end of *sushumna*.

BUDDHI Intellect, seat of intelligence.

CERVICAL SPINE The vertebrae of the neck.

CHAKRA Subtle energy center.

CHARAKA SAMHITA Treatise on *Ayurveda*. The author, Charaka, is said to be an incarnation of Patanjali.

COGNITION Effort of the mind to identify and interpret data supplied by the senses.

COGNITIVE *SAMADHI* *Samadhi* whose arising depends on cognition of an object; objective *samadhi*.

CONSCIOUSNESS That which is conscious, the observer, awareness.

DARSHANA View, system of philosophy. The *darshana*s are divided into orthodox and heterodox, depending on whether they accept or reject the authority of the Vedas. The orthodox *darshana*s are Samkhya (rational inquiry), Yoga (science of the mind), Mimamsa (science of action), Nyaya (logic), Vaiseshika (categorization), Vedanta (analysis of the *Upanishad*s). These *darshana*s ideally do not compete with each other but solve different problems. The Yoga master T. Krishnamacharya had degrees in all six systems. The heterodox *darshana*s are Jaina (Jainism), Baudha (Buddhism), and Charvaka (materialism). A special case is Tantra, which is neither accepted as orthodox nor seen as heterodox. Shankara was probably the last human being to have mastered all ten systems of philosophy.

DHARANA Concentration.

DHARMA 1. Characteristic, attribute. 2. Righteousness, virtue.

DHARMIN Object-as-such, such-ness of an object, essence of an object.

DHYANA Meditation.

DRISHTI Focal point.

EKAGRA CHITTA Single-pointed mind, the mind fit to practice higher yoga.

ENTROPY Amount of disorder in a system.

EXTENSION Returning from flexion.

FEMUR Thigh bone.

FLEXION To bind, to bring bones together.

FULL-*VINYASA* SYSTEM Practice in which one does a *vinyasa* to standing between sitting postures.

GUNAS *Rajas*, *tamas*, and *sattva*, the qualities or strands of *prakrti* which form, through their various intertwinings, all phenomena.

HALF-*VINYASA* SYSTEM Practice in which one transits through *Chaturanga Dandasana*, Upward Dog, and Downward Dog between sitting postures.

HATHA YOGA Tantric school of yoga that was founded approx. 1100 CE by the master Ghoraknath. Literally sun/moon yoga, the emphasis is on balancing the solar and lunar energy channels in the body. Hatha Yoga shifted the focus away from the mysticism and philosophy of the older upanishadic types of yoga toward using the body as a tool.

HATHA YOGA PRADIPIKA A tantric treatise authored by Svatmarama.

HEART Sanskrit *hrdaya*, referring to the core of all phenomena, which according to the Vedanta is consciousness. If the term is used in an anatomical instruction it refers to the core of the ribcage.

HUMERUS Arm bone.

HYPEREXTENSION Extension beyond 180°.

IDA Lunar energy channel.

INSERTION OF A MUSCLE End of the muscle that is distant from the center of the body.

INTELLECT Seat of intelligence.

ISHTADEVATA Meditation deity, personal projection that enables one to establish a devotional relationship to the Supreme Being

ISHVARA The Supreme Being, Brahman with form.

ISOMETRIC EXERCISE Exercise in which the muscle does not get shortened.

ISOTONIC EXERCISE Exercise that involves shortening of a muscle.

ITIHASA Scriptures that deal with what once was, history: the *Mahabharata*, the *Ramayana*, and the *Yoga Vashishta*.

JIVA Phenomenal self, image of oneself that is formed through contact with the phenomena, not the true self.

JNANA Knowledge, here knowledge of the self.

JNANIN Knower, here a knower of the self.

KAIVALYA Freedom, independence; the goal of yoga.

KALI YUGA Current age, age of darkness; started 3102 BCE with the death of Lord Krishna; thought to last for another 400,000 years.

KAPHA One of the three ayurvedic humors, sometimes translated as phlegm.

KARMA Action.

KARMA, LAW OF Law of cause and effect.

KARMASHAYA Storehouse where the effects of our actions are stored.

KLESHA Mode of suffering. The modes are ignorance, egoism, desire, hatred, and fear of death.

KRAMA Sequence of moments, succession of moments.

KRISHNA, LORD A form of the Supreme Being, *avatara* of Lord Vishnu, teacher in the *Bhagavad Gita*.

KSHANA Instant, moment, smallest time unit.

KSHIPTA CHITTA Restless mind, unfit to do yoga.

KUMBHAKA Breath retention.

KUNDALINI 1. The obstacle that closes the mouth of *sushumna*. 2. Sometimes used to refer to the rising of *shakti* in the *sushumna*.

KYPHOSIS Forward curvature of the spine.

LATERAL Sideways, away from the body midline.

LATERAL ROTATION External rotation.

LIBERATION To recognize one's true nature as the eternal, immutable consciousness.

LORDOSIS Backward curvature of the spine.

LUMBAR SPINE The vertebrae of the low back.

MAHABHARATA Largest piece of literature created by man, *dharma shastra* (scripture dealing with right action), authored by Rishi Vyasa; contains the *Bhagavad Gita*.

MAHABHUTA Gross element, i.e., ether, air, fire, water, or earth.

MANDALA Circular drawing, sacred geometry, a meditation object.

MANDUKYA KARIKA Commentary on the *Mandukya Upanishad*, authored by Acharya Gaudapada, which constitutes the beginning of the philosophical school of Advaita Vedanta. Gaudapada contends that the three states of waking, dreaming, and deep sleep have no reality of their own and are dependent on the fourth state (*turiya*), the consciousness.

MEDIAL Toward the body midline.

MEDIAL ROTATION Internal rotation.

MOKSHA Liberation from bondage.

MOKSHA SHASTRA Scripture dealing with liberation.

MUDHA CHITTA Mind infatuated with materialistic stupor, unfit to do yoga.

MUDRA Seal, usually a combination of *asana*, *pranayama*, and *bandha*.

MULA BANDHA Root lock.

NADI Literally river; energy channel.

NIRGUNA BRAHMAN Formless Brahman, deep reality, infinite consciousness.

NIRODHA CHITTA Suspended mind, the natural state, the goal of yoga.

OBJECT Everything that is not the subject (consciousness); includes ego, intelligence, and the universe.

OBJECT OF MEDITATION Any object of sattvic quality, such as a mantra, the symbol OM, a *yantra* or *mandala* (sacred geometry), a lotus flower, the breath, one's meditation deity, emptiness, the light or sound in the heart, the intelligence, the subtle elements.

OBJECTIVE SAMADHI *Samadhi* that depends for its arising on an object.

OBJECTLESS SAMADHI *Samadhi* that does not depend for its arising on an object, and therefore can reveal the subject, the consciousness.

ORIGIN OF A MUSCLE End of the muscle that is closer to the body center.

PARAVAIRAGYA Supreme surrender, total letting go, supreme detachment.

PARINAMA Transformation, change.

PINGALA Solar energy channel.

PITTA One of the three ayurvedic humors, sometimes translated as bile.

POSTERIOR Backward, opposite of anterior.

PRAJNA Complete knowledge of the phenomena produced by *prakrti*.

PRAKRTI Procreatress, procreativeness, nature, the matrix or womb that produces the entire subtle and gross universe apart from consciousness.

PRANA Life force or inner breath; refers sometimes to anatomical or outer breath.

PRANAYAMA Breath extension, breathing exercises to harmonize the flow of life force.

PRATYAHARA Independence from sensory stimuli.

PURANAS Literally ancients. Sacred texts that relate mysticism and philosophy, in the form of allegories and stories, to common man.

PURUSHA Pure consciousness, which is eternal and immutable; term used by Samkhya and Yoga instead of *atman*.

RAJAS Frenzy, energy, dynamics; one of the *guna*s of *prakrti*.

RAMAYANA Literally Rama's way. Ancient epic (*itihasa*) that describes the life of Rama, an *avatara* of Lord Vishnu.

RISHI Vedic seer, liberated sage, one who through suspension of mind can see to the bottom of his or her heart.

SAGUNA BRAHMAN The Supreme Being, Brahman, with form.

SAMADHI Absorption.

SAMAPATTI Identity of the mind with an object; state of the mind during objective *samadhi*.

SAMKHYA The oldest system of philosophy, founded by Rishi Kapila.

SAMKHYA KARIKA Treatise authored by Ishvarakrishna describing the Samkhya system of philosophy. The Karika is of great importance, since it is the oldest surviving text describing the Samkhya on which Yoga is based. One needs to keep in mind, however, that this text is younger than the *Yoga Sutra* and is not representative of older and more original forms of Samkhya.

SAMPRAJNATA Objective *samadhi*, cognitive *samadhi*.

SAMSARA Conditioned existence, the endless round of rebirths.

SAMSKARA Subconscious imprint.

SAMYAMA Combined application of *dharana*, *dhyana*, and objective *samadhi*.

SATTVA Light, wisdom, intelligence; one of the *guna*s of *prakrti*.

SHAIVITE A worshiper of Shiva.

SHAKTI 1. Mother Goddess, consort of Shiva, personification of *prakrti*. 2. Energy, life force, *prana*.

SHASTRA Scripture, path to truth.

SHATKRIYA Literally six actions, a set of purifying actions used in Hatha Yoga to restore the balance between the three humors (*dosha*s) of the body.

SHIVA, LORD A name of the Supreme Being, pure consciousness, Brahman with form.

SHRUTI *Veda*s and *Upanishad*s, revealed scriptures of divine origin, which are seen or heard by a *rishi*.

SHUNYATA Emptiness, void.

SHUNYAVADIN Adherent of the Buddhist Shunyavada school of thought, which holds that the inherent nature of all phenomena is emptiness (*shunyata*).

SIDDHA Perfected being.

SIDDHIS Perfections, supernatural powers.

SMRTI 1. Sacred tradition, scriptures conceived by the human mind that explain the revealed *shruti*.
2. Memory, one of the five fluctuations of the mind.

SUBCOMMENTARY A commentary that further explains an already existing commentary on an original treatise. Since Indian masters very much respected those that thought before them, they often compiled texts that added another layer of explanation and interpretation, rather than starting their own school of thought.

SUBTLE Something real but not perceptible to the senses. It can be perceived directly in objective *samadhi*. The word appears in many expressions such as subtle body, subtle element, subtle anatomy.

SUPERCOGNITIVE SAMADHI *Samadhi* beyond cognition of object, objectless *samadhi*, *samadhi* that reveals the subject, the consciousness.

SUSHUMNA Central energy channel, Hatha Yoga's metaphor for the heart.

SVADHYAYA Study of sacred texts.

TAMAS Dullness, inertia, mass; one of the *gunas* of *prakrti*.

TANMATRA Subtle element, infra atomic potential, smallest particle of matter.

TANTRA 1. System that focuses on the precise performance of actions rather than mystical speculation. 2. Treatise in which this system is described.

THORACIC SPINE The vertebrae of the rib cage.

TIBIA Shin bone.

UDDIYANA One of the *Shatkriyas* of Hatha Yoga; sucking of the abdominal contents up into the thoracic cavity during *Kumbhaka*.

UDDIYANA BANDHA Elevating lock, lower abdominal lock, drawing of the lower abdominal contents in against the spine.

UJJAYI PRANAYAMA Victorious stretching of life force.

UPANISHADS Ancient scriptures out of which all systems of Indian philosophy developed. The *Upanishads* are conceived by the heart (*shruti*).

UPVEDA Ancilliary Veda, of which there are four: *Ayurveda* (medicine), *Arthaveda* (economy), *Dhanurveda* (military science), and *Gandharvaveda* (music).

VAISHNAVITE A worshiper of Vishnu.

VASANA Conditioning, an accumulation of subconscious imprints.

VATA One of the three ayurvedic humors, sometimes translated as wind.

VAYU Literally wind, vital air current.

VEDANTA Literally end of the *Veda*. Analysis of the content of the *Upanishads*, main treatise being the *Brahma Sutra*. Several schools developed (Advaita Vedanta, Visishtadvaita Vedanta, Dvaita Vedanta).

VEDAS Oldest sacred texts of humankind. Vyasa divided the one *Veda* into four, the *Rig*, *Yajur*, *Sama*, and *Atharva Vedas*, all of which are subdivided into *Samhita* (hymns), *Brahmana* (ritual), *Aranyaka* (worship), and *Upanishad* (mysticism). There are four anciliary *Vedas* (*Upvedas*), which are *Ayurveda* (medicine), *Arthaveda* (economy), *Dhanurveda* (military science), and *Gandharvaveda* (music). The *Veda* has six limbs (*Vedangas*), which are *Vyakarana* (Sanskrit grammar), *Jyotisha* (astrology), *Nirukta* (etymology), *Shiksha* (phonetics), *Chandas* (meter), and *Kalpa* (ritual, duty). Early hymns of the *Rig Veda* are in excess of 8000 years old. According to tradition the *Vedas* are eternal and are seen at the beginning of each world age by the *rishis*.

VIDYA Correct knowledge, opposite of ignorance (*avidya*).

VIKALPA Conceptualization, a word without an object that it refers to.

VIKSHIPTA CHITTA Confused mind, the mind fit to commence practice of yoga.

VINYASA Sequential movement that interlinks postures to form a continuous flow. It creates a movement meditation that reveals all forms as being impermanent and for this reason are not held on to.

VIPARYAYA Wrong cognition, error, wrong identification of the perceived object.

VISHNU, LORD A name of the Supreme Being; Brahman with form.

VISISHTADVAITA VEDANTA Upanishadic philosophy propounding qualified monism, developed by the Acharya Ramanuja. Holds that the individual self (*atman*) and the deep reality (Brahman) are identical yet different.

VIVEKA KHYATEH Discriminative knowledge, knowledge of the difference between the seer and the seen.

VIVEKINAH A knower of the difference, one who has gained discriminative knowledge.

VRTTI Literally whirls, fluctuations, modifications (of the mind).

YANTRA Sacred drawing that is eventually visualized; meditation object used in the school of Tantra.

YOGA KORUNTA Treatise on sequential yoga authored by Rishi Vamana.

YOGA VASHISHTA Ancient treatise in which the nondualistic teachings of the Rishi Vasishta are rendered in 30,000 stanzas.

BIOGRAPHIES
OF YOGA MASTERS AND *RISHIS* MENTIONED IN THE TEXT

ARANYA, SWAMI HARIHARANANDA Late abbot of the Kapila Math in Bihar; author of a subcommentary on the *Yoga Sutra*.

ASHTAVAKRA, RISHI "The eightfold-bent," compiler of the *Ashtavakra Gita*. When Ashtavakra was still in his mother's womb, he once overheard his brahmin father recite the *Veda*s incorrectly, whereupon he called out from inside his mother's body and rebuked him. His father then angrily cursed Ashtavakra to be born bent in eight places, which indeed he was. Having been called to the court of the king to engage in learned dispute, his father was defeated by a famed *pandit* of the king and thrown into a dungeon. When Ashtavakra was only twelve years old he went and defeated the great *pandit* in disputation and had his father released. His father retracted the curse and asked him to bathe in a holy river, which made his body straight again.

GAUDAPADA, ACHARYA Master who developed Advaita Vedanta as a systematic philosophy; author of the *Mandukya Karika* and the commentary on the *Samkhya Karika*.

ISHVARA KRISHNA Author of the oldest remaining text on Samkhya, the *Samkhya Karika*.

KAPILA, RISHI Founder of Samkhya, the first systematic philosophy, noted in the *Bhagavad Gita* and *Bhagavata Purana* as a manifestation of the Supreme Being.

KRISHNAMACHARYA, SHRI T. Master of Shri Krishna Pattabhi Jois, student of Ramamohan Brahmachary.

MAHARSHI, RAMANA Liberated sage, modern master of Advaita Vedanta.

PANCHASIKHA, RISHI Ancient Samkhya master who further developed the teachings of the Rishi Kapila, author of a lost treatise on Samkhya.

PANINI Ancient Sanskrit grammarian, author of *Ashtadyayi*.

PATANJALI Author of the *Yoga Sutra*, the *Great Commentary* on Panini's grammar, and the *Charaka Samhita*, a text on *Ayurveda*. Thought to be a manifestation of the serpent of infinity.

PATTABHI JOIS, SHRI KRISHNA Modern master of Ashtanga Yoga, student of Shri T. Krishnamacharya.

RAMANUJA, ACHARYA Authored a commentary on the *Brahma Sutra* among other texts; developed the Visishtadvaita Vedanta; taught the identity-in-difference (*beda abeda*) between the individual self (*atman*) and the infinite consciousness (Brahman); advocate of Bhakti Yoga.

SHANKARA, ACHARYA Main protagonist of the Advaita Vedanta; mystic, philosopher, yogi; often believed to be of divine origin; author of commentaries on *Upanishads*, *Bhagavad Gita,* and *Brahma Sutra*. Probably the most influential of all Indian masters.

VACHASPATI MISHRA Tenth-century scholar who obtained fame by writing commentaries on all six orthodox systems of Indian philosophy; author of *Tattva-Vaisharadi* (subcommentary on the *Yoga Sutra*).

VAMANA, RISHI Author of the *Yoga Korunta*.

VASISHTA, RISHI Author of portions of the *Veda* and the *Yoga Vashishta*, court priest of King Dasharatha, the father of Lord Rama in the *Ramayana* epic.

VIJNANABHIKSHU Fourteenth-century yoga master and philosopher, author of *Yogavarttika*, a subcommentary on the *Yoga Sutra*.

VISHVAMITRA, RISHI Seer who saw the *Gayatri*, the most sacred of all mantras. Vishvamitra never hesitated to take hardship on himself, performing the severest and longest austerities of all the *rishi*s. He could never say no if approached for help by the downtrodden; this earned him his name, which means "friend of the world."

VYASA, RISHI Divider of the *Veda*, author of the *Mahabharata, Brahma Sutra, Yoga Commentary,* and *Purana*s, born as Krishna Dvaipayana.

YAJNAVALKYA, RISHI Most prominent of the upanishadic *rishi*s, he formulated the core doctrine of the *Upanishads*: that all appearances are nothing but Brahman.

BIBLIOGRAPHY

Adams, G. C., Jr., translator and commentator, *Badarayana's Brahma Sutras*, Motilal Banarsidass, Delhi, 1993.

Agehananda Bharati, Sw., *The Light at the Center*, Ross-Erickson, Santa Barbara, 1976.

Agehananda Bharati, Sw., *The Ochre Robe*, 2nd rev. ed., Ross-Erickson, Santa Barbara, 1980.

Agehananda Bharati, Sw., *The Tantric Tradition*, Anchor Books, New York, 1970.

Aranya, Sw. H., *Yoga Philosophy of Patanjali with Bhasvati*, 4th enlarged ed., University of Calcutta, Kolkata, 2000.

Ashokananda, Sw., translator and commentator, *Avadhuta Gita of Dattatreya*, Sri Ramakrishna Math, Madras.

Ashtavakra Gita, 8th ed., Sri Ramanasramam, Tiruvannamalai, 2001.

Baba, B., translator and commentator, *Yogasutra of Patanjali*, Motilal Banarsidass, Delhi, 1976.

Bachhofer, J., *Milarepa Meister der Verrueckten Weisheit*, Windpferd.

Bader, J., *Meditation in Sankara's Vedanta*, Aditya Prakashan, New Delhi, 1990.

Balantyne, J. R., translator and commentator, *Yoga Sutra of Patanjali*, Book Faith India, Delhi, 2000.

Banerjea, A. K., *Philosophy of Gorakhnath*, 1st Indian ed., Motilal Banarsidass, Delhi, 1983.

Bernard, T., *Heaven Lies Within Us*, Charles Scribner's Sons, New York, 1939.

Bernard, T., *Hindu Philosophy*, Jaico Publishing House, Mumbai, 1989.

Bhatt, G. P. (ed.), *The Skanda Purana*, part 1, trans. G. V. Tagare, Motilal Banarsidass, Delhi, 1992.

Bhattacharya, V., editor and translator, *The Agamasastra of Gaudapada*, Motilal Banarsidass, Delhi, 1943.

Bose, A. C., *The Call of the Vedas*, Bharatiya Vidya Bhavan, Mumbai, 1999.

Bouanchaud, B., *The Essence of Yoga*, Rudra Press, Portland, Oregon, 1997.

Briggs, G. W., *Goraknath and the Kanphata Yogis*, 1st Indian ed., Motilal Banarsidass, Delhi, 1938.

Calais-Germaine, B., *Anatomy of Movement*, rev. ed., Eastland Press, Seattle, 1991.

Calasso, R., *Ka — Stories of the Minds and Gods of India*, Vintage Books, New York, 1999.

Chaitow, L., *Positional Release Techniques*, 2nd ed., Churchill Livingstone, London, 2002.

Chandra Vasu, R. B. S., translator, *The Gheranda Samhita*, Sri Satguru Publications, Delhi, 1986.

Chandra Vasu, R. B. S., translator, *The Siva Samhita*, Sri Satguru Publications, Delhi, 1984.

Chang, G. C. C., translator, *Teachings and Practice of Tibetan Tantra*, Dover Publications, Mineola, New York, 2004.

Chapple, C., translator, *The Yoga Sutras of Patanjali*, Sri Satguru Publications, Delhi, 1990.

Clemente, C. D., *Anatomy — A Regional Atlas of the Human Body*, 4th ed., Williams & Wilkins, Baltimore, Maryland, 1997.

Cole, C. A., *Asparsa Yoga — A Study of Gaudapada's Mandukya Karika*, Motilal Banarsidass, Delhi, 1982.

Coulter, D., *Anatomy of Hatha Yoga*, Body and Breath Inc., Honesdale, Pennsylvania, 2001.

Dahlke, P., translator, *Buddha — Die Lehre des Erhabenen*, Wilhelm Goldmann Verlag, Munich, 1920.

Dasgupta, S., *A History of Indian Philosophy*, 1st Indian ed., 5 vols., Motilal Banarsidass, Delhi, 1975.

Dasgupta, S., *Yoga as Philosophy and Religion*, Motilal Banarsidass, Delhi, 1973.

Desikachar, T. K. V., *Health, Healing and Beyond*, Aperture, Denville, New Jersey, 1998.

Desikachar, T. K. V., *The Heart of Yoga*, Inner Traditions, Rochester, Vermont, 1995.

Desikachar, T. K. V., translator, *Yoga Taravali*, Krishnamacharya Yoga Mandiram, Chennai, 2003.

Deussen, P., *The Philosophy of the Upanishads*, translated by A. S. Geden, Motilal Banarsidass, Delhi, 1997.

Deussen, P., editor, *Sixty Upanisads of the Veda*, translated by V. M. Bedekar & G. B. Palsule, 2 vols., Motilal Banarsidass, Delhi, 1997.

Deutsch, E., *Advaita Vedanta — A Philosophical Reconstruction*, University of Hawaii Press, Honululu, 1973.

Digambarji, Sw., editor and commentator, *Vasishta Samhita*, Kaivalyadhama, Lonavla, 1984.

Doniger O'Flaherty, W., *Siva — The Erotic Ascetic*, Oxford University Press, London & New York, 1973.

Douglas, N., *Tantra Yoga*, Munshiram Manoharlal, New Delhi, 1971.

Dvivedi, M. N., translator and commentator, *The Yoga Sutras of Patanjali*, Sri Satguru Publications, Delhi, 1890.

Egenes, T., *Introduction to Sanskrit*, part 1, 3rd rev. ed., Motilal Banarsidass, Delhi, 2003.

Egenes, T., *Introduction to Sanskrit*, part 2, Motilal Banarsidass, Delhi, 2000.

Eliade, M., *Yoga — Immortality and Freedom*, 2nd ed., Princeton University Press, Princeton, New Jersey, 1969.

Evans-Wentz, W. Y., editor, *The Tibetan Book of the Dead*, Oxford University Press, London, 1960.

Evans-Wentz, W. Y., editor, *Tibetan Yoga and Secret Doctrines*, Oxford University Press, Oxford, 1958.

Evans-Wentz, W. Y., editor, *Tibet's Great Yogi Milarepa*, 2nd ed., Munshiram Manoharlal, Delhi, 2000.

Feldenkrais, M., *Awareness through Movement*, HarperCollins, San Francisco, 1990.

Feuerstein, G., *The Shambhala Encyclopedia of Yoga*, Shambhala, Boston, 1997.

Feuerstein, G., *The Yoga Tradition*, Hohm Press, Prescott, Arizona, 2001.

Feuerstein, G., translator and commentator, *The Yoga-Sutra of Patanjali*, Inner Traditions, Rochester, Vermont, 1989.

Frawley, D., *Ayurvedic Healing — A Comprehensive Guide*, 1st Indian ed., Motilal Banarsidass, Delhi, 1992.

Frawley, D., *From the River of Heaven*, 1st Indian ed., Motilal Banarsidass, Delhi, 1992.

Frawley, D., *Gods, Sages and Kings*, 1st Indian ed., Motilal Banarsidass, Delhi, 1993.

Frawley, D., *Tantric Yoga and the Wisdom Goddesses*, 1st Indian ed., Motilal Banarsidass, Delhi, 1996.

Frawley, D., *Wisdom of the Ancient Seers*, Motilal Banarsidass, Delhi, 1994.

Frawley, D., *The Yoga of Herbs*, 1st Indian ed., Motilal Banarsidass, Delhi, 1994.

Freeman, R., *The Yoga Matrix* (audio casettes), Sounds True, Boulder, Colorado, 2001.

Freeman, R., *Yoga with Richard Freeman* (video and handbook), Delphi Productions, Boulder, Colorado, 1993.

Friend, J., *Anusara Yoga — Teacher Training Manual*, Anusara Press, Spring 1999.

Gambhirananda, Sw., *Bhagavad Gita with Commentary of Sankaracarya*, Advaita Ashrama, Kolkata, 1997.

Gambhirananda, Sw., translator, *Brahma Sutra Bhasya of Sri Sankaracarya*, Advaita Ashrama, Kolkata, 1965.

Gambhirananda, Sw., translator, *Eight Upanisads*, Advaita Ashrama, Kolkata, 1996.

Ganganatha, J., translator, *Yoga-Sara-Sangraha of Vijnana — Bhiksu*, rev. ed., Parimal Publications, Delhi, 1995.

Ganguli, K. M., translator, *The Mahabharata*, 12 vols., Munshiram Manoharlal, New Delhi, 1998.

Gharote, M. L., translator, *Brhadyajnavalkyasmrti*, Kaivalyadhama, Lonavla, 1982.

Godman, D., editor, *Be As You Are — The Teachings of Ramana Maharshi*, Penguin Books India, New Delhi, 1985.

Gopal, L., *Retrieving Samkhya History*, D. K. Printworld (P) Ltd., New Delhi, 2000.

Gosh, S., translator, editor, and commentator, *The Original Yoga*, 2nd rev. ed., Munshiram Manoharlal, New Delhi, 1999.

Govinda, L. A., *Der Weg der weissen Wolken*, Scherz Verlag, Bern, 1975.

Grabowski, T., *Principles of Anatomy and Physiology*, 10th ed., John Wiley & Sons, Hoboken, New Jersey, 2003.

Guenther, H.v., translator, *Juwelenschmuck der geistigen Befreiung*, Eugen Diederichs Verlag, Munich, 1989.

Guenther, H.v., translator and commentator, *The Life and Teaching of Naropa*, Shambala, Boston, 1995.

Gupta, A. S., *The Evolution of the Samkhya School of Thought*, 2nd rev. ed., Munshiram Manoharlal, New Delhi, 1986.

Gupta, S. R., translator and commentator, *The Word Speaks to the Faustian Man*, vol. 2, *A Translation and Interpretation of the Prasthanatrayi*, Motilal Banarsidass, Delhi, 1995.

Gurdjieff, G. I., *Beelzebub's Erzaehlungen fuer seinen Enkel*, Sphinx Verlag, Basel, 1981.

Gurdjieff, G. I., *Begnungen mit bemerkenswerten Menschen*, Aurum Verlag, Freiburg, 1978.

Gurdjieff, G. I., *Das Leben ist nur dann wirklich wenn ich bin*, Sphinx Verlag, Basel, 1987.

Hamill, S. & Seaton, J. P., translators and editors, *The Essential Chuang Tzu*, Shambala, Boston, 1998.

Isayeva, N., *From Early Vedanta to Kashmir Shaivism*, 1st Indian ed., Sri Satguru Publications, Delhi, 1997.

Iyengar, B. K. S., *Light on Pranayama*, HarperCollins Publishers India, New Delhi, 1993.

Iyengar, B. K. S., *Light on the Yoga Sutras of Patanjali*, HarperCollins Publishers India, New Delhi, 1993.

Iyengar, B. K. S., *Light on Yoga*, 2nd ed., Allen & Unwin, London, 1976.

Iyengar, B. K. S., *The Tree of Yoga*, HarperCollins Publishers India, New Delhi, 1995.

Jacobsen, A. J., *Prakrti in Samhkya-Yoga*, 1st Indian ed., Motilal Banarsidass, Delhi, 2002.

Jagadananda, Sw., translator, *Upadesa Sahasri of Sri Sankaracarya*, Sri Ramakrishna Math, Madras.

Jagadananda, Sw., translator, *Vakyavrtti of Sri Sankaracarya*, Sri Ramakrishna Math, Madras.

Jois, K. P., *Ashtanga Yoga with K. Pattabhi Jois*, 1st series (video), Yoga Works Productions, Santa Monica, California, 1996.

Jois, K. P., *Yoga Mala*, 1st English ed., Eddie Stern / Patanjala Yoga Shala, New York, 1999.

Kale, M. R., *A Higher Sanskrit Grammar*, Motilal Banarsidass, Delhi, 1972.

Kalu Rinpoche, *The Gem Ornament*, Snow Lion, Ithaca, New York, 1986.

Kanshi, R., *Integral Non-Dualism*, Motilal Banarsidass, Delhi, 1995.

Kendall, F. P., *Muscles Testing and Function*, 4th ed., Lippincott Williams & Wilkins, Philadelphia, 1993.

Krishnamacharya the Purnacharya, Krishnamacharya Yoga Mandiram, Chennai.

Krishnamurti, J., *The Awakening of Intelligence*, HarperCollins, San Francisco, 1987.

Krishnamurti, J., *The First and Last Freedom*, HarperCollins, San Francisco, 1975.

Krishnamurti, J., *Krishnamurti's Journal*, 2nd rev. ed., Krishnamurti Foundation Trust India, Chennai, 2003.

Krishnamurti, J., *Krishnamurti to Himself*, HarperCollins, San Francisco, 1993.

Kumar, S., translator and annotator, *Samkhyasara of Vijnanbhiksu*, Eastern Book Linkers, Delhi, 1988.

Kunjunni Raja, K., editor, *Hathayogapradipika of Swatmarama*, The Adyar Library and Research Centre, Madras, 1972.

Kuvalayananda, Sw., *Asanas*, Kaivlayadhama, Lonavla, 1933.

Kuvalayananda, Sw., *Pranayama*, 7th ed., Kaivlayadhama, Lonavla, 1983.

Lad, V., *Ayurveda, The Science of Self-Healing*, 1st Indian ed., Motilal Banarsidass, Delhi, 1994.

Larson, G. J., *Classical Samkhya*, 2nd rev. ed., Motilal Banarsidass, Delhi, 1979

Larson, G. J. & Bhattacharya, R. S., *Encyclopedia of Indian Philosophies*, vol. 4, *Samkhya*, 1st Indian ed., Motilal Banarsidass, Delhi.

Leggett, T., *Realization of the Supreme Self*, New Age Books, New Delhi, 2002.

Leggett, T., translator, *Sankara on the Yoga Sutras*, 1st Indian ed., Motilal Banarsidass, Delhi, 1992.

Lester, R. C., *Ramanuja on the Yoga*, Adyar Library and Research Centre, Madras, 1976.

Long, R. A., *The Key Muscles of Hatha Yoga*, Bandha Yoga Publications, 2005.

Lorenzen, D. N., *Kabir Legends and Ananta Das's Kabir Parachai*, 1st Indian ed., Sri Satguru Publications, Delhi, 1992.

Lorenzen, D. N., *The Kapalikas and Kalamukhas*, 2nd rev. ed., Motilal Banarsidass, Delhi, 1991.

Madgula, I. S., *The Acarya*, 2nd rev. ed., Motilal Banarsidass, Delhi, 2001.

Madhavananda, Sw., translator, *The Brhadaranyaka Upanisad*, Advaita Ashrama, Kolkata, 1997.

Madhavananda, Sw., translator and commentator, *Minor Upanisads*, Advaita Ashrama, Kolkata, 1996.

Madhavananda, Sw., translator and annotator, *Vedanta Paribhasa*, Advaita Ashrama, Kolkata, 1997.

Mahadevan, T. M. P., *The Hymns of Sankara*, Motilal Banarsidass, Delhi, 1980.

Mani, V., *Puranic Encyclopedia*, 1st English ed., Motilal Banarsidass, Delhi, 1975.

Mascaro, J., translator, *The Upanishads*, Penguin Books, New Delhi, 1994.

Miele, L., *Ashtanga Yoga*, International Federation of Ashtanga Yoga Centres, Rome.

Mitchiner, J. E., *Tradition of the Seven Rsis*, Motilal Banarsidass, Delhi, 2000.

Mohan, A. G., *Yoga for Body, Breath and Mind*, Shambala, Boston & London, 2002.

Mohan, A. G., *Yoga Therapy*, Shambala, Boston & London, 2004.

Mohan, A. G., translator, *Yoga Yajnavalkya*, Ganesh & Co, Madras.

Monier-Williams, M., *A Sanskrit English Dictionary*, Motilal Banarsidass, Delhi, 2002.

Mueller, M., editor, *The Sacred Books of the East*, vol. 38, *Vedanta Sutras*, trans. G. Thibault, Motilal Banarsidass, Delhi, 1962.

Muktananda, Sw., *Der Weg und sein Ziel*, Deutsche Erstausgabe, Droemersche Verlagsanstalt, Munich, 1987.

Muktibodhananda, Sw., translator and commentator, *Hatha Yoga Pradipika*, 2nd ed., Yoga Publications Trust, Munger, 1993.

Nalanda Translation Committee, *The Life of Marpa the Translator*, Shambala, Boston, 1982.

Natarajan, A. R., *Ramana Maharshi — The Living Guru*, Ramana Maharshi Centre for Learning, Bangalore, 1996.

Natarajan, A. R., *Timeless in Time — A Biography of Sri Ramana Maharshi*, 2nd ed., Ramana Maharshi Centre for Learning, Bangalore, 2000.

Natarajan, N., translator and annotator, *Tirumantiram*, Sri Ramakrishna Math, Madras.

Neumann, D. A., *Kinesiology of the Muskuloskeletal System*, Mosby, St Louis, 2002.

Nikhilananda, Sw., translator, *The Mandukya Upanishad with Gaudapada's Karika and Sankara's Commentary*, Advaita Ashrama, Kolkata, 1987.

Nikhilananda, Sw., translator, *Vedanta-sara of Sadananda*, Advaita Ashrama, Kolkata, 1997.

Niranjanananda, P., *Yoga Darshan*, Sri Panchdashnam Paramahamsa Alakh Bara, Deoghar, 1993.

Norbu, N., *Dream Yoga*, Snow Lion, Ithaca, New York, 1992.

Pandey, K. C., editor, *Isvara Pratyabhijna Vimarsini — Doctrine of Divine Recognition*, 3 vols., Motilal Banarsidass, Delhi, 1986.

Panoli, V., translator and commentator, *Gita in Shankara's Own Words*, Shri Paramasivan, Madras, 1980.

Percheron, M., *Buddha*, Rowohlt Verlag, Hamburg, 1958.

Perry, E. D., *A Sanskrit Primer*, 4th ed., Motilal Banarsidass, Delhi, 1936.

Powell, R., editor, *The Experience of Nothingness — Sri Nisargadatta Maharaj's Talks on Realizing the Infinite*, 1st Indian ed., Motilal Banarsidass, Delhi, 2004.

Powell, R., editor, *The Nectar of Immortality — Sri Nisargadatta Maharaj's Discourses on the Eternal*, 1st Indian ed., Motilal Banarsidass, Delhi, 2004.

Prabhavananda, Sw., *Yoga and Mysticism*, Vedanta Press, Hollywood, 1969.

Prabhavananda, Sw., translator, *Bhagavad Gita*, Vedanta Press, Hollywood, 1987.

Prabhavananda, Sw., translator, *The Upanishads*, Vedanta Press, Hollywood, 1983.

Prabhavananda, Sw., translator and commentator, *Patanjali Yoga Sutra*, Sri Ramakrishna Math, Madras.

Prakashanand Saraswati, Sw., *The True History and the Religion of India*, 1st Indian ed., Motilal Banarsidass, Delhi, 2001.

Prasada, R., translator, *Patanjali's Yoga Sutras*, Munshiram Manoharlal, New Delhi, 2003.

Pungaliya, G. K., *Yoga Sastra*, Yoga and Allied Research Institute, Pune, 1998.

Radhakrishnan, S., *Indian Philosophy*, Indian ed., 2 vols., Oxford University Press, New Delhi, 1940.

Radhakrishnan, S., editor, *The Principal Upanisads*, HarperCollins Publishers India, New Delhi, 1994.

Radhakrishnan, S., translator and commentator, *The Bhagavad Gita*, HarperCollins Publishers India, New Delhi, 2002.

Rajneesh, O., *The Book of the Secrets*, 2nd ed., Rajneesh Foundation International, Antelope, Oregon, 1982.

Rajneesh, O., *Tantra: The Supreme Understanding*, The Rebel Publishing House, Portland, Oregon, 1997.

Ram Das, *Miracle of Love,* Munshiram Manoharlal, New Delhi, 1999.

Rama, Sw., *Path of Fire and Light*, vol. 1, The Himalayan Institute Press, Honesdale, Pennsylvania, 1988.

Rama, Sw., translator and commentator, *The Mystical Poetry of Kabir*, The Himalayan International Institute of Yoga, Honesdale, Pennsylvania, 1990.

Ramachandra Rao, S. K., *Yoga and Tantra in India and Tibet*, Kalpatharu Research Academy, Bangalore, 1999.

Ramakrishnananda, Sw., *Life of Sri Ramanuja*, Sri Ramakrishna Math, Madras.

Ramanasramam, S., *Sri Ramana Gita*, 8th ed., Sri Ramanasram, Tiruvannamalai, 1998.

Ramaswami, S., *Yoga for the Three Stages of Life*, Inner Traditions, Rochester, Vermont, 2000.

Reich, W., *Die Massenpsychologie des Faschismus*, Kiepenheuer & Witsch, Cologne, 1971.

Rieker, H. U., commentator, *Hatha Yoga Pradipika*, Aquarian/ Thorsons, London, 1992.

Rolf, I. P., *Rolfing — The Integration of Human Structures*, Dennis-Landman, Santa Monica, 1977.

Rukmani, T. S., translator, *Yogavarttika of Vijnanabhiksu*, 4 vols., Munshiram Manoharlal, New Delhi, 1998–2001.

Sangharakshita, *The Thousand-Petalled Lotus: The Indian Journey of an English Buddhist*, Sutton Pub. Ltd., 1988.

Satyananda Saraswati, Sw., *Moola Bandha*, 2nd ed., Bihar School of Yoga, Munger, 1996.

Scott, J., *Ashtanga Yoga*, Simon & Schuster, Roseville, NSW, 2000.

Sharma, A., *Advaita Vedanta*, Motilal Banarsidass, Delhi, 1993.

Sharma, C., *The Advaita Tradition in Indian Philosophy*, Motilal Banarsidass, Delhi, 1996.

Sharma, V. S., *Essentials of Ayurveda*, 2nd ed., Motilal Banarsidass, Delhi, 1998.

Shastri, J. L., editor, *The Kurma Purana*, trans. G. V. Tagare, 2 vols., Motilal Banarsidass, Delhi, 1981.

Shastri, J. L., editor, *The Linga Purana*, 2 vols., Motilal Banarsidass, Delhi, 1973.

Shastri, J. L., editor, *The Narada Purana*, trans. G.V. Tagare, 5 vols., Motilal Banarsidass, Delhi, 1980.

Shastri, J. L., editor, *The Siva Purana*, 4 vols., Motilal Banarsidass, Delhi, 1970.

Shrikrishna, *Essence of Pranayama*, 2nd ed., Kaivalyadhama, Lonavla, 1996.

Silburn, L., *Kundalini Energy of the Depths*, State University of New York Press, Albany, 1988.

Singh, J., translator and annotator, *Para Trisika Vivarana of Abhinavagupta*, Motilal Banarsidass, Delhi, 1988.

Singh, J., translator and annotator, *Siva Sutras — The Yoga of Supreme Identity*, Motilal Banarsidass, Delhi, 1979.

Singh, J., translator and annotator, *Spanda Karikas — The Divine Creative Pulsation*, Motilal Banarsidass, Delhi, 1980.

Singh, J., translator and annotator, *Vijnanabhairava*, Motilal Banarsidass, Delhi, 1979.

Sinh, P., translator, *The Hatha Yoga Pradipika*, Sri Satguru Publications, Delhi, 1915.

Sinha, N., *The Samkhya Philosophy*, Munshiram Manoharlal, New Delhi, 2003.

Sivananda Radha, Sw., *Kundalini Yoga*, 1st Indian ed., Motilal Banarsidass, Delhi, 1992.

Sjoman, N. E., *The Yoga Tradition of the Mysore Palace*, Abhinav Publications, New Delhi, 1996.

Sparham, G., *Dzog Chen Meditation*, Sri Satguru Publications, Delhi, 1994.

Sri Yukteswar, Sw., *Die Heilige Wissenschaft*, Otto Wilhelm Barth Verlag, Munich, 1991.

Stiles, M., *Structural Yoga Therapy*, Samuel Weiser, York Beach, Maine, 2000.

Stoler Miller, B., translator, *Yoga Discipline of Freedom*, Bantam Books, New York, 1998.

Subramaniam, K., translator, *Mahabharata*, Bharatiya Vidya Bhavan, Mumbai, 1999.

Subramaniam, K., translator, *Srimad Bhagavatam*, 7th ed., Bharatiya Vidya Bhavan, Mumbai, 1997.

Subramaniam, V. K., translator, *Saundaryalahari of Sankaracarya*, Motilal Banarsidass, Delhi, 1977.

Sullivan, B. M., *Seer of the Fifth Veda*, 1st Indian ed., Motilal Banarsidass, Delhi, 1999.

Swahananda, Sw., translator, *Chandogya Upanisad*, Sri Ramakrishna Math, Madras, 1956.

Swenson, D., *Ashtanga Yoga "The Practice Manual,"* Ashtanga Yoga Productions, Houston, 1999.

Taimni, I. K., translator and commentator, *The Science of Yoga*, The Theosophical Publishing House, Adyar, 1961.

Tapasyananda, Sw., translator, *Prasnottara-ratna-malika of Sri Sankaracarya*, Sri Ramakrishna Math, Madras.

Tapasyananda, Sw., translator, *Sankara-Dig-Vijaya*, Sri Ramakrishna Math, Chennai.

Tapasyananda, Sw., translator, *Sivanandalahari of Sri Sankaracarya*, Sri Ramakrishna Math, Madras.

Tapasyananda, Sw., translator and annotator, *Srimad Bhagavad Gita*, Sri Ramakrishna Math, Madras.

Thie, J. F., *Touch for Health*, rev. ed., DeVorss & Co., Marina del Rey, California, 1979.

Thurman, R., translator, *The Tibetan Book of the Dead*, HarperCollins Publishers India, New Delhi, 1998.

Tola, F., & Dragonetti, C., translators, *The Yogasutras of Patanjali*, Motilal Banarsidass, Delhi, 1987.

Torwesten, H., *Ramakrishna — Schauspieler Gottes*, Fischer Taschenbuch Verlag, Frankfurt, 1981.

Tsogyal, Y., *The Lotus Born — The Life Story of Padmasambhava*, trans. E. Pema Kunsang, Shambala, Boston, 1993.

Turiyananda, Sw., translator, *Vivekacudamani of Sri Sankaracarya*, Sri Ramakrishna Math, Madras.

Tyagisananda, Sw., translator and annotator, *Narada Bhakti Sutras*, Sri Ramakrishna Math, Madras.

Van Lysbeth, A., *Die grosse Kraft des Atems*, O. W. Barth Verlag, Munich, 1991.

Veda Bharati, Sw., *Meditation and the Art of Dying*, The Himalayan Institute Press, Honesdale, Pennsylvania, 1979.

Veda Bharati, Sw., translator and commentator, *Yoga Sutras of Patanjali*, vol. 2, Motilal Banarsidass, Delhi, 2001.

Venkatesananda, Sw., translator, *The Supreme Yoga* [*Yoga Vashishta*], 2 vols., The Divine Life Society, Shivanandanagar, 1995.

Venkatesananda, Sw., translator and commentator, *The Yoga Sutras of Patanjali*, The Divine Life Society, Shivanandanagar, 1998.

Verma, V., *Ayurveda — der Weg des gesunden Lebens*, Taschenbuchausgabe, Heyne Verlag, Munich, 1995.

Vimalananda, Sw., translator and annotator, *Mahanarayanopanisad*, Sri Ramakrishna Math, Madras.

Vimuktananda, Sw., translator, *Aparokshanubhuti of Sri Sankaracharya*, Advaita Ashrama, Kolkata, 1938.

Vireswarananda, Sw., translator, *Brahma Sutras According to Sri Sankara*, Advaita Ashrama, Kolkata, 1936.

Vireswarananda, Sw., translator, *Srimad Bhagavad Gita*, Sri Ramakrishna Math, Madras.

Virupakshananda, Sw., translator, *Samkhya Karika of Isvara Krsna*, Sri Ramakrishna Math, Madras.

Wasson, R. G., *Soma: Divine Mushroom of Immortality*, Harcourt Brace Jovanovich, 1970.

Whicher, I., *The Integrity of the Yoga Darsana*, 1st Indian ed., D. K. Printworld, New Delhi, 2000.

White, D. G., *The Alchemical Body*, The University of Chicago Press, Chicago, 1996.

Woodroffe, J., *Sakti and Sakta*, 10th ed., Ganesh & Co., Madras, 1994.

Woods, J. H., translator, *The Yoga System of Patanjali*, Motilal Banarsidass, Delhi, 1914.

Wu, J. C. H., translator, *Tao Teh Ching*, Shambala, Boston, 1990.

Yoga Journal, San Francisco, November / December 1995.

INDEX

abdominal breathing, 10, 13
abdominal muscles, 89
abductors, 55
active balancing, 39
active release, 73
active stretching, 20
adductors, 101
adhyatma, 181
Adishesha, 226
afflictions. *See kleshas*
Agastya, Rishi, 250
ahamkara, 144, 270
ahimsa. See nonviolence
Ajna chakra, 136
aloneness, 207
amrita, 123
Anahatta chakra, 136
ananta, 12, 134, 289
anger, 3
Angulimala, 219
antahkarana, 144
anterior cruciate ligament, 41
apana, 103, 260
aparigraha, 221
Aparokshanubhuti, 226
Aranya, Sw. Hariharananda, 136, 230, 253
Ardha Baddha Padma Pashimottanasana, 73
Ardha Baddha Padmottanasana, 56
Ardha Siddhasana, 58
armor, 3
asamprajnata samadhi. See objectless samadhi
asana, 3, 225ff.
Ashtavakra, Rishi, 288
asmita, 189, 270
atman, 205
austerity. *See tapas*
aversion, 191
avidya, 187ff.
awareness, 146, 203, 281
backbending, 111ff.
Baddha Konasana, 100
Baddha Padmasana, 126
Bakasana, 91
Balasana, 124–125
bandhas, 11

belief, 163, 277
Bhagavad Gita, 2, 5, 141, 192, 201, 207, 224, 226, 269
Bhagavata Purana, 163
Bhakti Yoga, 162, 166
Bhishma, 213, 221
Bhujapidasana, 90
biceps femoris, 40
body, 263
bondage, 156
boredom, 178, 210, 218
Brahma, Lord, 47, 63
Brahma Sutra, 15, 142, 256
Brahma Sutra commentary, 239
Brahmachary, Ramamohan, 1, 209, 260
brahmacharya, 214, 221
Brahman, 165, 235, 292
brahmarandhra, 123
brain-wave pattern, 4
breath, 3, 4, 9ff., 27
Brhad Aranyaka Upanishad, 3, 214
Buddha, Gautama, 15, 219, 221
buddhi. See intellect
cataleptic trance, 233
cerebral glands, 50
cerebrospinal fluid, 112
Chakrasana, 107
Chandogya Upanishad, 15, 256
Chaturanga Dandasana, 28
chitta. See mind
Chuang Tzu, 152
cognitive *samadhi. See* objective samadhi
concentration. *See dharana*
conceptualization, 151
conditioning, 194
confused mind. *See vikshipta chitta*
consciousness, 146, 202ff., 206, 257, 264ff., 272, 281, 284, 288, 291
conviction, 160, 163
correct perception, 149
cruciate ligaments, 42, 102
Daksha, 63
Dasgupta, S., 144, 146
dating the *Yoga Sutra*, 284
deities, 235
deliberative *samapatti*, 177

desire, 190
desires, fulfilling, 155
detachment, 153, 155, 156
devotion, 162
dharana, 4, 232, 235
dharma, 276, 288
dharma-megha-samadhi, 183, 287
dhyana. See meditation
direct experience, 236
disc bulges, 37–38
discriminative knowledge, 183, 208, 265, 286
doubt, 167
Downward Dog, 30
dreams, 173
dreamstate, 278
drishti, 14ff., 83
drug addiction, 190
dualism, 277
dvadashanta, 230
eccentric lengthening, 68
ecstasy, 291–292
ego, 255, 270
egomania, 211
eight limbs, 2
ekagra chitta, 133, 143, 275
Eliade, Mircea, 123
emotions, 13, 69, 198
erector spinae, 24
ethics, 196–197, 212, 275
experience, 182, 257
external rotators, 78
false views, 167
fasting, 231
fear, 191
feet, fallen arches, 53
Feldenkrais, M., 19
Feuerstein, G., 144, 185, 222
flexibility, 3
foot position, correct, 35
freedom, 183, 207, 291–292
freedom from doing, 209
freedom from the mind, 210
Freeman, R., 12
full *vinyasa*, 16, 21, 61
Garbha Pindasana, 95ff.
Garuda, 251
Gaudapada, 152, 165

303

About the Author

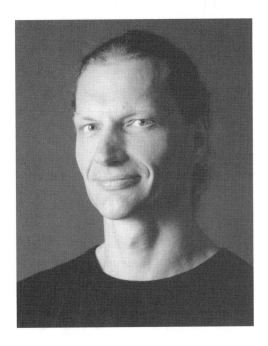

A student of history, philosophy, and comparative religion, Gregor Maehle has traveled to India every year since 1984 to study yoga, meditation, and philosophy with various masters. Meanwhile, he gained anatomical understanding through completing the requirements for a German health practitioner (Heilpraktiker) licence. Since 1990 Ashtanga Yoga has been his main form of yoga practice.

His passion is the study of Sanskrit.

Gregor is cofounder and director of 8limbs Ashtanga Yoga in Perth, Australia.
www.8limbs.com
www.ashtangayogabooks.com